Handbook of HIV/AIDS

Handbook of HIV/AIDS

Edited by Ivy Monroe

AMERICAN
MEDICAL PUBLISHERS
www.americanmedicalpublishers.com

American Medical Publishers,
41 Flatbush Avenue,
1st Floor, New York,
NY 11217, USA

Visit us on the World Wide Web at:
www.americanmedicalpublishers.com

ISBN: 978-1-63927-203-7

Cataloging-in-Publication Data

Handbook of HIV/AIDS / edited by Ivy Monroe.
p. cm.
Includes bibliographical references and index.
ISBN 978-1-63927-203-7
1. HIV infections. 2. AIDS (Disease). 3. HIV-positive persons. 4. AIDS (Disease)--Patients. I. Monroe, Ivy.

RC606.6 .H36 2022
616.979 2--dc23

Table of Contents

Preface

Human immunodeficiency virus (HIV) infection and acquired immune deficiency syndrome (AIDS) refer to a set of conditions in humans caused due to infection with HIV. The initial infection with the virus causes little or no symptoms, followed by a brief period of influenza-like illness. This period is succeeded by a long period with no symptoms. However, with the progression of the illness, a gradual shift in the immune response of the body emerges which is expressed with the incidence of common infections like tuberculosis, certain opportunistic infections and tumors which rarely affect people with a well-functioning immune system. HIV is contracted through unprotected sex, use of hypodermic needles, exposure to contaminated blood transfusions and mother to child HIV transmission during pregnancy, breast feeding and delivery. A patient may survive up to an average of 11 years without treatment. The disease can however be slowed down and patients can have a near-normal life expectancy, with antiretroviral therapies. This book brings forth some of the most innovative concepts and elucidates the unexplored aspects of HIV/AIDS. The various studies that are constantly contributing towards advancing the understanding and management of this disease are examined in detail. With state-of-the-art inputs by acclaimed experts of this field, this book targets students and professionals.

After months of intensive research and writing, this book is the end result of all who devoted their time and efforts in the initiation and progress of this book. It will surely be a source of reference in enhancing the required knowledge of the new developments in the area. During the course of developing this book, certain measures such as accuracy, authenticity and research focused analytical studies were given preference in order to produce a comprehensive book in the area of study.

This book would not have been possible without the efforts of the authors and the publisher. I extend my sincere thanks to them. Secondly, I express my gratitude to my family and well-wishers. And most importantly, I thank my students for constantly expressing their willingness and curiosity in enhancing their knowledge in the field, which encourages me to take up further research projects for the advancement of the area.

Editor

1

Characterization of occult hepatitis B virus infection among HIV positive patients

George Gachara[1,2], Tshifhiwa Magoro[1], Lufuno Mavhandu[1], Emmaculate Lum[3,4], Helen K. Kimbi[3,5], Roland N. Ndip[6,7] and Pascal O. Bessong[1*]

Abstract

Purpose: Occult hepatitis B infection (OBI) among HIV positive patients varies widely in different geographic regions. We undertook a study to determine the prevalence of occult hepatitis B infection among HIV infected individuals visiting a health facility in South West Cameroon and characterized occult HBV strains based on sequence analyses.

Methods: Plasma samples (n = 337), which previously tested negative for hepatitis B surface antigen (HBsAg), were screened for antibodies against hepatitis B core (anti-HBc) and surface (anti-HBs) antigens followed by DNA extraction. A 366 bp region covering the overlapping surface/polymerase gene of HBV was then amplified in a nested PCR and the amplicons sequenced using Sanger sequencing. The resulting sequences were then analyzed for genotypes and for escape and drug resistance mutations.

Results: Twenty samples were HBV DNA positive and were classified as OBI giving a prevalence of 5.9%. Out of these, 9 (45%) were anti-HBs positive, while 10 (52.6%) were anti-HBc positive. Additionally, 2 had dual anti-HBs and anti-HBc reactivity, while 6 had no detectable HBV antibodies. Out of the ten samples that were successfully sequenced, nine were classified as genotype E and one as genotype A. Three sequences possessed mutations associated with lamivudine resistance. We detected a number of mutations within the major hydrophilic region of the surface gene where most immune escape mutations occur.

Conclusions: Findings from this study show the presence of hepatitis B in patients without any of the HBV serological markers. Further prospective studies are required to determine the risk factors and markers of OBI.

Keywords: Hepatitis B virus, Occult hepatitis B infection, HIV, Cameroon

Background

Hepatitis B, a potentially life-threatening liver infection caused by the hepatitis B virus (HBV) is a major global health problem. Of the two billion people infected with the virus, more than 240 million are chronic carriers [1], and more than 686,000 die annually from HBV-related complications, including cirrhosis and hepatocellular carcinoma [2]. A growing body of evidence is emerging showing that the prevalence of HBV is significantly higher amongst HIV-positive individuals, presumably because of the shared transmission risks and risk factors [3, 4]. HIV generally accelerates the natural course of HBV infection and facilitates faster progression of liver disease to cirrhosis and hepatocellular carcinoma (HCC) [5].

Traditionally, HBV is diagnosed by serological techniques to detect antigens or antibodies. The hepatitis B surface antigen (HBsAg) is often used for routine diagnosis since it is considered as the hallmark of infection. During acute infection, antibodies to HBV core antigens (anti-HBc) (initially both IgM and IgG) appear 1–2 weeks after the appearance of HBsAg, while IgG persists during

*Correspondence: bessong@univen.ac.za; pascal.bessong@gmail.com
[1] HIV/AIDS & Global Health Research Program, Department of Microbiology, University of Venda, Private Bag X5050, Thohoyandou 0950, Limpopo, South Africa

chronic infection. The presence of antibodies to HBsAg (anti-HBs) represents immunity to HBV infection [6].

In the advent of molecular diagnostics, it has been shown that a number of individuals may harbour HBV-DNA at very low levels in their liver and/or serum despite the absence of detectable HBsAg by currently available assays [7]. This is termed occult hepatitis B infection (OBI), characterized by the presence of HBV DNA in the blood and liver in HBsAg-negative individuals, who may or may not have anti-HBc and anti-HBs [6]. There are several mechanisms that have been hypothesized to lead to development of OBI. These include development of HBV S gene mutants that affect the detectability of the virus by conventional HBsAg assays, strong suppression of viral replication and reduced expression of HBsAg, epigenetic mechanisms and co-infection with other viruses [8].

OBI is frequent in persons with HIV, and its prevalence varies considerably in different geographic regions [9]. It has been shown that immunosuppression due to HIV infection could lead to low antibody response to HBsAg and also HBV reactivation [10, 11]. Consequently, among HIV patients who test HBsAg negative, HBV DNA should be determined before starting highly active antiretroviral therapy (HAART) so that anti-HBV antiretrovirals can be included if necessary. The prevalence of OBI however, has been shown to vary in different demographic settings. A recent study in Cameroon reporting on OBI focused on patients from a health centre in the capital Yaoundé [12]. It would be expected therefore that the two regions of Cameroon from where the patients in the current study were derived would provide added information on OBI in this country where both HBV and HIV are endemic.

Methods

Study design and setting

This was a cross-sectional retrospective study using 337 HBsAg negative plasma samples from 455 HIV positive outpatient clients of the Mutengene Baptist Health Centre located in the South West Region of Cameroon. The health centre offers HIV/AIDS treatment, prevention, medical, spiritual and psychosocial care in the Tiko Health District. The hospital attends to at least 8000 patients per month. Patients come from various towns such as Buea, Limbe, Tiko, Kumba in the South West Region, and Douala, Nkongsamba, in the Littoral Region. Details of the study setting have been reported [13].

Sample collection and processing

All consenting participants completed a questionnaire regarding their socio-demographic characteristics. Five millilitres of venous blood was collected once from each consenting HIV positive adult individual using EDTA vacutainer tubes while two ml of blood was collected from young children (<5 years). Blood was centrifuged for 5 min at 3578×*g*. Following centrifugation, plasma was aspirated aseptically and aliquoted into sterile labelled cryotubes and stored at −80 °C. These were then transported on dry ice to the HIV/AIDS & Global Health Research laboratories at the University of Venda, South Africa where they were stored at −80 °C until used.

Serological testing

Initially, all samples were screened for HBsAg using a commercially available direct enzyme-linked immunosorbent assay (ELISA) kit (Bioelisa, Biokit, Barcelona, Spain). In this study, samples that were HBsAg negative were further screened for anti-HBc and anti-HBs using another ELISA commercial kit (DRG Instruments GmbH, Germany).

DNA extraction

DNA from HBsAg negative samples was extracted from 100 µl of plasma using the Quick-gDNA mini prep kit (Zymo research, USA) according to the manufacturer's instructions. The extracted DNA was amplified immediately after extraction or stored at −20 °C awaiting subsequent amplification.

Polymerase chain reaction (PCR) for HBV surface/polymerase gene

A nested PCR was performed in order to amplify the overlapping surface/polymerase gene covering nucleotides 403–768 from the EcoR1 site using primers and protocols described previously [14]. This generates a 366 bp product (Additional file 1: Figure S1). The first round reaction was conducted in a 50 µl volume containing 10 mM Tris-HCI pH 8.3, 50 mM potassium chloride, 0.2 mM dNTP mix, 2.5 mM magnesium chloride, 0.2 ng/µl of each primer, and 2 units of *Taq* polymerase (Applied Biosystems, PE, Italia). The thermocycling conditions involved 35 cycles of denaturation at 95 °C for 1 min, annealing at 55 °C for 1 min, and extension at 72 °C for 1 min. Five microlitre of the first round PCR product was used as a template for the nested PCR under the same reaction conditions, but performing only 20 cycles. The PCR products were then resolved by 1.5% agarose gel electrophoresis stained with ethidium bromide. PCR amplicons were then purified using the QiAquick PCR Purification Kit (Qiagen, Hilden; Germany) according to the manufacturer's instructions.

Sequencing and sequence analysis

Purified PCR amplicons were directly sequenced at Inqaba Biotech (Pretoria, South Africa) according to the Sanger protocol. Contiguous nucleotide sequences (contigs) were assembled from resulting forward and reverse reactions using the SeqMan Pro® module of the Lasergene (version 8.1.5) sequence analysis software suite (DNASTAR. Madison, WI.).

The resulting nucleotide sequences were aligned using the Clustal W program implemented in MEGA 6.06 [15]. They were also translated and checked for HBsAg mutations in the S gene and drug resistance associated mutations in the P gene. Phylogenetic reconstruction was carried out using the MrBayes program version 3.1.2 [16]. The Bayesian tree was inferred by running a Markov-chain Monte Carlo (MCMC) algorithm for 1 million generations, sampling at every 100th generation with a burn in setting of 10% of generations. The GTR+G+I model (general time-reversible model with gamma distributed rates of variation among sites and a proportion of invariable sites) was found to be the best-fit model for our dataset. The resulting phylogenetic tree was visualized using FigTree, version 1.3.1 (http://tree.bio.ed.ac.uk/software/figtree/) and used to determine the HBV genotype.

Statistical analysis

A database was prepared and processed using SPSS 20 (IBM, Chicago, IL, USA). Fisher's exact test was used to analyze the socio-demographic and clinical variables associated with OBI. A p value of less than 0.05 was considered statistically significant.

Results

Prevalence of occult HBV infection

HBV DNA was detected in 20 out of the 337 HBsAg negative samples giving an OBI prevalence of 5.9% in this study. OBI was higher among females, the unemployed, patients with low hemoglobin, those with normal white blood cell count and malaria negative individuals. However none of these variables were statistically associated with OBI (Table 1).

Serological profile of occult HBV infection

All the study samples were assayed for anti-HBs and anti-HBc serological markers. Out of the OBI positive samples, 9 (45%) were anti-HBs positive while 10 (52.6%) were anti-HBc positive (Table 2). Additionally, 2 individuals had dual anti-HBs and anti-HBc reactivity while 6 had no detectable HBV antibodies.

Molecular and genetic characterization of occult HBV DNA

Sequencing of the overlapping surface/polymerase gene was done for 10 out of the 20 OBI positive DNA samples. Phylogenetic analyses indicated that HBV genotype E and A occurred in 9 (90%) and 1 (10%) individuals respectively (Fig. 1).

Table 1 The prevalence of occult hepatitis B infection (OBI), demographic variables, and associated risk factors among HIV/HBV infected patients in Cameroon

Variable	OBI negative (%)	OBI positive (%)	p value
Gender			0.303
Male	85 (26.8)	3 (15.0)	
Female	232 (73.2)	17 (85.0)	
Age-group (years)			0.382
<15	30 (9.5)	4 (20.0)	
15–24	14 (4.4)	0 (0.0)	
25–35	140 (44.2)	6 (30.0)	
36–45	85 (26.8)	6 (30.0)	
>45	48 (15.1)	4 (20.0)	
Employment status			0.776
Employed	67 (21.1)	3 (15.0)	
Unemployed	250 (78.9)	17 (85.0)	
Malaria infection			1.00
Malaria positive	107 (33.8)	7 (35.0)	
Malaria negative	210 (66.2)	13 (65.0)	
WHO clinical stage			0.179
Stage 1	67 (21.7)	3 (15.0)	
Stage 2	87 (28.1)	7 (35.0)	
Stage 3	100 (32.4)	7 (35.0)	
Stage 4	55 (17.8)	3 (15.0)	
CD4 count			1.00
<350	174 (54.9)	11 (45.0)	
>350	143 (45.1)	9 (55.0)	
Haemoglobin level			1.00
Low Hb	220 (69.4)	14 (70.0)	
Normal Hb	97 (30.6)	6 (30.0)	
White blood cell count			0.193
Low WBC count	82 (25.9)	8 (40.0)	
Normal WBC count	235 (74.1)	12 (60.0)	

Table 2 Serological characterization of OBI individuals among HIV/HBV infected patients in Cameroon

OBI status	Anti-HBs status[a]		Anti-HBc status[b]	
	Anti-HBs$^+$	Anti-HBs$^-$	Anti-HBc$^+$	Anti-HBc$^-$
OBI positive[c]	5	14	10	9
OBI negative	104	201	176	134

[a] This was done for 324 patients due to insufficient sample volume

[b] This was done for 329 patients due to insufficient sample volume

[c] There was insufficient sample volume to conduct both anti-HBs and anti-HBc screening for one patient who was OBI positive

Mutations in the *"a"* determinant within the major hydrophilic region (MHR) of the S gene may cause a conformational change in HBsAg, leading to undetectability of HBsAg (diagnostic-escape) as well as evading

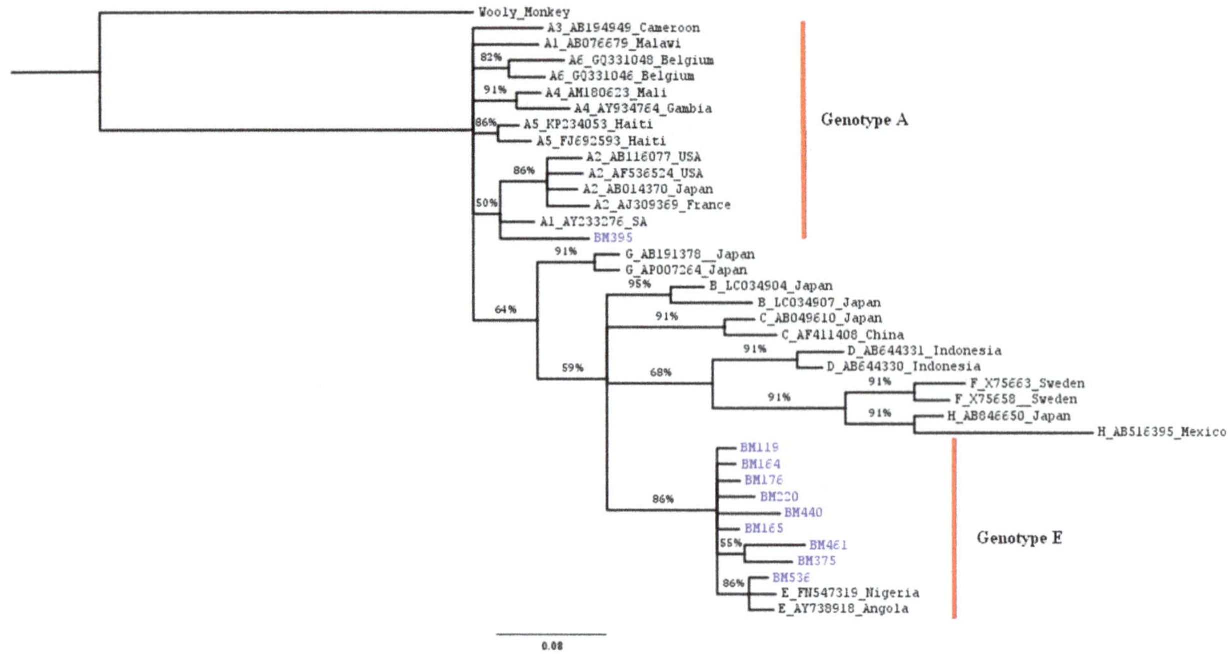

Fig. 1 A bayesian rooted phylogenetic tree constructed using MrBayesver 3.1.2 of the Cameroon OBI sequences from HBV/HIV co-infected individuals. Twenty-eight global sequences obtained from GenBank were included to support tree topology and genotype identification. The ten viruses characterised in this study are named with a prefix BM and highlighted in *blue* at the taxa

the host's immune response (immune-escape). The main mutation observed in this region was the G159A mutation observed in eight (80%) of the samples compared to 41.3% among HBsAg positive samples previously observed. Also, nine of the samples possessed leucine at amino acid 127. Examination of the RT domain of the polymerase gene indicated that three of the sequences had mutations associated with drug resistance. These mutations V173L, L180M, T184S and M204V/I are associated with resistance to lamivudine, entecavir and telbivudine (Fig. 2). The three patients harboring these mutations had treatment experience with Lamivudine as part of their antiretroviral therapy.

Discussion

Laboratory detection of Hepatitis B virus infection is crucial for global control and prevention of HBV disease. Among HIV infected individuals under HAART, the increased longevity may facilitate emergence of chronic liver disease which is often a cause of increased

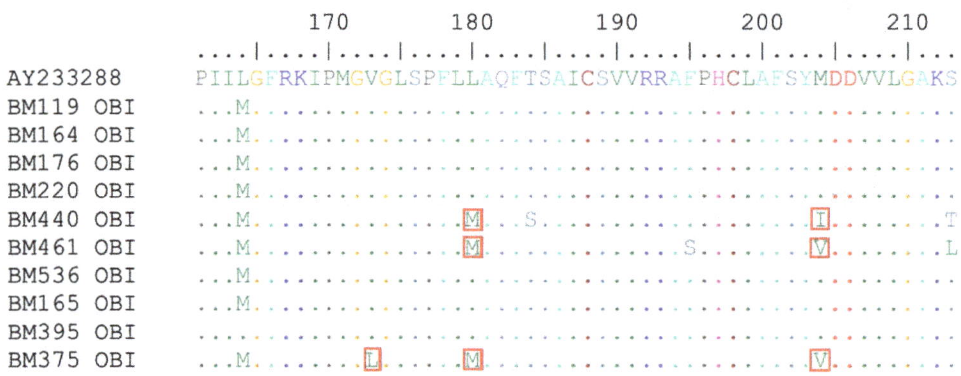

Fig. 2 Amino acid alignment of the RT domain (aa 161–213) of the P gene of HBV/HIV co-infected individuals from Cameroon. The Cameroon samples are named with a prefix BM and the drug resistance conferring mutations V173L, L180M, and M204V/I are shown. The numbering on *top* indicates the amino acid position

morbidity and mortality. A significant proportion of this burden may be attributed to occult hepatitis B virus infection since it has been shown to have hepatopathogenic potential. Furthermore, HAART creates immune reconstitution that can result in immune mediated liver injury and elevation of liver enzymes [17]. This may easily be misclassified as HAART-associated liver toxicity.

In this study, we have found a 5.9% prevalence of OBI among a group of HIV positive individuals in Cameroon and no significant association between the studied demographic parameters and risk factors of the participants and OBI was found.

The prevalence of OBI in this study is similar to the 5.9% found among HIV individuals in Sicily, Italy [18]. However, the observed prevalence is slightly lower than the 6.9 and 9.8% reported in Yaoundé, Cameroon and Khartoum, Sudan respectively [12, 19]. It should be noted however that the prevalence of OBI is dependent on the sensitivity of the DNA assay used, demography and the population studied [7]. Thus, the Sudan study used a more sensitive real time PCR method compared to the conventional PCR method used in this study. We propose that the difference in prevalence with the Yaoundé study may be due to demographics. Among HIV patients, several studies conducted worldwide have reported prevalence of OBI ranging from 0% to more than 90% [20, 21].

The current study did not find any association between OBI and the studied variables. This finding has also been made among Cuban HIV patients [22]. Generally, previous studies have made conflicting findings regarding factors associated with OBI. For example, Stuart et al. [20] have reported a significant association between low CD4 and OBI among HIV patients while other studies have not made this finding [22, 23]. Perhaps this may be due to the different diagnostic algorithms used to define OBI in the various studies.

Slightly more than half (52.6%) of the OBI positive individuals were anti-HBc positive, while 45% were anti-HBs positive. Our findings on the anti-HBc status is consistent with several studies that indicate the role of the anti-HBc profile as the most common serological surrogate of OBI although higher prevalence of anti-HBc alone does not necessarily reflect significantly higher frequency of OBI [24, 25]. Dual anti-HBc and anti-HBs reactivity was observed in 2 (20%) of the samples. Additionally, we identified six OBI positive individuals with no serologic evidence of infection (negative for HBsAg, anti-HBc, and anti-HBs). This is an indication that occult HBV can occur either in patients with serological evidence of past "apparently resolved" HBV infection, or also in individuals with no evident history of exposure to HBV [25]. Indeed this finding has epidemiological implications in that the burden of HBV in Cameroon, often determined by serological assays, is significantly underestimated. This 'silent' infection also has clinical implications since it leads to an increased risk of hepatocellular carcinoma [26].

The ten HBV strains sequenced in this study showed the circulation of both genotype E and A with genotype E predominating. Our findings are in agreement with previous studies in Cameroon that have documented the circulation of these two genotypes [12, 27]. Drug resistant patterns indicate that three of the strains had mutations associated with resistance to lamivudine, telbivudine and entecavir. Further, that the individuals harboring viruses with these mutations were all lamivudine experienced. Importantly though, none of the viruses harbored mutations associated with tenofovir and adefovir resistance. This finding is in agreement with the recommendation to include tenofovir as part of HAART among HIV/HBV co-infected patients [28]. Regarding mutations in the *"a"* determinant of the S gene, majority of the viruses had a G159A mutation. In addition, all the viruses had 127Lin this region. The 127L mutation has previously been associated with OBI [29], while the role of G159A in OBI is unclear.

The findings in this study should be interpreted in the light of several limitations. First, the HBV viral loads which are also often used as a marker of OBI were not available. Secondly, the study utilized a qualitative and not quantitative ELISA format, thus antibody titres were not determined. Thirdly, owing to resource constraints only 50% of the OBI positive samples were sequenced and lastly, the lack of liver enzyme levels precludes our ability to correlate the results reported here with clinical outcomes.

Conclusion

In conclusion, we report a 5.9% prevalence of OBI among HIV infected individuals in Cameroon and the dominance of HBV genotype E. We also show the occurrence of OBI in the absence of any serologic evidence of infection; and the presence of mutations associated with lamivudine drug resistance in the study cohort. Further prospective studies in a larger cohort are needed to determine the clinical implications of OBI in this region.

Authors' contributions

PB, HKK and RNN designed the study, EL recruited study subjects, collected samples and demographic data, TM and LM performed the laboratory analyses, GG analyzed the data and prepared the manuscript with contributions from all the authors. All authors read and approved the manuscript.

Author details

[1] HIV/AIDS & Global Health Research Program, Department of Microbiology, University of Venda, Private Bag X5050, Thohoyandou 0950, Limpopo, South Africa. [2] Department of Medical Laboratory Sciences, Kenyatta University, Nairobi, Kenya. [3] Department of Zoology and Animal Physiology, Faculty of Science, University of Buea, Buea, Cameroon. [4] Department of Biological Sciences, Higher Teachers' Training College, University of Yaounde, Yaounde, Cameroon. [5] Department of Medical Laboratory Science, Faculty of Health Sciences, University of Bamenda, Bambili, Bamenda, Cameroon. [6] Department of Biochemistry and Microbiology, Faculty of Science and Agriculture, University of Fort Hare, Alice, South Africa. [7] Department of Microbiology and Parasitology, University of Buea, Buea, Cameroon.

Acknowledgements

The authors would like to thank the study subjects for their participation.

Competing interests

The authors declare that they have no competing interests.

Funding

The study was not specifically funded. TM was supported by the National Research Foundation. PB is supported by the National Research Foundation and Medical Research Council of South Africa. GG is supported by award number D43 TW009359 from the Fogarty International Center, National Institutes of Health. None of the supporting funding bodies played a role in the execution of the study, data analysis, or writing of the manuscript. The information presented here is solely the responsibility of the authors.

References

1. WHO. Hepatitis B fact sheet. 2016. http://www.who.int/mediacentre/factsheets/fs204/en/. Accessed 20 Sept 2016.
2. Global, regional, and national age–sex specific all-cause and cause-specific mortality for 240 causes of death, 1990–2013: a systematic analysis for the global burden of disease study 2013. Lancet. 2014;385(9963):117–171. doi:10.1016/S0140-6736(14)61682-2.
3. Diop-Ndiaye H, Toure-Kane C, Etard JF, Lo G, Diaw P, Ngom-Gueye NF, et al. Hepatitis B, C seroprevalence and delta viruses in HIV-1 Senegalese patients at HAART initiation (retrospective study). J Med Virol. 2008;80(8):1332–6. doi:10.1002/jmv.21236.
4. Alter MJ. Epidemiology of viral hepatitis and HIV co-infection. J Hepatol. 2006;44(1 Suppl):S6–9. doi:10.1016/j.jhep.2005.11.004.
5. Vallet-Pichard A, Pol S. Natural history and predictors of severity of chronic hepatitis C virus (HCV) and human immunodeficiency virus (HIV) co-infection. J Hepatol. 2006;44(1 Suppl):S28–34. doi:10.1016/j.jhep.2005.11.008.
6. Trepo C, Chan HL, Lok A. Hepatitis B virus infection. Lancet. 2014;384(9959):2053–63. doi:10.1016/S0140-6736(14)60220-8.
7. Chemin I, Trepo C. Clinical impact of occult HBV infections. J Clin Virol. 2005;34(Suppl 1):S15–21. doi:10.1016/S1386-6532(05)80005-8.
8. Sood AK, Pangotra C, Manrai M. Prevalence of occult hepatitis B infection in patients visiting tertiary care hospital. Med J Armed Forces India. 2016;72(2):140–4. doi:10.1016/j.mjafi.2016.02.006.
9. Ramezani A, Banifazl M, Eslamifar A, Sofian M, Aghakhani A. Occult hepatitis B infection in different high risk patients. Hepat Mon. 2012;12(7):467–8. doi:10.5812/hepatmon.7094.
10. Burnett RJ, François G, Kew MC, Leroux-Roels G, Meheus A, Hoosen AA, et al. Hepatitis B virus and human immunodeficiency virus co-infection in sub-Saharan Africa: a call for further investigation. Liver Int. 2005;25(2):201–13. doi:10.1111/j.1478-3231.2005.01054.x.
11. Sagnelli C, Macera M, Pisaturo M, Zampino R, Coppola M, Sagnelli E. Occult HBV infection in the oncohematological setting. Infection. 2016. doi:10.1007/s15010-016-0891-1.
12. Salpini R, Forkam J, Ceccareilli L, Santoro MM, Nanfack A, Sosso SM, et al. High burden of HBV-infection and atypical HBV strains among HIV-infected Cameroonians. Curr HIV Res. 2016;14(2):165–71.
13. Magoro T, Gachara G, Mavhandu L, Lum E, Kimbi H, Ndip R. Serologic and genetic characterization of hepatitis B virus in HIV infected individuals from the South and Littoral Regions of Cameroon. Virol J. 2016;13:178. doi:10.1186/s12985-016-0636-x.
14. Marrone A, Zampino R, Karayannis P, Cirillo G, Cesaro G, Guerrera B, et al. Clinical reactivation during lamivudine treatment correlates with mutations in the precore/core promoter and polymerase regions of hepatitis B virus in patients with anti-hepatitis B e-positive chronic hepatitis. Aliment Pharmacol Ther. 2005;22(8):707–14. doi:10.1111/j.1365-2036.2005.02653.x.
15. Tamura K, Stecher G, Peterson D, Filipski A, Kumar S. MEGA6: molecular evolutionary genetics analysis version 6.0. Mol Biol Evol. 2013;30(12):2725–9. doi:10.1093/molbev/mst197.
16. Ronquist F, Huelsenbeck JP. MrBayes 3: Bayesian phylogenetic inference under mixed models. Bioinformatics. 2003;19(12):1572–4.
17. Shire NJ, Rouster SD, Stanford SD, Blackard JT, Martin CM, Fichtenbaum CJ, et al. The prevalence and significance of occult hepatitis B virus in a prospective cohort of HIV-infected patients. JAIDS J Acquir Immune Defic Syndr. 2007;44(3):309–14. doi:10.1097/QAI.0b013e31802e29a9.
18. Tramuto F, Maida CM, Colomba GME, Di Carlo P, Vitale F. Prevalence of occult hepatitis B virus infection in a cohort of HIV-positive patients resident in Sicily, Italy. Biomed Res Int. 2013;2013:859583. doi:10.1155/2013/859583.
19. Yousif M, Mudawi H, Hussein W, Mukhtar M, Nemeri O, Glebe D, et al. Genotyping and virological characteristics of hepatitis B virus in HIV-infected individuals in Sudan. Int J Infect Dis. 2014;29:125–32. doi:10.1016/j.ijid.2014.07.002.
20. Cohen Stuart JW, Velema M, Schuurman R, Boucher CA, Hoepelman AI. Occult hepatitis B in persons infected with HIV is associated with low CD4 counts and resolves during antiretroviral therapy. J Med Virol. 2009;81(3):441–5. doi:10.1002/jmv.21422.
21. Gupta S, Singh S. Occult hepatitis B virus infection in ART-naive HIV-infected patients seen at a tertiary care centre in north India. BMC Infect Dis. 2010;10:53. doi:10.1186/1471-2334-10-53.
22. Marite B, Montalvo MC, Rodriguez Lde L, Sariego S, Verdasquera D, Vincent M, et al. Occult hepatitis B in Cuban HIV patients. MEDICC Rev. 2011;13(2):32–7.
23. Fabris P, Biasin MR, Giordani MT, Berardo L, Menini V, Carlotto A, et al. Impact of occult HBV infection in HIV/HCV co-infected patients: HBV-DNA detection in liver specimens and in serum samples. Curr HIV Res. 2008;6(2):173–9.
24. Mphahlele MJ, Lukhwareni A, Burnett RJ, Moropeng LM, Ngobeni JM. High risk of occult hepatitis B virus infection in HIV-positive patients from South Africa. J Clin Virol. 2006;35(1):14–20. doi:10.1016/j.jcv.2005.04.003.
25. Firnhaber C, Chen CY, Evans D, Maskew M, Schulz D, Reyneke A, et al. Prevalence of hepatitis B virus (HBV) co-infection in HBV serologically-negative South African HIV patients and retrospective evaluation of the clinical course of mono- and co-infection. Int J Infect Dis. 2012;16(4):e268–72. doi:10.1016/j.ijid.2011.12.007.
26. Chen JD, Yang HI, Iloeje UH, You SL, Lu SN, Wang LY, et al. Carriers of inactive hepatitis B virus are still at risk for hepatocellular carcinoma and liver-related death. Gastroenterology. 2010;138(5):1747–54. doi:10.1053/j.gastro.2010.01.042.
27. Kouanfack C, Aghokeng AF, Mondain AM, Bourgeois A, Kenfack A, Mpoudi-Ngole E, et al. Lamivudine-resistant HBV infection in HIV-positive patients receiving antiretroviral therapy in a public routine clinic in Cameroon. Antivir Ther. 2012;17(2):321–6. doi:10.3851/IMP1911.
28. Soriano V, Puoti M, Bonacini M, Brook G, Cargnel A, Rockstroh J, et al. Care of patients with chronic hepatitis B and HIV co-infection: recommendations from an HIV-HBV International Panel. AIDS. 2005;19(3):221–40.
29. Svicher V, Cento V, Bernassola M, Neumann-Fraune M, Van Hemert F, Chen M, et al. Novel HBsAg markers tightly correlate with occult HBV infection and strongly affect HBsAg detection. Antiviral Res. 2012;93(1):86–93. doi:10.1016/j.antiviral.2011.10.022.

2

Transition into adult care: factors associated with level of preparedness among adolescents living with HIV

Siyan Yi[1,2*], Chanrith Ngin[1], Khuondyla Pal[1], Vohith Khol[3], Sovannary Tuot[1], Sokunmealiny Sau[3], Pheak Chhoun[1], Gitau Mburu[4], Sok Chamreun Choub[1], Kolab Chhim[1] and Penhsun Ly[3]

Abstract

Background: Preparing adolescents for transition into adult care and supporting their acquisition of self-health care management skills is a critical determinant of their post-transition HIV care outcomes. However, there is a scarcity of research on effective transition strategies. This study explores factors associated with adolescent preparedness for transition into adult care in Cambodia.

Methods: In August 2016, a cross-sectional study was conducted among 223 adolescents living with HIV aged 15–17, randomly selected from 11 antiretroviral therapy clinics, utilizing a structured questionnaire. The level of preparedness was determined using a pre-existing scale, and adolescents were categorized as having a high- or low level of preparedness for transition. Bivariate and multivariate analyses were conducted.

Results: Of 223 adolescents, 55.2% were male, and their mean age was 15.8 years. Overall, 53.3% had a high level of preparedness for transition. As part of the transition protocol, 2.7% had completed a transfer form, 24.7% had a transition case manager, 29.6% had been counselled about the transition, and 19.7% had visited an adult ART clinic. In multivariate analysis, a higher level of preparedness for transition was independently associated with older age (AOR 2.44, 95% CI 1.34–4.46; $p = 0.004$), family having received social support for their health (AOR 5.32, 95% CI 1.97–14.36; $p = 0.001$), knowing the kind of treatment they received (ART) (AOR 12.67, 95% CI 2.91–15.19; $p = 0.001$), trust in friends or family for HIV treatment (AOR 7.82, 95% CI 1.13–8.89; $p = 0.008$), receiving counseling on transition (AOR 3.17, 95% CI 1.15–8.76; $p = 0.03$), having a 'Case Manager' identified to support them during the preparation process for transition (AOR 3.89, 95% CI 1.08–13.96; $p = 0.04$), and satisfaction with preparation process for transition in general (AOR 0.35, 95% CI 0.03–0.87; $p = 0.01$).

Conclusions: A range of individual, social and health system and services factors may determine successful transition preparedness among adolescents in Cambodia. Strengthening implementation of age-appropriate and individualized case management transition at all sites, while creating supportive family, peer, and healthcare environments for adolescent transition is required.

Keywords: Adolescents, HIV, AIDS, Care and treatment, Transition, Cambodia

Background

Globally, adolescents and young people represent a growing share of people living with human immunodeficiency virus (HIV). Latest available data suggests that adolescents account for 12% of new HIV infections globally [1]. Approximately 670,000 young people between the ages of 15–24 were newly infected with HIV in 2015 alone, of whom 250,000 were adolescents between the ages of 15 and 19 [1]. About 1.8 million adolescents between the ages of 10 and 19 were living with HIV worldwide in 2015 [1], and this number is projected to increase further due

*Correspondence: siyan@doctor.com

[1] KHANA Center for Population Health Research, No. 33, Street 71, Phnom Penh, Cambodia

to rising access to antiretroviral therapy (ART) and ongoing new horizontal infections [2, 3]. The Pacific and South East Asia regions have the highest number of adolescents living with HIV outside of Sub-Saharan Africa, accounting for 11% of the global population of adolescents living with HIV [4]. As in other contexts [3, 5], majority of these adolescents have been vertically infected [4].

Although data on adolescents living with HIV are limited globally [6], concerns have emerged regarding their HIV-related clinical outcomes. While the overall mortality among people living with HIV in all other age groups had decreased by 32% during the period between 2005 and 2012, the overall mortality of adolescents living with HIV increased by 50% from 71,000 in 2005 to 110,000 in 2012 [6]. Adolescents are the only age group in which HIV-related mortality is rising [7].

Compared to adults, adolescents often have poorer rates of viral suppression [8, 9] and long-term immunologic recovery [10]. They face unique developmental, psychological, and sexuality challenges as they are still maturing physically, mentally, and sexually [5, 11], often in the context of restrictive parental consent laws and policies [12]. This is in addition to common contextual challenges encountered by most people living with HIV regardless of age, including stigma [13], disclosure difficulties [13], challenges with adherence [14], and economic hardships [15], all of which prevent attainment of optimal health outcomes. As a consequence, adolescents are considerably less likely to receive HIV services compared to adults. In 2013, less than one in four (24%) children up to 15 years living with HIV had received ART globally [16].

Recent research has identified transition to adult care as a significant determinant of HIV care outcomes among adolescents living with HIV [17]. For instance, studies have demonstrated that transition to adult HIV care is associated with worsening or reversal of immunological recovery [18], unsuppressed viral load [19, 20], and high rates of attrition and loss to follow up [20, 21] among transitioned adolescents. These concerns have led to calls for programs and policies to improve adolescent transition processes, data and outcomes [17, 22].

According to the World Health Organization (WHO), transition preparedness is determined by adolescents' ability to demonstrate basic health-care awareness, awareness of their status, understanding their disease, and development of own health management skills [23]. Few data exist on what approaches are most effective for preparing and implementing transition [17]. Meanwhile, there is consensus that adolescents cannot self-manage a chronic illness when they do not understand its nature and clinical management [24], and that there is a need for programs for adolescents that are empowering, continuous, coordinated, culturally appropriate, integrated and family-centered [17, 25].

Recent studies have also revealed a lack of consensus and consistency regarding specific elements of an ideal transition program [26]. Even in the contexts where transition is being implemented, there has been a pervasive lack of mechanisms to assess the impact of different transition approaches [26, 27]. Studies involving adolescents and health care providers have also demonstrated differing perceptions of readiness for transition [28] amid calls to assess adolescent readiness for transition [29]. These difficulties are not surprising. The issue of transition has unexpectedly been brought to fore due to increasing survival of perinatally-infected children, against a prior assumption that they would not survive into adulthood [30]. Although studies looking at survival of adolescents after transition have emerged prompted by the rising numbers of this population, most focus on experiences, retention and retrospective clinical outcomes in developed countries [27, 31–34], leaving a gap of information related to transition processes in low and middle income countries.

In Cambodia, where HIV prevalence in pregnant women attending antenatal care was 0.28% in 2015 [35], there were 8512 children and adolescents living with HIV at the end of 2013 [36], who accessed care from 37 ART clinics across the country. A previous exploratory study conducted in 2012 suggested that the majority of these adolescents were reluctant to transition into adult services [37] due to anticipated stigma, lack of familiarity with adult clinics, current relationship with pediatric health providers, negative perception of adult service quality, and concerns regarding confidentiality [37, 38]. These factors, combined with inability of adult health care providers to receive adolescents revealed in the above study formed the basis for calls to increase attention to adolescent transition in Cambodia, including better data analyses and operational research around transition [39].

To address these needs and imperatives, a study was conducted in 2016 to explore potential factors associated with level of preparedness for transition to adult care among adolescents living with HIV in Cambodia.

Methods

Study design and population

This overall study constituted of a cross-sectional survey and follow on in-depth interviews complemented by routine HIV care data retrieved from medical records in ART clinics. This study included adolescents living with HIV aged 15–17, who were accessing services from pediatric ART clinics in the capital city and 12 provinces. In this paper, we report the findings from the quantitative arm. Qualitative results have been reported separately.

Selection of study sites and participants

In Cambodia, 90% of adolescents living with HIV access services from 18 clinics, while the remaining 10% are distributed across 21 sites, each with less than 10 adolescents living HIV clients. At the time of the study, the number of adolescents per ART clinic varies from 1 to 116. Against this background, participants were selected in three stages. First, a two-stage 30 × 10 cluster sampling method was used to select clusters to sample participants from, using a methodology developed by the WHO [40]. A comprehensive list of all ART sites in the country with adolescents living with HIV population estimates was created and used to select the clusters after excluding ART clinics with less than 10 adolescents. This left a universe of 598 adolescents receiving treatment and care from the 18 major ART clinics. To minimize costs of data collection, additional seven clinics with less than 20 adolescents living with HIV clients aged 15–17 were excluded.

In the second stage the required sample size was determined taking into account population size, confidence interval, and estimated proportion of the population with the characteristics of interest [41], in this case being prepared for transition to adult care. Assuming 60% of adolescents had a high level of preparedness, a finite population size of 598, a design effect of 1.4 and a 10% drop-out or refusal rate, a minimum sample size of 220 was required for the study to measure variables among selected adolescents with a confidence interval of 4.3%.

Third, the number of participants that needed to be recruited from each cluster was determined. Because the size of the ART clinics varied, probability proportional to size sampling method [41] was used to ensure that adolescents in larger sites had the same probability of being included in the sample as those in smaller sites. Cumulative population size of each ART clinic was calculated; sampling interval was determined; and potential participants were randomly selected from the database using a random number table.

Finally, a list of selected adolescents was prepared and assigned a unique identification number based on the clinic ID code. Selected adolescents were then contacted on phone, screened for eligibility, and informed about the research objectives as well as place, date, and time of the interview by local study coordinators. A written consent was obtained from parents or guardians of selected adolescents before the interview. Potential participants were included if they were aged between 15 and 17 years, receiving treatment and care services from the selected ART clinics, able to communicate in Khmer, allowed by a parent or guardian to participate, able to present themselves on the day of the interview, and physically and mentally stable to assent and participate in the study. Recruitment continued until the required sample sizes for each cluster and clinics were achieved.

Questionnaire development

In reference to exiting literature [28, 42], a structured questionnaire was developed. The first part of the questionnaire collected information on socio-demographic characteristics, parental or caregiver information, and clinical and immunological data of participants obtained from health records. The second part collected information on adolescents' HIV knowledge, substance use and sexual behaviors. The third part assessed the level of preparedness for transition to adult care, using a questionnaire developed by the New York State Department of Health AIDS Institute [43]. This 11-item scale asked whether the adolescents: (1) could recognize when they are getting sick, (2) knew when they need to call the doctor, (3) were responsible for making appointments, (4) were responsible for refilling medications, (5) felt comfortable asking questions at appointments, (6) had a copy of your health records, doctor contact number, and address, (7) had a method of keeping track of healthcare appointments, (8) found it difficult to remember to take medicines, (9) would stop taking your medicine when they felt better, (10) would stop taking if they felt worse after taking medicines, and (11) had missed taking any medicines in the past 4 days. A total score of the scale, which ranged from 0 to 11, was calculated for each participant, with a Cronbach's alpha of 0.86. The final part of the questionnaire collected information on coping strategies and the maturity of the adolescents.

Data collection training

Data were collected by two teams of interviewers and moderators who were trained on the study protocol, research ethics, confidentiality and interview and questionnaire administration skills. Tool pre-testing was conducted among 20 adolescents living with HIV recruited from an ART clinic in Phnom Penh and 10 parents/guardians, followed by revision of contents and language based on feedbacks from the pre-test.

Data analyses

Data were coded and scaled continuously or categorically as dictated by the variables and entered into a computerized database using Epi Data version 3 (Odense, Denmark). Double data entry was performed to minimize errors. Descriptive analyses were conducted to determine proportions of variables, frequency distribution of responses, and means and standard deviation (SD) of continuous variables.

Because there was no recommended cut-off for determining level of preparedness for transition to adult care in the scale employed in this study [43], the mean score was used to categorize participants into two groups: one with a low level of readiness (with a total score of ≤ 7) and another group with a high level of readiness (with a total score of >7). Chi square test, Fisher's exact test, or *t* test were used as appropriate based on the nature of variables being analyzed to compare variables among adolescents with a low and high level of preparedness for transition to adult care. *p* values of less than 0.05 were considered significant.

A multivariate logistic regression model was constructed to identify factors associated with a high level of preparedness for transition. Age, gender, and all other variables associated with a high level of readiness in bivariate analyses at a level of *p* value <0.05 were simultaneously included in the model, followed by a backward selection to identify independent predictors. SPSS v22 (IBM Corporation, New York, USA) was used for all statistical analyses.

Ethics statement

This study was approved by the National Ethics Committee for Health Research, Ministry of Health in Cambodia (Ref: 297NECHR). All participants were required to assent to the study in writing and a written consent from their parent(s) or caregiver giver was obtained. All data were collected in private locations, and confidentiality strictly protected by removing all personal identifiers from the questionnaires, field notes, and the sampling frame. Participants were assigned a unique code. Researchers and data collectors were trained on confidentiality prior to data collection. All participants were provided with a token of 2.5–5 USD for transportation.

Results

Socio-demographic characteristics

Socio-demographic characteristics are shown in Table 1. A total of 223 adolescents were included in this study. Of these 55.2% were male, and their mean age was 15.8 years (SD = 0.8). 29.6% had completed primary school, and 50.7% had completed secondary school. Although 47.5 and 42.6% reported having a living mother and father, respectively, only 40.8% were living with parents, and the remaining were living with grandparents (15.7%) and with other relatives (33.6%). Almost 10% lived in an orphanage, with Buddhist monks, neighbors, or foster parents. Main caregivers included parents (55.6%), relatives (32.2%), siblings (6.7%), orphanage/NGO staff (3.3%), and grandparents (2.2%). About one-fifth (22.0%) were working for pay, and 48.4% came from families that received social support for their health care, in the form of food support (78.7%), school allowance (64.8%), transport allowance for going to ART clinic (55.6%), emotional counseling (32.4%), vocational training (25.9%), or home visit (10.2%).

Immunological and adherence characteristics

As shown in Table 2, based on their medical records obtained at the ART clinic, participants had received services from an ART clinic for an average of 114 (SD = 39) months, and had received ART for 101 (SD = 40) months. The mean initial CD4 count was 632 (SD = 506) cells/mm^3, and the most recent was 672 (SD = 295) cells/mm^3. The mean viral load at the first test was 44,691 (SD = 161,304) copies/ml, and at the most recent was 7686 copies/ml (SD = 48,682) copies/ml.

Awareness and disclosure of HIV status

Majority (93.7%) of the participants in this study were aware that they were living with HIV, and 78.9% reported that they had acquired it from their mothers. Half (50.7%) had never disclosed their HIV status to anyone, and the remaining 49.3% had disclosed it to their siblings (24.2%), friends (13.0%), school teachers (2.4%), or other persons (5.8%). Based on self-reported visual adherence scale, 95.6% were adherent to ART (Table 3).

HIV and health information sources

Table 4 shows that 60.1% of the adolescent participants reported ART clinic to be the main source of health information. Family (45.3%), and health providers (22.4%), were preferred by most adolescents to discuss issues of health, sexual life, or daily life, compared to friends (16.6%), counselors/peer educators (4.0%), or caregivers, relatives, and school teachers (11.7%). However, health care providers (78.9%) were most trusted in regard to HIV treatment and care, compared to family (12.1%), counselors/peer educators (4.5%), caregivers and relatives (4.5%).

Preparation process for transition into adult care

Table 4 shows that a total of 29.6% had received counseling on transition into adult services, of which majority were counselled by health care providers (36.9%) and counselors/peer educators (47.7%). However, only 19.7% had visited an adult ART clinic to prepare for the transition with friends/family (69.8%), counselors/peer educators (4.7%), or other including NGO staff (25.5%). In addition, only 2.7% of them had completed a transfer form. Most of the adolescents who had visited the adult facility (88.4%) reported that the visit was helpful in preparing for the transition. In addition, 24.7% reported that a 'Case Manager' had been identified to support them for the transition. When asked about their preparedness to manage their treatment going onward, 13.0% said they

Table 1 Socio-demographic characteristics of adolescents living with HIV with a low and high level of preparedness for transition to adult care

Socio-demographic characteristics	Total ($n = 223$)	Level of preparedness for transition[a]		
		Low (≤7) ($n = 104$)	High (>7) ($n = 119$)	p value[†]
	n (%)	n (%)	n (%)	
Age (in years)	15.8 ± 0.8	15.7 ± 0.8	15.9 ± 0.8	0.16
Gender				0.09
Male	123 (55.2)	51 (49.0)	72 (60.5)	
Female	100 (44.8)	53 (51.0)	47 (39.5)	
Currently living with				0.004
Parents	91 (40.8)	30 (28.8)	61 (51.3)	
Grandparents	35 (15.7)	18 (17.3)	17 (14.3)	
Relatives	75 (33.6)	47 (45.2)	28 (23.5)	
In an orphanage	18 (8.1)	7 (6.7)	11 (9.2)	
Other	4 (1.8)	2 (1.9)	2 (1.7)	
Mother is still alive				0.04
No	117 (52.5)	62 (59.6)	55 (46.2)	
Yes	106 (47.5)	42 (40.4)	64 (53.8)	
Mother's level of formal education				0.59
No education	12 (11.7)	5 (12.5)	7 (11.1)	
Primary school	26 (25.2)	9 (22.5)	17 (27.0)	
Secondary school	14 (13.6)	8 (20.0)	6 (9.5)	
High school or higher	20 (19.4)	8 (20.0)	12 (19.0)	
Don't know	31 (30.1)	10 (25.0)	21 (33.3)	
Father is still alive				0.37
No	128 (57.4)	63 (60.6)	65 (54.6)	
Yes	95 (42.6)	41 (39.4)	54 (45.4)	
Father's level of formal education				0.62
No education	4 (4.4)	1 (2.6)	3 (5.6)	
Primary school	21 (23.1)	10 (25.6)	11 (21.2)	
Secondary school	11 (12.1)	4 (10.3)	7 (13.5)	
High school or higher	19 (20.9)	20 (15.4)	13 (25.0)	
Don't know	36 (39.6)	18 (46.2)	18 (34.6)	
Main daily caregiver				0.003
Parent	124 (55.6)	48 (46.2)	76 (63.9)	
Grand parent	5 (2.2)	2 (1.9)	3 (2.5)	
Sibling	15 (6.7)	4 (3.8)	11 (9.2)	
Relatives	72 (32.3)	47 (45.2)	25 (21.0)	
Orphanage/NGO staff	7 (3.1)	3 (2.9)	4 (3.4)	
Main caregiver's level of formal education				0.08
Primary school or lower	7 (5.0)	6 (7.9)	1 (1.6)	
Secondary school	29 (20.9)	13 (17.1)	16 (25.4)	
High school	9 (6.5)	7 (9.2)	2 (3.2)	
University or higher	21 (15.1)	14 (18.4)	7 (11.1)	
Don't know	73 (52.5)	36 (47.4)	37 (58.7)	
Your level of formal education				0.49
Primary school or lower	66 (29.6)	32 (30.8)	34 (28.6)	
Secondary school	113 (50.7)	55 (52.9)	58 (48.7)	
High school or higher	44 (19.7)	17 (16.3)	27 (22.7)	

Table 1 continued

Socio-demographic characteristics	Total ($n = 223$)	Level of preparedness for transition[a]		
		Low (≤7) ($n = 104$)	High (>7) ($n = 119$)	p value[†]
	n (%)	n (%)	n (%)	
Currently working for pay				0.03
No	174 (78.0)	88 (84.6)	86 (72.3)	
Yes	49 (22.0)	16 (15.4)	33 (27.7)	
Family received social support for your health				0.03
No	115 (51.6)	62 (59.6)	53 (44.5)	
Yes	108 (48.4)	42 (40.4)	66 (55.5)	
Types of social support				
Transportation allowance	60 (55.6)	26 (61.9)	34 (51.5)	0.29
Food support	85 (78.7)	37 (88.1)	48 (72.7)	0.06
School allowance	70 (64.8)	28 (66.7)	42 (63.6)	0.75
Emotional counseling	35 (32.4)	21 (50.0)	14 (21.2)	0.002
Vocational training	28 (25.9)	18 (42.9)	10 (15.2)	0.001
Home visit	11 (10.2)	3 (7.1)	8 (12.1)	0.52

Values are number (%) for categorical variables and mean (±SD) for continuous variables

ART antiretroviral therapy, *HIV* human immunodeficiency virus, *NGO* non-governmental organization

[†] Chi square or Fisher's exact test was used for categorical outcome variables and Student's *t* test was used for continuous outcome variables

[a] Mean score of preparedness for transition scale was used to divide participants into two groups—adolescents with low level of readiness (≤7) and adolescents with high level of readiness (>7)

Table 2 Medical history among adolescents living with HIV with a low and high level of preparedness for transition to adult care

Medical history	Total ($n = 223$)	Level of preparedness for transition[a]		
		Low (≤7) ($n = 104$)	High (>7) ($n = 119$)	p value[†]
	n (%)	n (%)	n (%)	
Type of ART site				
Pediatric	206 (92.8)	67 (95.7)	139 (92.1)	0.59
Adult	10 (4.5)	2 (2.86)	7 (4.6)	
Other	6 (2.7)	1 (1.4)	5 (3.3)	
Type of current treatment				0.87
First line	183 (82.4)	58 (84.1)	124 (81.6)	
Second line	36 (16.2)	11 (15.9)	25 (16.4)	
Opportunistic infections	3 (1.4)	0 (0.0)	3 (2.0)	
Time since first ART clinic visit (in months)	114 ± 39	111 ± 38	116 ± 39	0.33
Time since first ART initiation (in months)	101 ± 40	100 ± 41	102 ± 41	0.66
Time from first visit to ART start (in months)	14 ± 25	12 ± 22	15 ± 26	0.50
First CD4 count	632 ± 506	623 ± 523	636 ± 502.4	0.86
Latest CD4 count	672 ± 295	717 ± 309	655 ± 286	0.15
First viral load count (copies)	44,691 ± 161,304	38,015 ± 139,375	47,922 ± 171,630	0.68
Latest viral load count (copies)	7686 ± 48,682	10,306 ± 77,534	6547 ± 27,418	0.61
Visual adherence scale (%)	95.6 ± 9.8	93.8 ± 10.7	97.1 ± 8.6	0.01

Values are number (%) for categorical variables and mean (± SD) for continuous variables

ART antiretroviral therapy, *HIV* human immunodeficiency virus

[†] Chi square or Fisher's exact test was used for categorical outcome variables and Student's *t* test was used for continuous outcome variables

[a] Mean score of preparedness for transition scale was used to divide participants into two groups—adolescents with low level of readiness (≤7) and adolescents with high level of readiness (>7)

Table 3 Assessment of HIV status disclosure among adolescents living with HIV with a low and high level of preparedness for transition to adult care

HIV status disclosure	Total ($n = 223$)	Level of preparedness for transition[a]		
		Low (≤7) ($n = 104$)	High (>7) ($n = 119$)	p value[†]
	n (%)	n (%)	n (%)	
Can you tell us, what is your disease?				0.17
HIV/AIDS	209 (93.7)	95 (91.3)	114 (95.8)	
Don't know	14 (6.3)	9 (8.7)	5 (4.2)	
Do you know how you have been infected?				0.78
Don't know	31 (14.8)	13 (13.7)	18 (15.8)	
Mother to child	165 (78.9)	77 (81.1)	88 (77.2)	
Other	13 (6.2)	5 (5.3)	8 (7.0)	
Do you know how is this disease transmitted?				
Don't know	7 (3.3)	7 (7.4)	0 (0.0)	0.004
Mother to child	142 (67.9)	65 (68.4)	77 (67.5)	0.89
Unprotected sex	156 (74.6)	66 (69.5)	90 (78.9)	0.12
Sharing needles	114 (54.5)	50 (52.6)	64 (56.1)	0.61
Blood transfusion	125 (59.8)	64 (57.4)	61 (53.5)	0.05
Do you know what kind of medicine you have received?				0.002
Pre-ART	3 (1.3)	1 (1.0)	2 (1.7)	
ART	183 (82.1)	76 (73.1)	107 (89.9)	
Don't know	37 (16.6)	27 (26.0)	10 (8.4)	
Have you ever disclosed your HIV status to anyone?				0.04
No	113 (50.7)	60 (67.7)	53 (44.5)	
Yes	110 (49.3)	44 (42.3)	66 (55.5)	
To whom have you ever disclosed your HIV status to?				0.06
Siblings	50 (24.2)	14 (14.9)	36 (31.9)	
School teachers	5 (2.4)	2 (2.1)	3 (2.7)	
Friends	27 (13.0)	12 (12.8)	15 (13.3)	
Other	12 (5.8)	6 (6.4)	6 (5.3)	

AIDS acquired immune deficiency syndrome, *ARV* antiretroviral, *HIV* human immunodeficiency virus

[†] Chi square or Fisher's exact test was used as appropriate

[a] Mean score of preparedness for transition scale was used to divide participants into two groups

were very prepared; 75.3% were somewhat prepared; 5.4% were somewhat unprepared; and 6.3% were very unprepared. The majority felt supported during the preparation process for transition with 14.5% feeling very supported, and 59.5% felt somewhat supported. However, 58.3% said that they were very dissatisfied, and 11.7% said that they were somewhat dissatisfied with the preparation process in general. Despite these findings, the majority (83.9%) of participants preferred to receive HIV treatment and care in a pediatric ART clinic.

Assessment of adolescents' preparedness for transition into adult care

Based on the scale employed in this study [43], 53.3% had a high level of preparedness for transition to adult care. As shown in Fig. 1, majority of the participants reported that they could recognize when they are getting sick (73.5%), knew when they needed to call a health care provider (82.5%), and had a method of keeping track of their clinic appointments (62.3%). However, smaller proportions reported being responsible for making their actual clinic appointments (48.4%), refilling their own medications (58.7%), or feeling comfortable asking questions during clinic appointments (15.2%). Less than half (46.6%) reported having a copy of their health records and contacts of health care providers. Regarding ART adherence, 24.2% found it difficult to remember to take medicines, but only a small proportion would stop taking medicines if they feel better (0.9%) or worse (9.9%). A total of 13.9% reported either having missed or being uncertain of whether they had missed their medicines over the past 4 days preceding

Table 4 Experience of preparation for transition among adolescents living with HIV with a low and high level of preparedness for transition to adult care

Experiences in preparation process for transition	Total ($n = 223$)	Level of preparedness for transition[a]		
		Low (≤7) ($n = 104$)	High (>7) ($n = 119$)	p value[†]
	n (%)	n (%)	n (%)	
Facility you prefer to receive HIV treatment and care				0.08
Pediatric ART services	187 (83.9)	92 (88.5)	95 (79.8)	
Adult ART services	36 (16.1)	12 (11.5)	24 (20.2)	
Preferred to discuss questions related to health, sexual life, or daily life with				0.78
Health care providers	50 (22.4)	21 (20.2)	29 (24.4)	
Counselors/peer educators	9 (4.0)	5 (4.8)	4 (3.4)	
Friends	37 (16.6)	20 (19.2)	17 (14.3)	
Family	101 (45.3)	45 (43.3)	56 (47.1)	
Other	26 (11.7)	13 (12.5)	13 (10.9)	
Person who you trust the most for your treatment				0.001
Health care providers	176 (78.9)	92 (88.5)	84 (70.6)	
Counselors/peer educators	10 (4.5)	5 (4.8)	5 (4.2)	
Friends/family	27 (12.1)	3 (2.9)	24 (20.2)	
Other	10 (4.5)	4 (3.8)	6 (5.0)	
Sources of information about health				0.90
ART clinic	134 (60.1)	61 (58.7)	73 (61.3)	
NGOs	17 (7.6)	8 (7.7)	9 (7.6)	
Family	51 (22.9)	26 (25.0)	25 (21.0)	
Other	21 (9.4)	9 (8.7)	12 (10.1)	
Received counseling on transition to adult services				0.01
No	157 (70.4)	82 (78.8)	75 (63.0)	
Yes	66 (29.6)	22 (21.2)	44 (37.0)	
Person who provided the counseling				0.43
Health providers	24 (36.9)	7 (33.3)	17 (38.6)	
Counselors/peer educators	31 (47.7)	9 (42.9)	22 (50.0)	
Other	10 (15.4)	5 (23.8)	5 (11.4)	
Ever completed a transfer form				0.14
No	217 (97.3)	103 (99.0)	114 (95.8)	
Yes	6 (2.7)	1 (1.0)	5 (4.2)	
Ever visited an adult clinic to prepare for transition				0.03
No	179 (80.3)	90 (86.5)	89 (74.8)	
Yes	44 (19.7)	14 (13.5)	30 (25.2)	
Person who took you to visit the adult clinic to prepare for transition				0.15
Counselors/peer educators	2 (4.7)	1 (7.7)	1 (3.4)	
Friends/family	30 (69.8)	11 (84.6)	19 (63.3)	
Other	11 (25.5)	1 (7.7)	10 (33.3)	
The visit was helpful for you to cope with the transition				0.61
No	5 (11.6)	2 (15.4)	3 (10.0)	
Yes	38 (88.4)	11 (84.6)	27 (90.0)	
A 'Case Manager' has been identified to support you during the transition				<0.001
No	168 (75.3)	91 (87.5)	77 (64.7)	
Yes	55 (24.7)	13 (12.5)	42 (35.3)	

Table 4 continued

Experiences in preparation process for transition	Total ($n = 223$)	Level of preparedness for transition[a]		
		Low (≤7) ($n = 104$)	High (>7) ($n = 119$)	*p* value[†]
	n (%)	*n* (%)	*n* (%)	
Preparedness to manage your treatment going forward				0.01
Very prepared	29 (13.0)	8 (7.7)	21 (17.6)	
Somewhat prepared	168 (75.3)	81 (77.9)	87 (73.1)	
Somewhat unprepared	12 (5.4)	4 (3.8)	8 (6.7)	
Very unprepared	14 (6.3)	11 (10.6)	3 (2.5)	
Feeling supported during preparation process for the transition to adult care				0.96
Very supported	11 (14.9)	2 (11.8)	9 (15.8)	
Somewhat supported	44 (59.5)	10 (58.8)	34 (59.6)	
Somewhat unsupported	7 (9.4)	2 (11.8)	5 (8.8)	
Very unsupported	12 (16.2)	3 (17.6)	9 (15.8)	
Satisfaction you with the preparation process for transition in general				<0.001
Very satisfied	16 (7.2)	2 (1.9)	14 (11.8)	
Somewhat satisfied	51 (22.9)	15 (14.4)	36 (30.3)	
Somewhat dissatisfied	26 (11.7)	11 (10.6)	15 (12.6)	
Very dissatisfied	130 (58.3)	76 (73.1)	54 (45.4)	

ART antiretroviral therapy, *HIV* human immunodeficiency virus

[†] Chi square or Fisher's exact test was used as appropriate

[a] Mean score of preparedness for transition scale was used to divide participants into two groups—adolescents with low level of readiness (≤7) and adolescents with high level of readiness (>7)

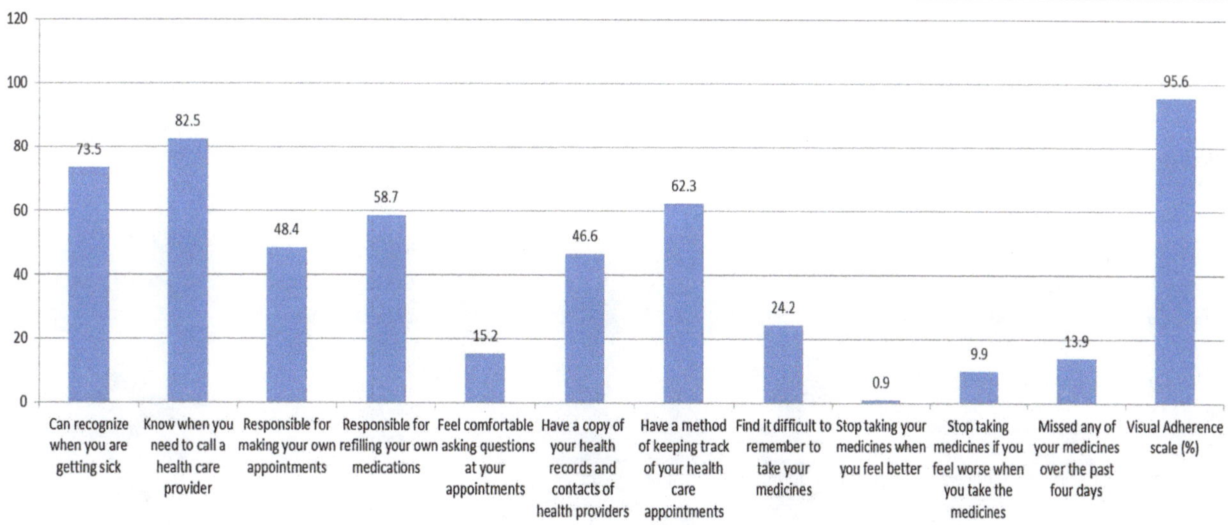

Fig. 1 Assessment of preparedness for the transition from pediatric to adult care among adolescents living with HIV

the interview, with a mean score of visual adherence scale of 95.6% (SD = 9.8%).

Factors associated with level of preparedness for transition into adult care

Bivariate analyses showed that adolescents with a higher level of preparedness were significantly more likely to live with their parents (28.8% vs. 51.3%, $p = 0.004$), to have a living mother (40.4% vs. 53.8%, $p = 0.04$), and to have their parent as their main caregiver (46.2% vs. 63.9%, $p = 0.003$), while adolescents with a lower level of preparedness were more likely to live with relatives (45.2% vs. 21.0%, $p = 0.003$) (Table 1). In addition, the level of adherence was significantly higher among adolescents with a higher level of preparedness on bivariate analysis (93.8 ± 10.7 vs. 97.1 ± 8.6, $p = 0.01$) (Table 2). Adolescents with a lower level of preparedness were significantly more likely to report that they did not know how their disease was transmitted (7.4% vs. 0.0%, $p = 0.004$), to not know the kind of medicines they were receiving (20.6% vs. 8.4%, $p = 0.002$), and to have disclosed their HIV status to someone (42.3% vs. 55.5%, $p = 0.04$). Conversely, adolescents with a higher level of preparedness knew that they were receiving ART (73.1% vs. 89.9%, $p = 0.002$) (Table 3).

Adolescents with a lower level of preparedness were significantly more likely to trust health care providers with their HIV treatment and care (88.5% vs. 70.6%, $p = 0.001$), while adolescents with a higher level of preparedness identified friends or family in this regard (2.9% vs. 20.2%, $p = 0.001$). A higher level of preparedness was associated with receiving counseling on transition into adult services (21.2% vs. 37.0%, $p = 0.01$) and having visited an adult clinic in preparation for transition (13.5% vs. 25.2%, $p = 0.03$). Presence of a 'Case Manager' to support adolescents during transition was also associated with a higher level of preparedness (12.5% vs. 35.3%, $p < 0.001$). Not surprisingly, adolescents with a higher level of preparedness perceived that they were very prepared for the transition (7.7% vs. 17.6%, $p = 0.01$), while those with a lower level of preparedness reported that they were very dissatisfied with the preparation process (73.1% vs. 45.4%, $p < 0.001$) (Table 4).

As shown in Table 5, multivariate logistic regression analysis found that a higher level of preparedness remained significantly associated with older age (AOR 2.44, 95% CI 1.34–4.46), family having received social support for their health (AOR 5.32, 95% CI 1.97–14.36),

Table 5 Factors associated with level of preparedness for transition to adult care in multivariate logistic regression model

Variables in the final model[a]	Level of preparedness for transition[b]	
	AOR (95% CI)	*p* value
Age	2.44 (1.34–4.46)	0.004
Family received social support for your health		
No	Reference	
Yes	5.32 (1.97–14.36)	0.001
Do you know what kind of medicine you have received?		
Don't know	Reference	
Pre-ART	4.20 (1.99–7.39)	0.02
ART	12.67 (2.91–15.19)	0.001
Person who you trust the most for your treatment		
Health providers	Reference	
Counselors/peer educators	2.41 (0.42–13.79)	0.33
Friends/family	7.82 (1.13–8.89)	0.008
Other	1.51 (0.23–9.78)	0.66
Received counseling on transition to adult services		
No	Reference	
Yes	3.17 (1.15–8.76)	0.03
A 'Case Manager' has been identified to support you during the transition		
No	Reference	
Yes	3.89 (1.08–13.96)	0.04
Satisfaction with preparation for transition in general		
Very satisfied	Reference	
Somewhat satisfied	0.21 (0.08–5.46)	0.35
Somewhat dissatisfied	0.32 (0.01–0.94)	0.04
Very dissatisfied	0.35 (0.03–0.87)	0.01

AOR adjusted odds ratio, *ART* antiretroviral therapy, *CI* confidence interval

[a] Age, gender and all variables associated with level of preparedness for transition to adult care at a level of $p < 0.05$ were simultaneously included in a multivariate logistic regression model

[b] Mean score of readiness for transition scale was used to divide participants into two groups—adolescents with low level of readiness (≤ 7) and adolescents with high level of readiness (>7)

knowing the kind of treatment received (ART) (AOR 12.67, 95% CI 2.91–15.19), trusting friends or family for HIV treatment (AOR 7.82, 95% CI 1.13–8.89), receiving counseling on transition to adult services (AOR 3.17, 95% CI 1.15–8.76), having a 'Case Manager' to support them for the transition (AOR 3.89, 95% CI 1.08–13.96), and satisfaction with preparation process for transition in general (AOR 0.35, 95% CI 0.03–0.87).

Discussion

Preparing adolescents for transition into adult care and supporting their acquisition of self-health care management skills is an essential part of transition protocols [44, 45], which affects outcomes after transition [31, 34, 45, 46]. This is the first study exploring factors associated with preparedness for transition from pediatric to adult care among adolescents living with HIV in Cambodia. A number of findings that merit program and policy attention.

First, the overall level of preparedness for transition from pediatric to adult care among adolescents living with HIV in this study was fairly good. The results indicated that although few were undertaking practical activities associated with taking control of their HIV management such as booking their own appointment, refilling their own medications, keeping a copy of their health cards, a good number of them felt confident that they could recognize when they are getting sick and know when they need to call a health care provider. It is, however, difficult to know for certain if adolescents will be comfortable with these practical tasks in the wake of transition. A good transition process enables adolescents to be autonomous and responsible for their own HIV care by the time they engage with adult services [46], and as such ongoing support is required until and after they start accessing adult care, and afterwards.

Second, this study provides important information regarding individual, social and health system determinants of preparedness to transition, which should be considered moving forward. As other researchers have asserted, the preparation for transition ought to take into account the characteristics and contexts of adolescents and their families; physical, sexual, and emotional maturity; complexity of their health needs; and access to health care professionals and services [25, 45, 49]. In a concentrated epidemic context such as Cambodia, being an adolescent from a key population can exacerbate stigma and other barriers to successful transition [20].

At the individual domain, a higher level of preparedness for transition into adult care was independently associated with older age and being aware of the kind of treatment received. While the prominence of age is not necessarily surprising, having been highlighted in other studies [34, 47], these findings do emphasize that tailored, age- and developmental appropriate transition should recognize the evolving capacity of adolescents [45]. This may have a gender-implication given that female adolescents, who generally mature earlier than their male counterparts were older in this study. In addition, this finding emphasizes the need to coordinate the processes of disclosure and transition, ensuring that adolescents are fully aware of the nature of disease and treatment before transition, which will require focussed and differentiated HIV and treatment literacy interventions for adolescents as they approach transition into adult care.

At the social level, a higher level of preparedness for transition into adult care was independently associated with trust in friends or family for HIV treatment, and receipt of health-related social support at the family level such as emotional counseling and vocational training. These findings are consistent with other studies showing the importance of supportive family members, peers, and friends and a communicative family environment in coping with both an HIV diagnosis [49] and transition to adult care [50]. These findings are particularly important given the high level of stigma [38], and the large proportion of adolescents not living with their parents in the study context, implying the necessity for interpersonal support.

In relation to health systems and services, receiving specific counseling on transition to adult services, having a Case Manager to support adolescents for transition preparation was associated with higher levels of preparedness. Other studies have consistently shown the importance of dedicated health and social workers to support transition in the United States [51–53], and having trusting relationships with health providers [25, 30], which may often require additional training to improve competency of health providers [30] to enable them to receive adolescents and create atmosphere which enables communication and questions from adolescents. Creating familiarity with adult clinics, including through visits has a significant impact in facilitating adolescents' connection to the adult clinic consistent with research from other settings [33]. In our study, 88% of participants who had visited an adult clinic as part of the preparation for transition reported that they found the visit helpful, although only a fifth of the study sample had been to the clinic. In addition, despite the importance of transition case management, less than a quarter (24.7%) of the participants had an identified Case Manager, and only a third (29.6%) had been counselled about the transition process.

Third, these results emphasize calls to take into account adolescents views and experiences regarding specific elements of the transition process [47, 54]. Failure to take adolescents' perspectives into account leads to routine problematization of adolescents as inadequately equipped to manage transition into adult clinical care [55], yet little research is focused on understanding perspectives of adolescents having difficulties with transition. In our study for instance, it is not surprising that adolescents with a higher level of preparedness reported satisfaction with preparation process for transition in general. However, notable proportions of adolescents reported being somewhat dissatisfied (11.7%) or very dissatisfied (58.3%) with the preparation process in general. Despite the preparation for transition, most adolescents expressed preference to continue accessing services in pediatric clinics. Although anxiety and reluctance to the transfer into adult clinics is not unusual [28, 37, 39, 51, 54], understanding the underlying reasons why adolescents were dissatisfied with the preparation process will be important in facilitating improvement of the transition preparedness process in the study context.

Fourth, an overarching strategy that contributed to the preparation for transition was having an agreed transition readiness protocol in place, whose distinct elements can be evaluated in depth. In this regards, it is particularly important to evaluate how the transition procedure is understood by adolescents, health providers, parents and guardians, and its uniformity which is implemented across different clinics. Despite the presence of a transition protocol, only a small proportion of adolescents had completed a transfer form (2.7%), been allocated with a Case Manager (24.7%), been counselled about the transition process (29.6%) or visited an adult ART clinic (19.7%) as part of the preparation for transition, suggesting that the transition process was not uniformly implemented. Availability and subsequent implementation of transition protocols is a key feature of transition quality [47]. In addition, variation between sites in terms of process implementation as well as conceptualization; e.g., viewing transition as an event rather than a process—can significantly affect the care quality and outcomes after the transition [26, 47].

Finally, results from this study generally indicate areas where additional support may be required by adolescents living with HIV to improve their disease management, coping mechanisms and outcomes, even if these factors did not necessarily affect transition preparedness independently. This includes support with adherence for the few that found it difficult to remember to take medicines, providing skills for the half that did not have a method of keeping track of their health care appointments, increasing HIV disclosure education for parents whose adolescents did not know what medicines they were taking, ongoing support with social and transport, vocational training, ongoing HIV and ART literacy, and information services for those who did not know the nature of their infection, support to cope with stigma, and ensuring adequate supplies of treatments to prevent unnecessary appointments. Although these are not unique challenges as they have been reported elsewhere [17, 24, 25], they could significantly affect ability of adolescents to stay in school instead of working, manage and keep their appointments, cope with HIV diagnosis in the long term, manage their own disclosure to sexual partners, and ultimately their ability to manage HIV on their own. Further data are useful in providing information regarding the best ways in which adolescents can be supported to meet the above needs comprehensively.

Limitations of the study

Data reported in this study were collected from a diverse sample of major ART clinics in 13 city and provinces with different socio-demographic and geographical characteristics. However, generalizability of these results may be limited by biases resulting from the use of self-reported measures, recall of events that had taken several months or years before the study. The study focused exclusively on large ART clinics, adolescents who could communicate in Khmer and adolescents who were with a parent or guardian available for consent and ability to transport themselves to the clinic. These criteria may limit the generalizability of the study findings to only adolescents who are more affluent, educated and living in urban areas where there tend to be more resources available. One may speculate that this population is more prepared for the transition into adult care. It is possible that factors influencing preparedness for transition could change over time; however, this cross-sectional study captured a snapshot of these factors. In addition, qualitative data will be useful in contextualizing findings reported in this paper.

Analyses and results reported in this paper was based on scale developed and validated elsewhere [43]. While, generalizable tools to assess transition preparedness are limited, different conclusions may have been reached had a different scale been use such as that used by Wiener et al., which classifies preparedness into four categories: poor, moderate, good and excellent [53]. In their study, Wiener et al. [53] assessed six variables: (1) whether a local health care provider had been identified and, if so, (i) whether the participant had made an appointment with this provider, (ii) who made the appointment, and (iii) how comfortable the participant felt calling the provider for advice or turning to this provider for medical care (8 items); (2) if the participant had medical insurance and whether they (i) would need to pay out of pocket for medications and (ii) have the financial ability to cover these costs (4 items); (3) whether the participant had transportation for medical appointments (1 item);

(4) whether a pharmacy had been identified and whether the participant had obtained medications and/or refills through this pharmacy (2 items); (5) knowledge of disease status, medication regimens and dosages (5 items); and (6) if they had or knew of a social worker who would be available for assistance with obtaining support and/or services (1 item). The scale yields one global readiness score, which is used to classify participants' preparedness as either poor, moderate, good or excellent.

It is notable that the self-reported perception of preparedness was somewhat higher than the assessment using the scale, as 13 and 75.3% of participants reported feeling very prepared and somewhat prepared, respectively on a 4-item Likert scale. These differences may be due to social desirability bias, or genuine shortcomings in how the scale used in this study assessed preparedness, especially given that it dichotomises preparedness into two categories as opposed to the scale used by Wiener et al. referred to above. Nevertheless, the overlap of some factors included in these two scales, together with our own pre-testing of the former scale suggested that the factors we focused on were highly relevant to the study setting. At the same time, transition preparedness could be affected by physiological, psychological or age-related developmental or factors. For instance, Wiener et al. [53] went further to include a separate assessment of anxiety within their study, and found that over time, transition preparedness improved, while the state of anxiety decreased. Although we did not examine the nature of psychological influences on transition preparedness in depth—which could be explored in future research, our study provided valuable information regarding the implementation of the transition protocol and highlighted areas that require attention.

Conclusions

This study reports individual, social, and health system and services factors that contribute to successful transition preparedness in the context of a clear and structured transition protocol for adolescents living with HIV in Cambodia, a substantial proportion of whom were prepared for the transition to adult services. Nevertheless, gaps were identified, which will require to be addressed to ensure that age-appropriate and individualized case management for transition is enhanced and uniformly implemented across different sites. Transition process and interventions will also need to concurrently address contextual issues facing adolescents living with HIV, by focusing on disclosure, sexuality, stigma, social protection, and social support, as well as HIV education and ART literacy, while at the same time creating supportive family, peer, and healthcare environments for adolescent transition. To achieve these goals, adolescents, parents, and health providers should be involved.

Abbreviations

AIDS: acquired immune deficiency syndrome; AOR: adjusted odds ratio; CI: confidence interval; HIV: human immunodeficiency virus infection; NECHR: National Ethics Committee for Health Research; NGO: non-governmental organization; SD: standard deviation; WHO: World Health Organization.

Authors' contributions

SY, ST, SS and VK conceived the study. KP, PC and ST were responsible for data collection and data entry. SY and KP analyzed data. SY, CN and GM wrote the manuscript. KC, SCC, VK and PL supervised all stages of the study and reviewed and provided critical inputs for writing the manuscript. All authors read and approved the final manuscript.

Author details

[1] KHANA Center for Population Health Research, No. 33, Street 71, Phnom Penh, Cambodia. [2] Center for Global Health Research, Touro University California, Vallejo, USA. [3] National Center for HIV/AIDS, Dermatology and STD, Phnom Penh, Cambodia. [4] Division of Health Research, Lancaster University, Lancaster, UK.

Acknowledgements

This study was conducted in collaboration between KHANA Center for Population Health Research and National Center for HIV/AIDS, Dermatology and STD. The authors thank staff members at participating ART clinics, implementing partners, community support volunteers, outreach workers as well as all the study participants and their family for the excellent contribution to the data collection.

Competing interests

The authors declare that they have no competing interests.

Funding

This study was funded by UNICEF Cambodia.

References

1. United Nations Children's Fund (UNICEF). Turning the tide against AIDS will require more concentrated focus on adolescents and young people. New York: UNICEF; 2016.
2. Slogrove AL, Mahy M, Armstrong A, Davies MA. Living and dying to be counted: what we know about the epidemiology of the global adolescent HIV epidemic. J Int AIDS Soc. 2017;20(Suppl 3):4–15.
3. Ferrand RA, Corbett EL, Wood R, Hargrove J, Ndhlovu CE, Cowan FM, et al. AIDS among older children and adolescents in Southern Africa: projecting the time course and magnitude of the epidemic. AIDS. 2009;23(15):2039–46.
4. Porth T, Suzuki C, Gillespie A, Kasedde S, Idele P. Disparities and trends in AIDS mortality among teenagers living with HIV in low- and middle-income countries. 20th International AIDS Conference, Melbourne, Australia; 2014.

5. Lowenthal ED, Bakeera-Kitaka S, Marukutira T, Chapman J, Goldrath K, Ferrand RA. Perinatally acquired HIV infection in adolescents from sub-Saharan Africa: a review of emerging challenges. Lancet Infect Dis. 2014;14(7):627–39.
6. Idele P, Gillespie A, Porth T, Suzuki C, Mahy M, Kasedde S, et al. Epidemiology of HIV and AIDS among adolescents: current status, inequities, and data gaps. J Acquir Immune Defic Syndr. 2014;66(Suppl 2):S144–53.
7. UNAIDS. Global report. UNAIDS report on the global AIDS epidemic 2013. Geneva: UNAIDS; 2013.
8. Cruz ML, Cardoso CA, Darmont MQ, Souza E, Andrade SD, D'Al Fabbro MM, et al. Viral suppression and adherence among HIV-infected children and adolescents on antiretroviral therapy: results of a multicenter study. J Pediatr. 2014;90(6):563–71.
9. Zanoni BC, Mayer KH. The adolescent and young adult HIV cascade of care in the United States: exaggerated health disparities. AIDS Patient Care STDS. 2014;28(3):128–35.
10. Nachega JB, Hislop M, Nguyen H, Dowdy DW, Chaisson RE, Regensberg L, et al. Antiretroviral therapy adherence, virologic and immunologic outcomes in adolescents compared with adults in southern Africa. J Acquir Immune Defic Syndr. 2009;51(1):65–71.
11. Brown LK, Lourie KJ, Pao M. Children and adolescents living with HIV and AIDS: a review. J Child Psychol Psychiatry. 2000;41(1):81–96.
12. Binagwaho A, Fuller A, Kerry V, Dougherty S, Agbonyitor M, Wagner C, et al. Adolescents and the right to health: eliminating age-related barriers to HIV/AIDS services in Rwanda. AIDS Care. 2012;24(7):936–42.
13. Siu GE, Bakeera-Kitaka S, Kennedy CE, Dhabangi A, Kambugu A. HIV serostatus disclosure and lived experiences of adolescents at the Transition Clinic of the Infectious Diseases Clinic in Kampala, Uganda: a qualitative study. AIDS Care. 2012;24(5):606–11.
14. Kim SH, Gerver SM, Fidler S, Ward H. Adherence to antiretroviral therapy in adolescents living with HIV: systematic review and meta-analysis. AIDS. 2014;28(13):1945–56.
15. Abubakar A, Van de Vijver FJ, Fischer R, Hassan AS, Gona JK, Dzombo JT, et al. 'Everyone has a secret they keep close to their hearts': challenges faced by adolescents living with HIV infection at the Kenyan coast. BMC Public Health. 2016;16:197.
16. Joint United Nations Programme on HIV/AIDS (UNAIDS). Gap report. Geneva, Switzerland: UNAIDS; 2015.
17. Lee S, Hazra R. Achieving 90–90–90 in paediatric HIV: adolescence as the touchstone for transition success. J Int AIDS Soc. 2015;18(Suppl 6):20257.
18. Judd A, Sohn AH, Collins IJ. Interventions to improve treatment, retention and survival outcomes for adolescents with perinatal HIV-1 transitioning to adult care: moving on up. Curr Opin HIV AIDS. 2016;11(5):477–86.
19. Evans D, Menezes C, Mahomed K, Macdonald P, Untiedt S, Levin L, et al. Treatment outcomes of HIV-infected adolescents attending public-sector HIV clinics across Gauteng and Mpumalanga, South Africa. AIDS Res Hum Retroviruses. 2013;29(6):892–900.
20. Bailey H, Cruz MLS, Songtaweesin WN, Puthanakit T. Adolescents with HIV and transition to adult care in the Caribbean, Central America and South America, Eastern Europe and Asia and Pacific regions. J Int AIDS Soc. 2017;20(Suppl 3):50–9.
21. Dahourou DL, Gautier-Lafaye C, Teasdale CA, Renner L, Yotebieng M, Desmonde S, et al. Transition from paediatric to adult care of adolescents living with HIV in sub-Saharan Africa: challenges, youth-friendly models, and outcomes. J Int AIDS Soc. 2017;20(Suppl 3):34–49.
22. Sohn AH, Vreeman RC, Judd A. Tracking the transition of adolescents into adult HIV care: a global assessment. J Int AIDS Soc. 2017;20(Suppl 3):1–3.
23. World Health Organization (WHO). HIV and adolescents: guidance for HIV testing and counseling and care for adolescents living with HIV: recommendations for a public health approach and considerations for policy-makers and managers. Geneva, Switzerland: WHO; 2013.
24. Agwu AL, Fairlie L. Antiretroviral treatment, management challenges and outcomes in perinatally HIV-infected adolescents. J Int AIDS Soc. 2013;16:18579.
25. Dowshen N, D'Angelo L. Health care transition for youth living with HIV/AIDS. Pediatrics. 2011;128(4):762–71.
26. Gilliam PP, Ellen JM, Leonard L, Kinsman S, Jevitt CM, Straub DM. Transition of adolescents with HIV to adult care: characteristics and current practices of the adolescent trials network for HIV/AIDS interventions. J Assoc Nurses AIDS Care. 2011;22(4):283–94.
27. Hussen SA, Chahroudi A, Boylan A, Camacho-Gonzalez AF, Hackett S, Chakraborty R. Transition of youth living with HIV from pediatric to adult-oriented healthcare: a review of the literature. Future Virol. 2015;9(10):921–9.
28. Sharma N, Willen E, Garcia A, Sharma TS. Attitudes toward transitioning in youth with perinatally acquired HIV and their family caregivers. J Assoc Nurses AIDS Care. 2014;25(2):168–75.
29. Fair CD, Goldstein B, Dizney R. Congruence of transition perspectives between adolescents with perinatally-acquired HIV and their guardians: an exploratory qualitative study. J Pediatr Nurs. 2015;30(5):684–90.
30. Boudreau ME, Fisher CM. Providing effective medical and case management services to HIV-infected youth preparing to transition to adult care. J Assoc Nurses AIDS Care. 2012;23(4):318–28.
31. Westling K, Naver L, Vesterbacka J, Belfrage E. Transition of HIV-infected youths from paediatric to adult care, a Swedish single-centre experience. Infect Dis. 2016;48(6):449–52.
32. Ryscavage P, Macharia T, Patel D, Palmeiro R, Tepper V. Linkage to and retention in care following healthcare transition from pediatric to adult HIV care. AIDS Care. 2016;28(5):561–5.
33. Tanner AE, Philbin MM, DuVal A, Ellen J, Kapogiannis B, Fortenberry JD. Transitioning HIV-positive adolescents to adult Care: lessons learned from twelve adolescent medicine clinics. J Pediatr Nurs. 2016;31(5):537–43.
34. Kakkar F, Van der Linden D, Valois S, Maurice F, Onnorouille M, Lapointe N, et al. Health outcomes and the transition experience of HIV-infected adolescents after transfer to adult care in Quebec, Canada. BMC Pediatr. 2016;16:109.
35. Mun M, Sopheab H, Tuot S, Morgan P, Pal K, Chhoun P, et al. National HIV sentinel survey among women attending antenatal care clinics in Cambodia in 2014. Phnom Penh: National Center for HIV/AIDS, Dermatology and STD (NCHADS); 2016.
36. National Center for HIV/AIDS Dermatology and STD (NCHADS). Diagnosis and treatment for HIV infected infant, children and adolescents in Cambodia. Phnom Penh: NCHADS; 2013.
37. National Center for HIV/AIDS Dermatology and STD (NCHADS). Factors affecting the transition from paediatric to adult HIV care services among children living with HIV aged 12–17 in Cambodia. Phnom Penh: NCHADS; 2012.
38. Seng SDT, Welle E, Mok S, Soch K, Tep S, et al. Stigma and discrimination as factors affecting the transition from paediatric to adult HIV care services by children living with HIV aged 12–17 in Cambodia: a qualitative exploratory study. Melbourne: International AIDS Conference; 2014.
39. Chandler C, Ngoksin A. Lost in transitions: current issues faced by adolescents living with HIV in Asia Pacific. Bangkok: UNICEF; 2013.
40. Henderson RH, Sundaresan T. Cluster sampling to assess immunization coverage: a review of experience with a simplified sampling method. Bull World Health Organ. 1982;60(2):253–60.
41. Skinner J. Probability proportional to size (PPS) sampling. London: Wiley; 2006.
42. Bakeera-Kitaka S, Nabukeera-Barungi N, Nostlinger C, Addy K, Colebunders R. Sexual risk reduction needs of adolescents living with HIV in a clinical care setting. AIDS Care. 2008;20(4):426–33.
43. New York State Department of Health AIDS Institute. Transitioning HIV-infected adolescents into adult care. NewYork: New York State Department of Health AIDS Institute; 2011.
44. White AJ, Howland L, Clark MJ. Enhancing acquisition of health care management skills in youth living with HIV prior to transition: a pilot study. J Assoc Nurses AIDS Care. 2015;26(3):296–300.
45. Wiener LS, Kohrt BA, Battles HB, Pao M. The HIV experience: youth identified barriers for transitioning from pediatric to adult care. J Pediatr Psychol. 2011;36(2):141–54.
46. Righetti A, Prinapori R, Nulvesu L, Fornoni L, Viscoli C, Di Biagio A. Transitioning HIV-infected children and adolescents into adult care: an Italian real-life experience. J Assoc Nurses AIDS Care. 2015;26(5):652–9.

47. Machado DM, Succi RC, Turato ER. Transitioning adolescents living with HIV/AIDS to adult-oriented health care: an emerging challenge. J Pediatr. 2010;86(6):465–72.
48. Mark D, Armstrong A, Andrade C, Penazzato M, Hatane L, Taing L, et al. HIV treatment and care services for adolescents: a situational analysis of 218 facilities in 23 sub-Saharan African countries. J Int AIDS Soc. 2017;20(Suppl 3):25–33.
49. Mburu G, Ram M, Oxenham D, Haamujompa C, Iorpenda K, Ferguson L. Responding to adolescents living with HIV in Zambia: a social–ecological approach. Child Youth Serv Rev. 2014;45:9–17.
50. Battles HB, Wiener LS. From adolescence through young adulthood: psychosocial adjustment associated with long-term survival of HIV. J Adolesc Health. 2002;30(3):161–8.
51. Valenzuela JM, Buchanan CL, Radcliffe J, Ambrose C, Hawkins LA, Tanney M, et al. Transition to adult services among behaviorally infected adolescents with HIV—a qualitative study. J Pediatr Psychol. 2011;36(2):134–40.
52. Betz CL, Smith KA, Van Speybroeck A, Hernandez FV, Jacobs RA. Movin' On Up: an innovative nurse-led interdisciplinary health care transition program. J Pediatr Health Care. 2016;30(4):323–38.
53. Wiener LS, Zobel M, Battles H, Ryder C. Transition from a pediatric HIV intramural clinical research program to adolescent and adult community-based care services: assessing transition readiness. Soc Work Health Care. 2007;46(1):1–19.
54. Machado DM, Galano E, de Menezes Succi RC, Vieira CM, Turato ER. Adolescents growing with HIV/AIDS: experiences of the transition from pediatrics to adult care. Braz J Infect Dis. 2016;20(3):229–34.
55. Persson A, Newman C. When HIV-positive children grow up: a critical analysis of the transition literature in developed countries. Qual Health Res. 2012;22(5):656–67.

3

Antiretroviral therapy supply chain quality control and assurance in improving people living with HIV therapeutic outcomes

M. P. Ngogang Djobet[1*], David Singhe[2], Julienne Lohoue[3], Christopher Kuaban[4], Jeanne Ngogang[1,5] and Ernest Tambo[1,5,6]

Abstract

Background: Evaluation of medication efficacy and safety is an essential guarantee to successful therapeutic outcome in public health practices. However, larger distribution chain supply in developing countries such as Cameroon is often challenged by counterfeit drugs, poor manufacturing, storage and degradation leading to health and patient adverse consequences. Yet, access to supply chain management in strengthening ARVs quality assurance and outcomes remains poorly documented. More than 53,000 patients have been enrolled on free ARVs medications, but little is documented on quality assurance and validity of safety for affected populations along the supply chain management since 2008.

Methods: The cross sectional study was conducted in ARVs distribution units and centers in central, littoral and south west regions of Cameroon. ARVs drugs samples included Nevirapine, Efavirenz, and fixed dose combinations of Zidovudine + Lamivudine, Lamivudine + Stavudine and Zidovudine + Lamivudine + Nevirapine. Drugs packaging and labeling was assessed and galenic assays were performed at National Laboratory of quality Control of Medications and Expertise (LANACOME), Yaoundé, Cameroon.

Results: The study covered 16 structures located in eight different towns including the central ARVs store, two regional pharmaceutical procurement centers and thirteen HIV approved treatment centers and management units. A total of 35 ARVs products were collected. Only eight ARVs drugs containing Lamivudine and Stavudine presented with white stains on tablets, however these drugs were standard for all other tests performed. The others 28 ARVs products were standards to all assays performed.

Conclusion: We concluded that ARVs drugs freely accessible and distributed to PLWHA are of good quality in Cameroon. However, with the increase number of patients under HAART since 2013, adoption of "Test and Treat" approach to reach the 90-90-90 goals and with the implementation of new national antiretroviral regimen guidelines and molecules such as boosted protease inhibitors, continuous quality control and assurance surveillance, monitoring and evaluation is recommended. Assessment of quality of formulations that are more susceptible to degradation such as pediatric formulations for averting the rising multidrug resistance trend is also desired.

Keywords: Quality, ARVs, HIV/AIDS, Therapeutic, Outcome, Medicine, Drugs

*Correspondence: mngogang@gmail.com
[1] LABOREB—Laboratoire de Recherche et d'Expertise Biomédicale, Yaoundé, Cameroon
Full list of author information is available at the end of the article

Background

Although scaling up of antiretroviral therapy (ART) is clearly documented across epidemics countries in Africa and elsewhere, ARVs supply chain quality control and assurance in terms of conformity, content, dosage as well as packaging and labeling instructions on use in most developing countries, and Africa in particular is still poorly understood [1–3]. Yet, it is also documented that counterfeit drugs, poor manufacturing and unregulated drugs are found or reported in most developing countries including Cameroon [4]. This situation is worsened by multifactorial challenges and issues including the lack of competent local regulatory authorities, lack or inexistent drugs quality control laboratories, and poverty related socio-economic factors [6–8]. These gaps explain why sub standards medications may also be found in legal drug supply chain [9, 10].

Prior findings have raised concern on presence of substandard antiretroviral drugs in some countries in Africa [11–14]. Sustained access to and use of such poor quality antimicrobial drugs may result in harmful consequences such as serious adverse effects impacting on patient's adherence as well as therapeutic failure and antimicrobial resistance rising disability, morbidity and mortality [15, 16]. While on the other hand, the effective use and compliance to highly active antiretroviral therapy (HAART) and HIV service delivery have shown to significantly reduce morbidity and mortality in people living with HIV/AIDS (PLHA) by preventing relapse and opportunistic infections as well as improvement of quality of life and productivity of patients [17–19]. In Cameroon, data and information related to ARVs quality is based on a 2005 joint project in seven African countries [20] with the adoption and implementation of free ARVs treatment since 2008, thousands of people living with HIV/AIDS (PLWHA) are under HAARVs in the country.

The study aimed at evaluating the quality control and assurance of antiretroviral (ARVs) drugs supply chain and distribution in order to improve therapeutic service delivery and outcomes in PLWHA in Cameroon.

Methods

Study site and population

In Cameroon, ARVs drugs are freely distributed in HIV approved treatment centers (ATC) and management units (MU) which are directly supplied by corresponding regional pharmaceutical procurement centers (RPPC). All regional procurement centers (10 all over the country) are supplied by unique Essential Drugs National Procurement Center (EDNPC). In this study antiretroviral drugs were collected in Central, Littoral and South West regions reported to have higher rates of follow up of HAART patients. In each region, five approved treatment centers or management units were randomly selected in both urban and semi-urban settings. The study lasted for 7 months from 2008 to Jan 2009.

Ethical clearance

The ethical authorization and clearance was obtained from the National AIDS Control Committee (NACC) committee and the Ministry of Health, Cameroon. All samples analyses were performed in LANACOME, Yaoundé Cameroon.

ARVs selection criteria and collection

Antiretroviral active principle selected were those frequently prescribed and consumed within the country as first line regimen for adults [21]. These included the following active principle: Efavirenz, Nevirapine and fixed dose combination containing Lamivudine + Zidovudine, Lamivudine + Stavudine or Zidovudine + Lamivudine + Nevirapine. An administrative authorization from the Ministry of Public Health allowed collection of one or a maximum of two boxes of medications containing the selected active principle within the selected facilities. ARVs medications were provided depending on the stocks available in each facility. A code containing the generic name of the drug as well as the site and date of collection was assigned to each medication box. Boxes were placed into a sterile sealed plastic bag with suitable conditioning and transported to LANACOME laboratory for further analysis.

Inspection of ARVs, packaging characteristics

Each medication box was inspected prior analysis to describe packaging characteristics. Primary and secondary containers and labeling information were verified namely: product's brand name, active principle(s) name(s) and quantity, number of tablets, manufacturer's reference number ,date of manufacturing and expiration, storage conditions, as well as manufacturer's or retailer address. Tablet's color uniformity, odor and presence or absence of powder at the bottom of the secondary container was also recorded on a sheet designed for the purpose of the study.

Determination of tablet weight uniformity, hardness and disintegration time

The determination of weight uniformity of each sample was done using 20 tablets randomly selected inside the secondary container. Analytical precision balance at 0.01 g METTLER PM 400® auto calibrated was used to weight serially one table after another and weight were recorded. The average weight was calculated as well as the standard deviation. Hardness testing was performed on 10 tablets using ERWEKA® TBH 28 and the crushing power of each tablet was expressed in mean Kp. Disintegration time was defined using Pharma test® PT2 Auto 3. Here six tablets of each ARVs was dropped in an apparatus containing distilled water at room temperature and the complete disintegration time was followed up over 15 min and/or repeated in case of failure at time lapsed using (6-6-6 = 18) tablets.

Identification and evaluation of ARVs quality and concentration

ARVs identification and dosage tests were based on European an American Pharmacopeia and all ARVs products analysis were conducted in LANACOME, Yaoundé, Cameroon.

For the purpose of identification of ARVs, thin layer chromatography (TLC) was used to identify each given ARVs active principle using silica gel F245 with 95% ethanol diluting solvent. The development solvent was composed by mixed n-Butanol (40 ml), cyclohexane (30 ml), acetone (30 ml) and ammonia (10 ml). For preparation of standards, 10 mg of each standard was mixed with 10 ml of diluting solvent and homogenized using a vortex. For drug samples, one tablet of drug sample was mixed with 10 ml diluting solvent and homogenized. 5 µl of each standard and sample solutions where placed at 2 cm from the edge of the plate which was then placed inside the chromatography box saturated with the development solvent. After 15 cm of migration, the migration plate was removed and dried at room temperature. Plate was revealed under 254 nm UV light. Identification was considered conform if samples migrated at the same position than standards. Position of migration for each active principle was drawn on an overlay sheet to keep as record.

For concentration (dosage) of active principle(s), it was done through spectrophotometry analyses based on American Pharmacopeia in line with manufacturers labeling specifications. For Nevirapine and Efavirenz samples, tablets were crushed and a quantity corresponding to half a tablet was introduced into a 50 ml graduated flask and then 95% ethanol was added. This S1 solution was sonicated and further diluted into a 1:25 ratio solution (S2) that was also sonicated. Absorbance of S2 solution was measured around 287 nm for Nevirapine and 265 nm for Efavirenz. Drug dosage content was calculated using the following formula:

C = (Standard specimen × optical density of sample × dilution rate of sample/dilution rate of standard × optical density of standard × sample specimen) × mean weight of the tablet in mg.

Drug content was expressed in mg.

For fixed dose combinations, standard were prepared following the steps stated above. For FDC samples, half a tablet of drugs was dissolved in 250 ml of diluted hydrochloric acid (1:62): S1 solution. This S1 solution was diluted into a 1:10 S2 solution that was sonicated again for 15 min. Absorbance of solutions was measured around 263 nm for Stavudine, 265 nm for Zidovudine and 280 nm for Lamivudine.

Data analysis

All data were reported, processed and analyzed on Microsoft office, Excel spreadsheet (version 2007). Results of the conformity and quality and labeling of ARVs drugs tested were expressed in percentage.

Results

Classification of active principles per structures

The study covered 16 structures of the supply chain distribution and storage in eight different towns, including the Essential Drugs National Procurement Center (EDNPC): Central level, two regional pharmaceutical procurement centers (RPPC): Intermediate level and 13 treatment centers: peripheral level including five approved treatment centers (ATC) and 08 management units (MU). The antiretroviral drugs collected were all generics. We assessed the quality of 35 ARVs drugs. From the 35 ARVs drugs collected, four were collected at the central level of the supply chain, seven at the intermediate level and 24 at peripheral level. 19 ARVs drugs were fixed dose combination. Table 1 summarized the distribution of active principle collected per structure (Table 1).

Assessment of packaging and labeling characteristics for collected ARVs

All the 35 collected ARVs were packed in two containers (primary and secondary container). None of these drugs had the expiration date due. All the tablets were stored in bottles (primary containers) made with vinylpolychloride and 80% of these bottles were sealed on top with aluminium foil. More than half (64%) of these bottles had both hydrophilic cotton, aluminium foil and a dryer. All tablets had a homogeneous colour and normal odour, except those of eight (8) Lamivudine + Stavudine fixed dose combination from the same manufacturer whose pink tablets presented with white stains. None of the boxes had broken tablets. All required information was available on the primary container leaflets or patients instructions.

Assessment of tablets hardness/shelf life, weight, and disintegration time

There was uniformity of weight for tablets for all these drugs. Friability and hardness testing as well as disintegration or residual degradation time was also conforming to general WHO pharmacopoeia standards.

Table 1 Classification of active principle (s) per local structure in the three regions

Name of active(s) ingredient(s)	Total numbers of samples	Structures			
		Central level (EDNPC)	Intermediate level (RPPC)	Peripheral level (ATC) (MU)	
Efavirenz tablet 200 mg	2	1	–	1	–
Efavirenz tablet 600 mg	7	–	2	2	3
Lamivudine 150 mg + Stavudine 30 mg tablets	9	1	2	2	4
Lamivudine 150 mg + Zidovudine 300 mg tablets	7	1	1	2	3
Nevirapine 200 mg tablets	7	1	1	2	3
Zidovudine 300 mg + Lamivudine 150 mg + Nevirapine 200 mg	3	–	1	–	2
Total	35	4	7	9	15

Identification of active ingredient(s)/principle(s)

Identification of active principle was performed using thin layer chromatography (TLC). Identification was in concordance for all the collected ARVs. For example, the identification of Efavirenz and fixed dose combination tablets containing Zidovudine, Lamivudine and Nevirapine is shown in Figs. 1 and 2.

In Fig. 1, the image shows on the left, the plate reveal under UV light for eight Efavirenz samples. Image on the right shows overlay sheets of the same plate. The standard position is indicated with the red arrow. All samples tested migrated at the same position as for the standard. There weren't additional spots along the migration way thus assuming purity of these medications (Fig. 1).

In Fig. 2, the image shows identification of active principle in six fixed dose combination containing Zidovudine and Lamivudine and three fixed dose combination containing Zidovudine, Lamivudine and Nevirapine. The black arrow indicates the position where samples were deposited. Red arrow indicates position of migration of

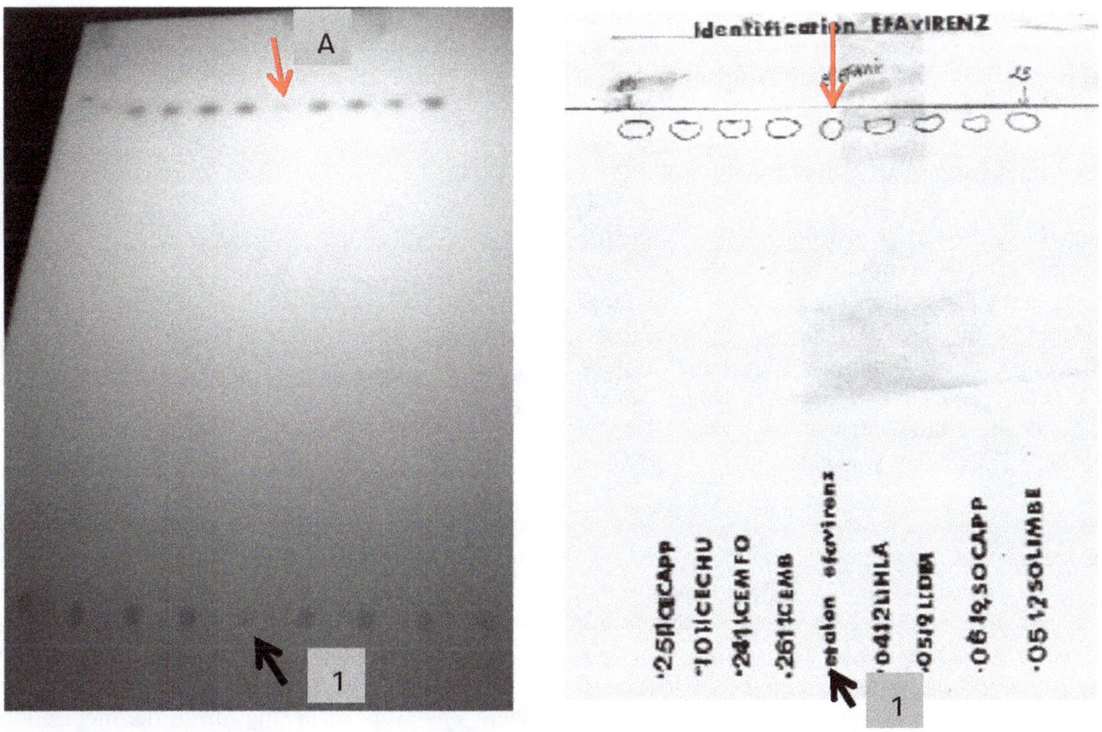

Fig. 1 TLC for Efavirenz samples, plate reveal under ultraviolet (UV) light. *1* Deposit site of standards and samples. *A* Migration site for efavirenz standard

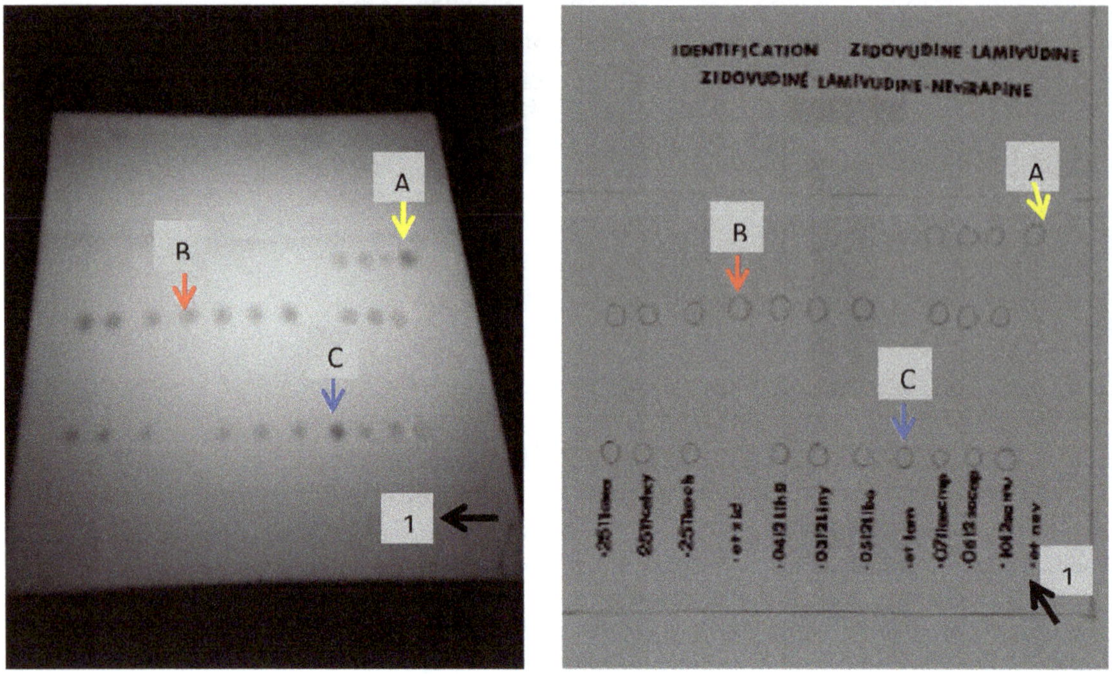

Fig. 2 TLC for fixed dose combinations containing Zidovudine, Lamivudine and Zidovudine, Lamivudine and Nevirapine, plate reveal under UV light. *1* Deposit site of standards and samples. *A* Migration site for nevirapine standard. *B* Migration site for zidovudine standard. *C* Migration site for lamivudine standard

Zidovudine standard, while blue and yellow arrows indicate position of lamivudine and Nevirapine standards respectively. Identification was in concordance for these nine fixed dose combinations. No additional spots were observed during this migration thus assuming purity of these medications (Fig. 2).

Assessment of the concentration of active principle per tablet

According to American's pharmacopeia, concentration of active principles should range between 90 and 110% of the dosage stated on the container. This range was respected for the 35 ARVs collected. Figure 3 shows range of content for Nevirapine and Efavirenz samples. Dosage of active principle in Nevirapine samples varied between 95.85 and 105.36% of the stated dose while for Efavirenz tablets, variation was between 95.9 and 103% (Fig. 3).

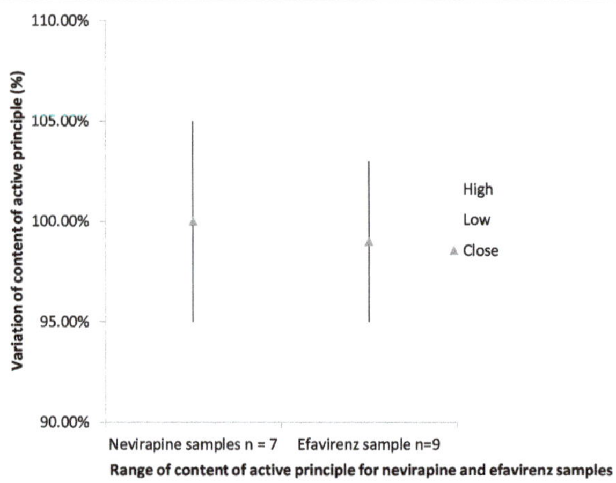

Fig. 3 Range of active principle concentration for Nevirapine and Efavirenz

Discussions

The study assessed the quality of 35 ARVs drugs collected; four were collected at the central level of the supply chain, seven at the intermediate level and 24 at peripheral level. 19 ARVs drugs were fixed dose combination. It also provided insights on ARVs supply chain adherence in Cameroon. It showed that ARVs tablets weight were uniform for all these drugs, while the hardness (friability) and hardness testing as well as disintegration time were also conforming. None of these drugs had the expiration date due. As packaging preserves the stability and quality of medicinal products, packaging of ARVs collected was primarily assessed using WHO recommendations [23]. There was proper labelling for all the medication boxes collected and specific description of containers revealed that all the tablets were stored in bottles (primary containers) made with vinyl-polychloride and 80% of these bottles were sealed on top with aluminium foil. More than half (64%) of these bottles had both hydrophilic cotton, aluminium foil and a dryer. Sealing with aluminium foil and combination of cotton, aluminium foil and dryer are elements of the manufacturing process that contribute to enhance drug stability. All tablets had a homogeneous colour and normal odour, except those of eight (8) Lamivudine + Stavudine fixed dose combination from the same manufacturer whose pink tablets presented with white stains. None of the boxes had broken tablets. Regarding classification of principles and structure, the selection of ARVs was based on rate of consumption of antiretroviral drugs obtained from the National Aids Control Committee report [21]. Only active principle from first line regimen were considered (nucleosidic and non nucleosidic inhibitors) because of their frequent use and also because by that time, not many people were under second line regimen including protease inhibitors. Since drugs are freely distributed, stocks of medications are strictly calculated for each region, management units and treatment centers from central level of the supply chain. Thus we were given ARVs drugs in such a way not to disrupt stocks in each structure and active principle depended on availability. This explains the variability in the number and the nature of active principle collected among the various structures. We could not obtain drugs from one of the structure at the intermediate level, because of additional administrative procedures requested in that structure.

Our findings from the assessment of formulation, labeling and packaging characteristics of different collected ARVs revealed that all these ARVs were properly packed according to WHO guidelines on packaging for pharmaceutical products [22]. Appropriate packaging of the generic drugs can be explained by the fact that all the medications were WHO prequalified products, meaning they were manufactured in sites audited and recognized by WHO to respect quality assurance during manufacturing process [23]. Use of prequalified drugs has been set up by the government to ensure good quality of ARVs available in the country.

During inspection procedure, Lamivudine and Stavudine fixed dose combination tablets from the same pharmaceutical company did not have a homogeneous colour. This lack of uniformity was observed on tablets of all the samples collected in the various regions. However, they conformed to all others tests performed, suggesting that this lack of uniformity of colour may be related to manufacturing process and was not a result of tablet's degradation. Nonetheless, Stavudine regimen have been progressively phased out in the country [24] and are not anymore used due to HIV patients severe toxicity widely reported [25, 26].

Findings from assessment of physico–chemical properties, identification and active principle dosage showed that all the drugs collected complied for the tests performed. Good quality of medications recorded could firstly be explained by the fact that procurement process for these free ARVs drugs in the country follow up strong regulations and secondly all brands collected were WHO prequalified products [23], guaranteeing the source of manufacturing. Our findings were consistent with previous assessment of antiretroviral drugs quality in seven African countries where Cameroon was the second country using pre-qualified drugs (68% of antiretroviral available) compared to Uganda, Nigeria and Zambia with respectively 32.33 and 34% of use [20].

Methods used for identification and active principle dosage in this study were those available at LANACOME. Although there are more sensitive methods such as high liquid performance chromatography that could be used [27], thin layer chromatography and spectrometry analyses have been demonstrated to remain good practices for identification and dosage of drugs, especially in country where accessibility to expensive equipment as for high performance liquid chromatography (HPLC) is not possible [28]. Baseline characterization of active principle(s) concentration per tablet and per class of ARV drugs were consistent with standard recommended by WHO guidelines and manufacturers labels/patients instructions. Good quality of antiretroviral drugs found in our study was consistent with other studies [29–31]. However, other relevant issues that rose from previous findings in other studies such as storage conditions and their impact on quality of medications were not documented [2–5, 32–34].

The findings limitations included limited access to other regions of Cameroon in assessing the quality of ARVs drugs, only tablets formulations could be tested and lack of equipment and facilities for liquid formulations assessment at LANACOME.

Conclusion

It was evident, ARVs supply chain distribution in terms of quality and conformity standards were consistent with international regulations in the three assessed regions. According to our findings, procurement of prequalified drugs is highly recommended to avoid distribution of fake medication, especially for ARVs, since manufacturing sites for these drugs are numerous. Also, conducting other assessment studies in different settings is advisable to gather insights that can help to ensure safe, efficient and effective use of safe ARVs. Importantly, coherent and coordinated supply chain harmonization and coordination as well as continuous quality control monitoring and evaluation of all forms of drugs seems to be crucial in maintaining efficacy and safety towards PLWHA patients' successful therapeutic care delivery and outcomes.

Abbreviations

ARVs: antiretroviral; ATC: approved treatment center; EDNPC: Essential Drugs National Procurement Center; FDC: fixed dose combination; HPLC: high performance liquide chromatography; LANACOME: Laboratoire Nationale de Contrôle de Qualité des Médicaments et d'Expertise; MU: management unit; NACC: National AIDS Control Committee; PLWHA: people living with HIV/AIDS; RPPC: regional pharmaceutical procurement center; TLC: thin layer chromatography; WHO: World Health Organization.

Authors' contributions

MAPND conducted the study, DS and JYN provided technical support, JL and CK supervised the study. MAPND and ET drafted and revised the manuscript. All authors read and approved the final manuscript.

Author details

[1] LABOREB—Laboratoire de Recherche et d'Expertise Biomédicale, Yaoundé, Cameroon. [2] LANACOME, National Laboratory for Drugs Quality Control, Ministry of Public Health, Yaoundé, Cameroon. [3] Faculty of Medicine and Biomedical Sciences, University of Yaoundé I, Yaoundé, Cameroon. [4] Faculty of Medicine, University of Bamenda, Bamenda, Cameroon. [5] Université des Montagnes, Bangangté, Cameroon. [6] Africa Disease Intelligence and Surveillance, Communication and Response (Africa DISCoR) Institute, Yaoundé, Cameroon.

Acknowledgements

We acknowledge the Ministry of Public Health of Cameroon and the National Aids Control Committee for authorizing this study and the collection of antiretrovirals among facilities.

Competing interests

The authors declare that they have no competing interests.

Funding

The study was funded by Centre International de Référence Chantal BIYA.

References

1. Fayorsey RN, Saito S, Cartser RJ, Gusmao E, Frederix K. Decentralization of pediatric HIV care and treatment in five sub-saharan african countries. J Acquir Immun Defic Syndr. 2013;62:e124–30.
2. Beker LG, Venter F, Cohen K, Goemare E, Van Cutsem G, Boulle A, Wood R. Provision of antiretroviral therapy in South Africa: the nuts and bolts. Antiretrovir Ther. 2014;19(Suppl 3):105–16.
3. Hoen ET. Assuring access to quality antiretroviral medicines: the WHO prequalification of medicines program and access to HIV treatment. Cad Saúde Pública. 2014;30(5):908–9.
4. Committee on Understanding the Global Public Health Implications of Substandard, Falsified, and counterfeit medical products; Board on Global Health; Institute of Medicine. In: Buckley GJ, Gostin LO, editors. Countering the problem of falsified and substandard drugs. Washington: National Academies Press; 2013.
5. The effects of falsified and substandard drugs. https://www.ncbi.nlm.nih.gov/books/NBK202526/. Accessed 12 Oct 2016.
6. Desale A, Taye B, Belay G, Nigatu A. Assessment of laboratory logistics management information system practice for HIV/AIDS and tuberculosis laboratory commodities in selected public health facilities in Addis Ababa, Ethiopia. Pan Afr Med J. 2013;8(15):46.
7. Rägo L, Sillo H, t Hoen E, Zweygarth M. Regulatory framework for access to safe, effective quality medicines. Antivir Ther. 2014;19(Suppl 3):69–77.
8. Windisch R, Waiswa P, Neuhann F, Scheibe F, de Savigny D. Scaling up antiretroviral therapy in Uganda: using supply chain management to appraise health systems strengthening. Glob Health. 2011;1(7):25.
9. Schneider H, Blaauw D, Gilson L, Chabikuli N, Goudge J. Health systems and access to antiretroviral drugs for HIV in Southern Africa: service delivery and human resources challenges. Reprod Health Matters. 2006;14(27):12–23.
10. Ondari C, Maponga C. The quality of antimalarials. A study in selected African countries. Geneva: WHO; 2003.
11. World Health Organization Regional Office for Africa. Medicines regulatory authorities: current status and the way forward. Report of the regional director. ARF/RC/56/11; 2006.
12. James S. Counterfeit drugs: check combivir, serostim, epogen. AIDS Treat News. 2001; issue 380. http://www.aegis.com/pubs/atn/2002/ATN38003.html. Accessed 24 Jun 2015.
13. Ravinetto R. Counterfeit ARVs in DRC. E- drug. 2004. http://www.essentialdrugs.org/edrug. Accessed 12 Oct 2016.
14. Penzak SR, Acosta EP, Turner M, Tavel JA, Masur H. Antiretroviral drug content in products from developing countries. Clin Infect Dis. 2004;38:1317–9.
15. Schuman M, Schneider S, Omes C, Wennig R, Fundira L, Tayari JC, Arendt V. HPLC analysis of generic antiretroviral drugs purchased in Rwanda. Bull Soc Sci Méd. 2005;3:317–25.
16. Johnston A, Holt DW. Substandard drugs: a potential crisis for public health. Br J Clin Pharmacol. 2014;78(2):218–43.
17. Kelesidis T, Falagas M. Substandard/counterfeit antimicrobial drugs. Clin Microbiol Rev. 2015;28(2):443–64.
18. Oguntibeju OO. Quality of life of people living with HIV and AIDS and antiretroviral therapy. HIV/AIDS (Auckl). 2012;4:117–24.
19. Candiani TMS, Pinto J, Cardoso CAA, Carvalho IR, Dias ACM, Carneiro M, Goulart EA. Impact of highly active antiretroviral therapy (HA) on the incidence of opportunistic infections, hospitalizations and mortality among children and adolescents living with HIV/AIDS in Belo Horizonte, Minas Gerais State Brazil. Cadernos de Saúde Pública. 2007;23(Suppl 3):S414–23.
20. Goga AE, Singh Y, Singh M, Noveve N, Magasana V, Ramraj T, Abdullah F, Coovadia AH, Bhardwaj S, Sherman GG. Enhancing HIV treatment access and outcomes amongst HIV infected children and adolescents in resource limited settings. Matern Child Health J. 2016. **(Epub ahead of print)**.
21. WHO quality assurance and safety medicines policy and standards. Survey of the quality of antiretroviral medicines circulating in selected African Countries; 2007. WHO/PSM/QSM/2007.9.
22. Comité National de Lutte contre le SIDA. Vers l'accès universel aux traitements et soins en faveur des adultes et enfants vivant avec le VIH/SIDA au Cameroun. Rapport de progrès N°11; 2008.
23. World Health Organization. Guidelines on packaging for pharmaceutical products. WHO technical report series. Geneva: World Health Organisation; 2002.
24. WHO Prequalification Programme: Access to quality control laboratories that meet recommended international norms and standards for the analysis of products in the prequalification programme. HIV/AIDS, malaria and tuberculosis products version: 5th ed. 2007. disponible à l'http://mednet3.who.int/prequal/lists/PQ_QCLabsList.pdf, consulté le 20 janvier 2009.
25. World Health Organization. Consolidated guidelines on the use of antiretroviral drugs for treating and preventing HIV infection WHO. Geneva: World Health Organisation; 2013.
26. van Oosterhout JJ, Mallewa J, Kaunda S, Chagoma N, Njalale Y, et al. (2012) Stavudine toxicity in adult longer-term ART patients in Blantyre, Malawi. PLoS ONE 7(7):e42029. doi:10.1371/journal.pone.0042029.
27. Palmer M, Chersich M, Moultrie H, Kuhn L, Fairlie L, Meyers T. Frequency of stavudine substitution due to toxicity in children receiving antiretroviral treatment in sub-Saharan Africa. AIDS. 2013;27(5):781–5.
28. Siddiqui MR, AlOthman ZA, Rahman N. Analytical techniques in pharmaceutical analysis: a review. Arabian J. Chem. 2017;10(Suppl 1):S1409–21.

29. Penzack S, Acosta E, Tavel J, Masur H. Analysis of generic Nevirapine products in developing countries. JAMA. 2003;289:2648–9.
30. Manji I, Manyara SM, Jakait B, Ogallo W, Hagedorn IC, Lukas S, Kosgei EJ, Pastakia SD. The revolving fund pharmacy model: backing up the ministry of health supply chain in western Kenya. Int J Pharm Pract. 2016;24(5):358–66.
31. Du Toit K, du Preez W, Padayachee S. Patents and the quality, safety and efficacy of medicines. S Afr Med J. 2015;105(11):905–6.
32. Anywaine Z, Abaasa A, Levin J, Kasirye R, Kamali A, Grosskurth H, Munderi P, Nunn A. Safety of discontinuing cotrimoxazole prophylaxis among HIV infected adults on anti-retroviral therapy in Uganda (COSTOP trial): design. Contemp Clin Trials. 2015;43:100–4.
33. Masimirembwa C, Dandara C, Leutscher PD. Rolling out Efavirenz for HIV precision medicine in Africa: are we ready for pharmacovigilance and tackling neuropsychiatric adverse effects? OMICS. 2016;20(10):575–80.
34. Phillips AN, Cambiano V, Miners A, Revill P, Pillay D, Lundgren JD, Bennett D, Raizes E, Nakagawa F, De Luca A, Vitoria M, Barcarolo J, Perriens J, Jordan MR, Bertagnolio S. Effectiveness and cost-effectiveness of potential responses to future high levels of transmitted HIV drug resistance in antiretroviral drug-naive populations beginning treatment: modelling study and economic analysis. Lancet HIV. 2014;1(2):e85–93.

4

The developmental effects of HIV and alcohol: a comparison of gestational outcomes among babies from South African communities with high prevalence of HIV and alcohol use

Kirsten A. M. Donald[1*], Anne Fernandez[2], Kasey Claborn[2,3,4], Caroline Kuo[2,5,6], Nastassja Koen[6], Heather Zar[1,7] and Dan J. Stein[6,8]

Abstract

Background: There is growing evidence of the negative impact of alcohol on morbidity and mortality of individuals living with HIV but limited evidence of in utero effects of HIV and alcohol on exposure on infants.

Methods: We conducted a population-based birth cohort study (N = 667 mother-infant dyads) in South Africa to investigate whether maternal alcohol use and HIV affected gestational outcomes. Descriptive data analysis was conducted for all variables using frequency distributions, measures of central tendency, and estimates of variance. Hierarchical multiple regression was conducted to determine whether maternal alcohol use, maternal HIV status and other risk factors (socioeconomic status, smoking, depression) predicted infant outcomes.

Results: Our results showed severity of recent alcohol use and lifetime alcohol use predicted low birth weight. Similarly lifetime alcohol use predicted shorter infant length, smaller head length, smaller head circumference, and early gestational age. However, HIV status was not a significant predictor of gestational outcomes.

Conclusions: The unexpected finding that maternal HIV status did not predict any of the gestational outcomes may be due to high rates of ART usage among HIV-infected mothers. The potentially negative effects of HIV on gestational outcomes may have been attenuated by improved maternal health due to high coverage of antiretroviral treatment in South Africa. Interventions are needed to reduce alcohol consumption among pregnant mothers and to support healthy growth and psychosocial development of infants.

Keywords: Gestational outcomes, Alcohol, HIV, South Africa, Pregnancy

Background

Alcohol use, including hazardous and harmful levels, remains a serious health problem among individuals living with HIV globally and in South Africa specifically. In South Africa, the country with the largest number of people living with HIV (PLWH) globally [1], alcohol consumption is among the highest in the world [2]. A national survey documented that 9% of the population engage in risky or hazardous drinking [3–5]. Even more concerning is a high proportion of individuals living with HIV struggle with alcohol abuse and dependence. While national estimates are unavailable, local studies in communities with high prevalence of HIV show rates of recent alcohol use as high as 51% as well as concerning levels of dependence or abuse among PLWH (7%) [6, 7].

*Correspondence: kirsty.donald@uct.ac.za
[1] Department of Paediatrics and Child Health, Institute of Child Health Building, Red Cross War Memorial Children's Hospital, 5th Floor, Klipfontein Road, Rondebosch, Cape Town 7700, South Africa

A growing body of literature highlights the synergistic and detrimental effects of alcohol on morbidity and mortality of individuals living with HIV [8]. Alcohol use accelerates disease progression via biological pathways. This includes both increased viral replication and diminished immune function. For example, alcohol use is associated with depletion of CD4 cells [9, 10] and has been shown to negatively affect performance of T and B lymphocytes and other important immune responses [11–15]. Alcohol use also accelerates disease progression via behavioral pathways for PLWH. A recent meta-analysis and a systematic review showed that alcohol use was linked to poorer adherence to antiretroviral therapy and lower utilization of health services [16, 17].

The negative health-related consequences of alcohol use among PLWH may be of even greater concern among pregnant women living with HIV. Several meta-analyses indicate that heavy alcohol use during pregnancy can increase risk for low birth weight, preterm birth, small gestational age [18] and long term growth impact including gross motor deficits [19]. Similarly, maternal HIV infection has been associated with poor fetal outcomes including low birth weight [20] and pre-term delivery [21, 22]. Maternal HIV infection, particularly mother-to-child transmission of HIV, can affect fetal development of the infant brain. For example, there is growing evidence that babies infected with HIV are at risk of significantly poorer performance of infant motor and cognitive development even if they do not meet criteria for HIV encephalopathy [23]. There may be synergistic effects of alcohol and HIV on health, particularly during the gestational period. As such, additional research is needed to determine whether HIV might interact with alcohol to negatively affect infant outcomes among babies born to mothers affected by HIV and using alcohol.

South Africa is an ideal setting to investigate whether living with HIV and using alcohol during pregnancy might have synergistic affects upon fetal outcomes. Rates of alcohol use during pregnancy have been well-documented in South Africa. South Africa has the highest global rates of fetal alcohol syndrome (FAS) [24]. However, only a handful of studies document rates of alcohol use among HIV-infected pregnant women in South Africa. One cross-sectional survey of pregnant women attending clinics documented that 18 percent engaged in drinking during pregnancy and 67% reported problem drinking (more than 3 drinks in one sitting) [25]. Another study analyzing a subset of data from a longitudinal cohort of female drinkers in Cape Town documented that 73% continued drinking after recognition of pregnancy [26]. However, no study to date has compared alcohol use patterns among HIV-positive and HIV-negative pregnant women or examined whether alcohol use among pregnant mothers living with HIV has any effect on gestational outcomes.

We conducted a population-based birth cohort study in the Western Cape Province, a region supported heavily by an agricultural economy centered on wine production. Our choice of this site was purposeful given the rates of alcohol abuse and dependence, and HIV prevalence in this region. Rates of alcohol use may be particularly problematic due to the historical legacy of the 'dop' system where farm workers were paid in crude wine [27]. Rates of FAS or Partial Fetal Alcohol Syndrome (PFAS) are alarmingly high, at 135–207 cases per 1000 people in certain high risk communities in the Western Cape [28]. Our analyses focused on determining whether there were differences in alcohol intake between HIV-positive and HIV-negative pregnant women and whether HIV or alcohol had any synergistic effects of gestational outcomes of birth weight percentile, length, head circumference, and gestational age.

Methods

Data was collected from an investigation of child health, called the Drakenstein Child Health Study (DCHS). The DCHS consisted of a multidisciplinary birth cohort study following mother–child dyads from the prenatal period through to five years of age [29, 30]. The aim of DCHS is to investigate the epidemiology, etiology, and risk factors of childhood respiratory disease and the determinants of child health in a low socioeconomic area of South Africa [30]. The study investigates the role and interaction of possible risk factors in 7 areas (environmental, infectious, nutritional, genetic, psychosocial, maternal and immunological risk factors) that may impact child health.

Design

Pregnant women were recruited from two primary care clinics in the Drakenstein sub-district near Cape Town, South Africa between March 2012 and September 2014. Data collection occurred at these two clinics (maternal data) and at a central hospital (newborn outcomes). Participants were enrolled in the study at 20–28 weeks gestation upon presenting for antenatal booking. The mothers were followed throughout pregnancy and mother–child dyads are followed until five years after birth. Data collection for the DCHS remains ongoing. Throughout the study, participants receive regular medical care as per the South Africa national program and expanded program for immunization (EPI) schedule.

Setting

The DCHS is located in the Drakenstein area, a peri-urban area, 60 km outside Cape Town, South Africa with a population of approximately 200,000. The community is stable, with low levels of immigration or emigration. The local economy is based around commercial agriculture and light industry. More than 90% of the population access health care in the public sector including antenatal and child health services [31]. This area has a well-established, free primary health care system, with high coverage for childhood immunizations. The public health system is comprised of 23 primary health care clinics and one centralized hospital where all births and all hospital-based pediatric care, including admissions occur [30].

Participants

To be eligible for the study, participants were: (a) over age 18, (b) pregnant, (c) 20–28 weeks gestation, and (d) receiving antenatal care at a participating study site. The two primary clinics were TC Newman clinic (serving a predominantly "Coloured" or mixed ancestry community) and Mbekweni clinic (serving a predominantly black African community). Exclusion criteria were minimal in order to maximize generalizability, and focused primarily on those individuals who did not live in the region (and could not readily complete follow-up assessments) or those who were intending to move out of the district within the following 2 years. The cohort comprised mothers presenting in an unfiltered manner to the antenatal services and were not selected for any clinical risk factors or exposures. The study was approved by the Faculty of Health Sciences, Human Research Ethics Committee, University of Cape Town (401/2009), and by the Western Cape Provincial Health Research committee. Written informed parental consent was obtained from all participants at the time of enrolment.

Measures

Demographics

Demographic data was collected regarding participant age, education, employment, and socioeconomic status (SES). For our purposes, a composite SES score was developed in order to categorize participants into quartiles based on their relative SES. This composite score is calculated based on current employment status and standardized scores of educational attainment, household income, and a composite asset index based on access to household resources, amenities, and market access. Participants were categorized as being of low, low-moderate, moderate-high, or high SES based on their relative composite SES score.

HIV status

Maternal HIV status was determined using an HIV ELISA test, which all mothers in South Africa receive during pregnancy due to the high prevalence of HIV. Those who tested positive for HIV self-reported whether she was prescribed antiretroviral therapy. Mothers who were newly diagnosed received a second confirmatory HIV ELISA test and were referred for counseling and evaluation for treatment initiation as per standard management guidelines.

Newborn birth outcomes

All babies were born at a central hospital that serves the communities of both clinics. Trained clinical staff recorded newborn birth weight (kilograms) at the time of delivery, using a digital scale with a precision level of 10 g. Gestational age (weeks), head circumference and length in centimeters were also recorded at birth. We defined low birth weight and very low birth weight according to World Health Organization's (WHO's) parameters for weight for age, with low birth weight defined as less than 2.5 kilograms and very low birth weight as less than 1.5 kg [32]. Percentile for infant birth weight was then calculated using the formula proposed by Mikolajcyzk et al. [33]. This formula enabled us to calculate the birth weight percentile based on gestational week of each infant. We used full-term, low-risk infants (N = 100) as the reference group for anchoring our percentile estimates. This method for estimating fetal weight percentiles has a better ability to predict adverse perinatal outcomes than other unadjusted and fully individualized formulas [33].

Alcohol use

Risk of substance use was assessed using the alcohol, smoking and substance involvement screening test (ASSIST) at the second antenatal visit (28–32 weeks gestation). This tool was developed by the WHO to detect psychoactive substance use and related disorders in primary care settings. It has shown good reliability, feasibility and validity in international, multisite studies [34, 35], and is useful for identifying risk of substance dependence in poly-substance abusers with varying degrees of psychopathology. Seven items are included to assess alcohol and other drug use across 10 categories (i.e., tobacco products; alcoholic beverages; cannabis; cocaine; amphetamine-type stimulants; inhalants, sedatives or sleeping pills; hallucinogens; opioids; and a general category entitled "other", in which the participant is required to specify the substance used). ASSIST scores from 0 to 10 for alcohol and 0–3 for illicit drugs indicating low-risk, scores from 11 to 26 for alcohol and 4–26 for illicit drugs indicate moderate-risk and scores above 26 indicate high risk of severe problems, with the likelihood of substance dependence. The higher the score, the greater substance-related risk. The ASSIST has good reliability scores and has been validated in numerous populations [36], as well as primary care settings [37]. For our purposes, only data for alcohol were extracted from the ASSIST, as reports of other substance use were negligible with the exception of tobacco where a biochemical measure of exposure was used as detailed below. Lifetime alcohol use was a dichotomous variable coded as 0, 1. Past 3 month alcohol use severity was calculated as a continuous variable using standard scoring techniques to calculate a sum score based on past 3-month alcohol use frequency, craving, consequences, and other symptoms of alcohol use disorders as detailed above [38].

Tobacco use

Biochemical verification of smoking status was determined through cotinine urine analysis collected on the same day as the baseline interview. Cotinine is a nicotine metabolite that is measurable among people who smoke, use smokeless tobacco, use nicotine products, or are exposed to environmental tobacco smoke. An antenatal urine cotinine cut-off value of 500 was used to distinguish active smokers from non-smokers [39].

Depression

The Beck Depression Inventory-II (BDI-II) [40] was used to assess depressive symptomatology. This is a widely used self-report measure of the severity of depressive symptoms with strong internal consistency and concurrent validity in clinical and non-clinical samples [41, 42]. Each item is assessed on a severity scale ranging from 0, "absence of symptoms", to 3 "severe, often with functional impairment". A total score was obtained by summing individual item responses, with higher scores indicative of more severe depressive symptoms.

Data analysis

Descriptive data analysis was conducted for all variables using frequency distributions, measures of central tendency, and estimates of variance. Hierarchical multiple regression was conducted to determine whether maternal HIV status, alcohol use, and other risk factors (socioeconomic status or SES, smoking, depression) predicted infant outcomes. Infant outcomes included birth weight percentile, length, head circumference, and gestational age. All outcomes were entered as continuous variables in regression analyses. The analyses were conducted in a step-wise fashion to examine the unique contributions for each block of predictor variables. The four steps/blocks of variables in the regression analyses included (in order): (1) HIV status, (2) SES score, BDI-II score, and smoking status, (3) alcohol use, and (4) interaction variables (HIV by alcohol use and HIV by smoking status). We examined separate models using the predictors past 3-month alcohol use severity and lifetime alcohol. All regression models were examined for violations of normality, linearity, homoscedasticity, redundancy, and multicollinearity. Data performed excellently on all criteria except for length of gestation. Length of gestation was non-normal (skew = −2.04, kurtosis = 7.38) and the log of this variable was used in the analysis. Statistical significance was set at the 0.05 level.

Results

Descriptive analyses

The sample included 667 mother-infant dyads of whom 19.6% (n = 131) of the maternal sample was HIV-positive (Table 1). All mothers with HIV were on ART; no infants were HIV-infected. A diverse range of socioeconomic backgrounds was represented, and 26.7% (n = 178) of mothers were categorized as low SES. In terms of depression as measured by the BDI-II, 25% (n = 167) of the mothers reported symptoms consistent with mild depression, 22.5% (n = 150) reported moderate depression, and 7.8% (n = 52) reported high/severe depression. With regards to alcohol use as measured by the ASSIST, 42.2% (n = 280) of mothers reported a lifetime history of alcohol use, and 21.54%, (n = 148) reported alcohol use in the past 3-months. Heavy alcohol use in the past 3-months was reported by a small percentage of mothers (3.1%; n = 21), moderate alcohol use was reported by 7.7% (n = 53), and light use by 10.8% (n = 74). In this cohort, HIV-infected mothers had significantly lower lifetime history of alcohol use (14.6%) compared to HIV-negative mothers (48.9%), χ^2 (1, N = 664) = 50.32, p < 001; lower 3-month alcohol use (light use: 12.8% vs. 10.8%, moderate use: 8.5% vs. 4.6%, heavy use: 2.9% vs. 3.8%, χ^2 (1, N = 148) = 7.78, $p < 0.020$. Approximately 1 in 3 mothers were current smokers (32.7%; n = 213).

Infant outcomes are presented in Table 2. The mean birth weight was 3.02 kilograms (SD = 0.58), with 3.3% (n = 22) of infants categorized as low birth weight (<10th percentile) and 4.8% (n = 32) of infants categorized as very low birth weight (<3rd percentile). The mean gestational age was 38.35 weeks (SD = 2.58). Pre-term infants (<37 weeks gestation) accounted for 15.6% (n = 104) of the infant sample. The mean head circumference was 33.55 cm (SD = 1.87). The mean length was 49.86 cm (SD = 3.8).

Hierarchical multiple regression analyses

Birth weight percentile

Model results for the hierarchical multiple regression analysis for birth weight percentile is presented in Table 3. Step 1 of the model, which included HIV status was not significant, and accounted for a very small proportion of variance in birth weight percentile, F (1, 648) = 2.92, p = 0.09, R^2 = 0.004. Step 2, which added smoking, SES, and depression, was significant, F (4,

Table 1 Maternal characteristics and risk factors by maternal HIV status

	HIV negative		HIV positive		Total		p value
	N = 556	%	N = 131	%	N = 667	%	
Socio-economic status							<0.000
Low	125	23.32	53	40.46	178	26.69	
Low-moderate	101	18.84	34	25.95	135	20.24	
Moderate-high	157	29.29	27	20.61	184	27.59	
High	153	28.54	17	12.98	170	25.49	
Depression							<0.095
Minimal	244	45.52	54	41.22	298	44.68	
Mild	137	25.56	30	22.90	167	25.04	
Moderate	120	22.39	30	22.90	150	22.49	
High	35	6.53	17	12.98	52	7.80	
Lifetime alcohol use							
Yes	261	48.88	19	14.62	280	42.17	<0.000
Past 3-month alcohol use severity score							<0.020
None	422	75.90	117	89.31	539	78.46	
Light	71	12.77	3	2.29	74	10.77	
Moderate	47	8.45	6	4.58	53	7.71	
Heavy	16	2.88	5	3.82	21	3.06	
Smoking (Cotinine)							
Yes	183	35.06	30	23.08	213	32.67	<0.009

Table 2 Infant characteristics by maternal HIV status

	HIV negative		HIV positive		Total		p value
	N (556)	%	N (131)	%	N (667)	%	
Birth weight percentile (%)							<0.748
<3	28	5.23	4	3.05	32	4.80	
3 to <10	20	3.74	2	1.53	22	3.30	
≥10	487	91.03	125	95.42	612	91.89	
Gestational age (full/pre-term)							
<37 weeks	80	14.93	24	18.32	104	15.59	<0.337
	HIV negative		**HIV positive**		**Total**		**p value**
	Mean	**SD**	**Mean**	**SD**	**Mean**	**SD**	
Infant birth weight (kg)	3.01	0.58	3.03	0.58	3.02	0.58	<0.729
Infant head circumference (cm)	33.50	1.80	33.76	2.08	33.55	1.87	<0.944
Infant length (cm)	49.87	3.63	49.84	4.48	49.86	3.8	<0.153
Length of gestation (weeks)	38.39	2.45	38.21	3.07	38.35	2.58	<0.489

cm centimeters, *kg* kilograms

648) = 10.88, p < 0.001, $R^2 = 0.06$, and increased the proportion of variance accounted for by 6% ($\Delta R^2 = 0.06$). Step 3, which added alcohol use severity was significant, F (5, 650) = 10.17, p < 0.001, $R^2 = 0.07$. The change in variance accounted for was 1% ($\Delta R^2 = 0.01$). Step 4, which added the interaction terms, HIV by alcohol and HIV by smoking, did not improve the model. Therefore Step 3 was chosen as the final model. The standardized beta weights for the final model are presented in Table 4. Alcohol use severity ($\beta = -0.10$), smoking ($\beta = -0.18$), and depression ($\beta = -0.09$) were significant predictors of birth weight percentile.

We ran a subsequent model using lifetime alcohol use as a predictor in Step 3 of the regression equation. Step

Table 3 Results of multiple regression analyses for birth weight percentile, length, head circumference, and gestational age

		df	Mean square	F value	p value	R2	Ä R2
Birth weight percentile							
Block 1	HIV status (pos/neg)	1	3004	2.92	0.088	0.00	
Block 2	Smoking, depression, SES	4	10,597	10.88	0.000	0.06	0.06
Block 3	3-month alcohol use severity	5	9816	10.17	0.000	0.07	0.01
Block 4	Interactions	7	7058	7.29	0.000	0.07	0.00
Length							
Block 1	HIV status (pos/neg)	1	0.001	0.001	0.992	0.00	
Block 2	Smoking, depression, SES	4	115.17	8.23	0.000	0.05	0.05
Block 3	3-month alcohol use severity	5	93.36	6.67	0.000	0.05	0.00
Block 4	Interactions	7	66.83	4.76	0.000	0.05	0.00
Head circumference							
Block 1	HIV status (pos/neg)	1	7.352	2.10	0.148	0.00	0.00
Block 2	3-month alcohol use severity	4	38.649	11.73	0.000	0.07	0.07
Block 3	3-month alcohol use severity	5	31.496	9.56	0.000	0.07	0.00
Block 4	Interactions	7	22.599	6.84	0.000	0.07	0.00
Gestational age (log)							
Block 1	HIV status (pos/neg)	1	0.003	0.60	0.439	0.00	
Block 2	Smoking, depression, SES	4	0.021	3.86	0.004	0.02	0.02
Block 3	3-month alcohol use severity	5	0.021	3.85	0.002	0.03	0.01
Block 4	Interactions	7	0.015	2.80	0.007	0.03	0.00

Table 4 Standardized beta weights and t test results for predictors of birth weight percentile

	Beta	SE	t	p value
Birth weight percentile				
Constant		2.34	24.39	<0.000
Mother's confirmed HIV status	0.057	3.14	1.47	0.143
SES	0.046	0.59	1.16	0.247
BDI score	−0.085	0.13	−2.18	0.030
Smoker (yes, no)	−0.184	2.68	−4.71	<0.000
3-month alcohol use severity	−0.103	0.17	−2.63	0.009

SES socioeconomic status, *BDI* Beck Depression Inventory

1 and Step 2 model results were identical. Step 3, which added lifetime alcohol use was also significant, F (5, 648) = 11.91, $p < 0.001$, $R^2 = 0.085$, and increased the proportion of variance accounted for by 2% ($\Delta R^2 = 0.02$). The standardized beta weight for lifetime alcohol use was −0.161 ($p < 0.001$). In Step 4, the interaction terms were not significant predictors of birth weight percentile.

Infant length

Model results for the hierarchical multiple regression analysis for infant length are presented in Table 3. Step 1 of the model, which included HIV status only was not significant, and accounted for no variance in infant length, $F(1, 647) = 0.001$, $p = 0.99$, $R^2 < 0.000$. Step 2, which added smoking, SES, and depression, was significant F (4, 647) = 8.23, $p < 0.001$, $R^2 = 0.05$, and increased the proportion of variance accounted for by 5% ($\Delta R^2 = 0.05$). Step 3 and Step 4 did not improve the model. Smoking ($\beta = -0.196$) was the only significant predictor of infant length.

We ran a subsequent model using lifetime alcohol use as a predictor in Step 3 of the regression equation. Step 1 and Step 2 model results were identical. Step 3, which added lifetime alcohol use was also significant, F (5, 645) = 7.14, $p < 0.001$, $R^2 = 0.053$, and increased the proportion of variance accounted for by 0.4% ($\Delta R^2 = 0.004$). The standardized beta weight for lifetime alcohol use was −0.07 ($p = 0.09$). In Step 4, the interaction terms were not significant predictors of infant length.

Head circumference

Model results for the hierarchical multiple regression analysis for head circumference are presented in Table 3. Step 1 of the model, which included HIV status only was not significant, and accounted for very little variance in head circumference, F (1, 645) = 2.10, $p = 0.148$, $R^2 = 0.003$. Step 2, which added smoking, SES, and depression, was significant F (4, 645) = 11.73, $p < 0.001$, $R^2 = 0.07$, and increased the proportion of variance accounted for by 7% ($\Delta R^2 = 0.07$). Step 3 and

Step 4 did not improve the model. Smoking (β = −0.21), and depression (β = −0.09) were significant predictors of head circumference.

We ran a subsequent model using lifetime alcohol use as a predictor in Step 3 of the regression equation. Step 1 and Step 2 model results were identical. Step 3, which added lifetime alcohol use was also significant, F (5, 645) = 10.35, $p < 0.001$, $R^2 = 0.068$, and increased the proportion of variance accounted for by 0.5% ($\Delta R^2 = 0.005$). The standardized beta weight for lifetime alcohol use was −0.08 (p = 0.06). In Step 4, the interaction terms were not significant predictors of head circumference.

Gestational age

Model results for the hierarchical multiple regression analysis for gestational age are presented in Table 3. Step 1 of the model, which included HIV status was not significant, and accounted for very little variance in gestational age, F (1, 651) = 0.60, p = 0.44, $R^2 = 0.001$. Step 2, which added smoking, SES, and depression, was significant F (4, 651) = 3.86, p = 0.023, $R^2 = 0.02$, and improved the model, ($\Delta R^2 = 0.02$). Step 3 and Step 4 did not improve the model. Only SES was significantly related to gestational age (β = 0.14).

We ran a subsequent model using lifetime alcohol use as a predictor in Step 3 of the regression equation. Step 1 and Step 2 model results were identical. Step 3, which added lifetime alcohol use was also significant, F (5, 648) = 11.91, $p < 0.001$, $R^2 = 0.085$, and increased the proportion of variance accounted for by 2% ($\Delta R^2 = 0.02$). The standardized beta weight for lifetime alcohol use was −0.161 ($p < 0.001$). In Step 4, the interaction terms were not significant predictors of birth weight percentile.

Discussion

This is the first study that examines the relationship between maternal HIV and alcohol use on infant birth outcomes in a setting with some of the highest global prevalence of HIV and alcohol use. Our results indicate that there were concerning levels of lifetime and recent alcohol use among pregnant women. In regards to alcohol use, we found lower lifetime and recent alcohol use reported by HIV-positive mothers. Recent and lifetime alcohol use predicted lower birth weight, and lifetime alcohol use predicted shorter infant length, smaller head circumference, and younger gestational age. The finding that alcohol use severity did not predict all gestational outcomes was unexpected, and is possibly due to relatively low rates of reported past 3-month alcohol use overall, and large percentages of light alcohol users among past 3-month alcohol users. The small number of heavy alcohol users documented on this self-report tool likely limited our ability to detect alcohol use on gestational outcomes. Regardless, the overall findings point towards the detrimental effects of alcohol on infant outcomes. The negative effects of alcohol on gestational outcomes borne out in our cohort are consistent with the existing literature [18].

We also examined whether maternal HIV and alcohol had any synergistic effects of gestational outcomes. Our results for this analyses showed that HIV and alcohol did not appear to have significant synergistic effects on gestational outcomes of birth weight percentile, length, head circumference, and gestational age. These findings were surprising, but should be interpreted with caution. Possible explanations for these unexpected findings might include that the limited number of heavy alcohol users in the sample as mentioned previously, or benefits of perinatal mother to child transmission (PMTCT) programs may be attenuating the synergistic effects of alcohol and HIV on gestational outcomes among HIV-infected mothers, nearly all who were on antiretroviral treatment. South Africa has successful PMTCT programs which have provided substantial HIV prevention benefits to both mothers and babies in South Africa. There may still be a synergistic negative effect of HIV and alcohol on the long-term developmental outcomes of children but this needs further investigation with larger samples of mothers with diverse adherence behaviours as well possible purposeful sampling of mothers using alcohol on the more moderate to severe end of the spectrum. Such type of future sampling would allow further exploration of the relationship between HIV status, varying ART adherence, and alcohol on gestational outcomes. Studies from elsewhere in Southern Africa indicate that antiretroviral treatment (ART) given to prevent mother-to-child transmission attenuates the negative effects of maternal HIV on fetal outcomes. For example, recent retrospective cohort data from a study in Malawi showed that HIV-infected children had significantly poorer health outcomes (development and functioning) than their uninfected peers [43].

Limitations

We recognize several study limitations that offer several areas for development in future studies. First, this study uses self-report for alcohol data. Social reporting bias may be an issue especially for recent alcohol use. This may be due in part, to low literacy which necessitated field-worker administered assessments. Although fieldworkers were trained carefully in sensitive interviewing techniques, future studies could be aided by audio computer assisted self-interviewing (A-CASI) techniques which has been shown to improve accuracy of reporting on sensitive behaviors including substance use [44, 45].

Improved methods for gathering substance use may also address possible issues of under-reporting due to social desirability bias so the use of audio computer assisted self-interviewing methods or bio-verifiable methods for use may be warranted. Future studies could also be aided by the use of biomarker verification of alcohol [46]. Self-report on other drugs use are extremely low in this community. While alcohol has relative social acceptability, mothers, particularly in the context of pregnancy remain reluctant to volunteer this information. Second, longitudinal data would have enhanced our ability to assess the temporal relationship between maternal HIV and alcohol use. Findings indicated that mother's HIV infection did not seem to adversely affect intra-uterine growth in regards to weight, length, head circumference, and gestational age. Future longitudinal studies could further develop our understanding of the role alcohol plays in risk of HIV infection among women desiring safe conception. Additional research should further explore why and how HIV infection might be linked to alcohol severity scores, and how differential alcohol use might impact ART adherence. The concerning levels of recent alcohol among HIV-infected mothers also suggests that future studies need to explore the temporal association between HIV, alcohol, and psychosocial outcomes among HIV-infected mothers, especially in relation to gestational outcomes. A particularly important focus of future studies is a better understanding of long-term growth outcomes among children born to HIV-infected mothers who are drinking at more severe levels. Even if children are not infected, or do not demonstrate poor gestational outcomes, there may be long-term developmental, growth, and psychosocial implications of maternal alcohol use among HIV-infected mothers. Despite these limitations which highlight areas to develop for future research, there are several strengths to this study. These include a population-based sample, use of dyadic data, and exploration of the effect of maternal HIV and alcohol use on gestational outcomes among a high risk population.

Summary and conclusions

Although the broader literature suggests that HIV and alcohol have detrimental synergistic effects on the mortality and morbidity of individuals living with HIV, findings from this study indicate that HIV exposure alone in this cohort does not confer risk of poor growth outcomes at birth. The effect of maternal HIV and alcohol use on gestational may be attenuated by ARTs with similar findings from several recent meta-analyses and systematic reviews showing good maternal and infant outcomes for HIV-infected mothers on ARTs [47, 48]. While such findings are positive, they do not negate the potentially harmful effects of HIV and alcohol on long-term developmental outcomes of children, which need to be explored further. Our study highlights the importance of South Africa's robust program of PMTCT of HIV. PMTCT is critical for supporting healthy mothers and protecting infants during the gestational period. However, mothers and their infants from high risk communities remain vulnerable to contextual factors which may impact individually and synergistically on gestational and developmental outcomes and meeting the needs of families is likely to require a broad approach.

While continued investment in PMTCT has provided immense benefits for mothers and children, and prevented adverse effects of HIV on mothers and their infants, additional investment is needed to develop interventions and provide policy and programmatic support to address the complex challenges faced by HIV-infected mothers including alcohol and nicotine use, poor mental health, and low SES. Indeed, our study highlights that these families face multiple risks that necessitate a strategic and intensive family approach that links together complementary intervention approaches to create what experts have termed, "a universal lattice of protection" [49]. At the foundation of these approaches is the understanding of HIV as a family disease that takes place against the complicated backdrop of overlapping epidemics of substance use, poor mental health, and poverty. Intervening at critical time points in the family trajectory, such as during gestation and early birth, offer important opportunities for prevention and building family resilience.

Abbreviations

HIV: human immunodeficiency virus; ART: antiretrovirals treatment; PLWH: people living with HIV; FAS: fetal alcohol syndrome; PFAS: partial fetal alcohol syndrome; DCHS: Drakenstein Child Health Study; EPI: expanded program for immunization; SES: socioeconomic status; WHO: World Health Organization; ASSIST: the alcohol, smoking and substance involvement screening test; BDI-II: The Beck Depression Inventory-II; PMTCT: perinatal mother to child transmission; A-CASI: audio computer assisted self-interviewing.

Authors' contributions

All authors have made substantial contribution to the conception, design, gathering, analysis and/or interpretation of data and a contribution to the writing and intellectual content of the article; and acknowledged that they have exercised due care in ensuring the integrity of the work. KD and CK formulated the research questions and the approach on analysis strategy. AF and KC analysed data, and interpreted the results. KD, CK, KC and AF all contributed to writing the draft of the manuscript and provided critical review of the manuscript. NK managed the co-ordination of data collection. HZ is the principal investigator of the umbrella study, the DCHS, and created the study design of the umbrella study. DS is principal investigator of the psychosocial component of the DCHS and contributed to the analysis strategy. All authors have read and approved the manuscript.

Author details

[1] Department of Paediatrics and Child Health, Institute of Child Health Building, Red Cross War Memorial Children's Hospital, 5th Floor, Klipfontein Road, Rondebosch, Cape Town 7700, South Africa. [2] Center for Alcohol and Addiction Studies, Brown University School of Public Health, Providence, RI, USA.

[3] Department of Medicine, Rhode Island Hospital, Providence, USA. [4] Department of Psychiatry and Human Behavior, Warren Alpert Medical School of Brown University, Providence, USA. [5] Department of Behavioral and Social Sciences, Brown University School of Public Health, Providence, RI, USA. [6] Department of Psychiatry and Mental Health, University of Cape Town, Cape Town, South Africa. [7] South African Medical Research Council Unit on Child & Adolescent Health, Cape Town, South Africa. [8] South African Medical Research Council Unit on Risk and Resilience in Mental Disorders, Cape Town, South Africa.

Acknowledgements
We thank the study staff and the staff at Paarl Hospital, Mbekweni and TC Newman clinics for their support of the study. We thank the families and children who participated in this study.

Competing interests
The authors declare that they have no competing interests.

Funding
The study was funded by the Bill and Melinda Gates Foundation [OPP 1017641]. Additional support for publication was provided to CK from the US National Institutes for Health Awards K01 MH096646, L30 MH098313, and R24 HD077976 and a Newton advanced fellowship to KAD and grants from the South African Medical Research Council and National Research Foundation provided to KAD. This research was also supported in part by Grant Number T32 AA0007459 from the National Institute of Alcohol Abuse and Alcoholism at the National Institute of Health. HJZ and DJS are supported by the South African Medical Research Council. The content is solely the responsibility of the authors. Authors have no conflict of interests to report.

References

1. UNAIDS. Global report: UNAIDS report on the global AIDS epidemic. Geneva: UNAIDS; 2013.
2. Rehm J, Rehn N, Room R, Monteiro M, Gmel G, Jernigan D, et al. The global distribution of average volume of alcohol consumption and patterns of drinking. Eur Addict Res. 2003;9:147–56.
3. Peltzer K, Davids A, Njuho P. Alcohol use and problem drinking in South Africa: findings from a national population-based survey. Afr J Psychiatr. 2011;14(1):30–7.
4. Peltzer K, Ramlagan S. Alcohol use trends in South Africa. J Soc Sci. 2009;18(1):1–12.
5. Van Heerden MS, Grimsrud AT, Seedat S, Myer L, Williams DR, Stein DJ. Patterns of substance use in South Africa: results from the South African stress and health study. S Afr Med J. 2009;99(5):358–66.
6. Simbayi LC, Kalichman SC, Strebel A, Cloete A, Henda N, Mqeketo A. Disclosure of HIV status to sex partners and sexual risk behaviours among HIV-positive men and women, Cape Town, South Africa. Sex Transm Infect. 2007;83(1):29–34.
7. Myer L, Smit J, Roux LL, Parker S, Stein DJ, Seedat S. Common mental disorders among HIV-infected individuals in South Africa: prevalence, predictors, and validation of brief psychiatric rating scales. AIDS Patient Care STDS. 2008;22(2):147–58.
8. Shuper PA, Neuman M, Kanteres F, Baliunas D, Joharchi N, Rehm J. Causal considerations on alcohol and HIV/AIDS–a systematic review. Alcohol Alcohol. 2010;45(2):159–66.
9. Pol S, Artru P, Thepot V, Berthelot P, Nalpas B. Improvement of the cd4 cell count after alcohol withdrawal in hiv-positive alcoholic patients. AIDS. 1996;10(11):1293–4.
10. Parsons M, Campa A, Lai S, Li Y, Martinez JD, Murillo J, Greer P, Martinez SS, Baum MK. Effect of GSTM1-polymorphism on disease progression and oxidative stress in HIV infection: modulation by HIV/HCV Co-infection and alcohol consumption. J AIDS Clin Res. 2013;4(9):10002337.
11. Neuman MG. First international symposium on the molecular pathology and clinical aspects of the inflamed liver: alcohol and cytokines. Clin Invest Med. 1998;21(6):283.
12. Bagasra O, Bachman SE, Jew L, Tawadros R, Cater J, Boden G, Ryan I, Pomerantz RJ. Increased human immunodeficiency virus type 1 replication in human peripheral blood mononuclear cells induced by ethanol: potential immunopathogenic mechanisms. J Infect Dis. 1996;173(3):550–8.
13. Conen A, Fehr J, Glass TR, Furrer H, Weber R, Vernazza P, Hirschel B, Cavassini M, Bernasconi E, Bucher HC. Self-reported alcohol consumption and its association with adherence and outcome of antiretroviral therapy in the Swiss HIV Cohort Study. Antivir Ther (Lond). 2009;14(3):349–57.
14. Chander G, Lau B, Moore RD. Hazardous alcohol use: a risk factor for non-adherence and lack of suppression in HIV infection. J Acquir Immune Defic Syndr. 2006;43(4):411–7.
15. Samet JH, Horton NJ, Traphagen ET, Lyon SM, Freedberg KA. Alcohol consumption and HIV disease progression: are they related? Alcohol Clin Exp Res. 2003;27(5):862–7.
16. Hendershot CS, Stoner SA, Pantalone DW, Simoni JM. Alcohol use and antiretroviral adherence: review and meta-analysis. J Acquir Immune Defic Syndr. 2009;52(2):180–202.
17. Azar MM, Springer SA, Meyer JP, Altice FL. A systematic review of the impact of alcohol use disorders on HIV treatment outcomes, adherence to antiretroviral therapy and health care utilization. Drug Alcohol Depend. 2010;112(3):178–93.
18. Patra J, Bakker R, Irving H, Jaddoe VW, Malini S, Rehm J. Dose–response relationship between alcohol consumption before and during pregnancy and the risks of low birthweight, preterm birth and small for gestational age (SGA)—a systematic review and meta-analyses. BJOG Int J Obstet Gynaecol. 2011;118(12):1411–21.
19. Lucas BR, Latimer J, Pinto RZ, Ferreira ML, Doney R, Lau M, Jones T, Dries D, Elliott EJ. Gross motor deficits in children prenatally exposed to alcohol: a meta-analysis. Pediatrics. 2014;134(1):e192–209.
20. Ndirangu J, Newell ML, Bland RM, Thorne C. Maternal HIV infection associated with small-for-gestational age infants but not preterm births: evidence from rural South Africa. Hum Reprod. 2012;27(6):1846–56.
21. Turner AN, Tabbah S, Mwapasa V, Rogerson SJ, Meshnick SR, Ackerman WE 4th, Kwiek JJ. Severity of maternal HIV-1 disease is associated with adverse birth outcomes in Malawian women: a cohort study. J Acquir Immune Defic Syndr. 2013;64(4):392–9.
22. Slyker JA, Patterson J, Ambler G, Richardson BA, Maleche-Obimbo E, Bosire R, Mbori-Ngacha D, Farquhar C, John-Stewart G. Correlates and outcomes of preterm birth, low birth weight, and small for gestational age in HIV-exposed uninfected infants. BMC Pregnancy Childbirth. 2014;14(1):1.
23. Walker SP, Wachs TD, Grantham-McGregor S, Black MM, Nelson CA, Huffman SL, Baker-Henningham H, Chang SM, Hamadani JD, Lozoff B, Gardner JMM, Powell CA, Rahman A, Richter L. Inequality in early childhood: risk and protective factors for early child development. Lancet. 2011;378(9799):1325–38.
24. May PA, Gossage JP, Kalberg K, Robinson L, Buckley D, Manning M. Prevalence and epidemiologic characteristics of FASD from various research methods with an emphasis on recent in-school studies. Dev Disabil Res Rev. 2009;15(3):176–92.
25. Desmond K, Milburn N, Richter L, Tomlinson M, Greco E, Van Heerden A, Van Rooyen H, Comulada WS, Rotheram-Borus MJ. Alcohol consumption among HIV-positive pregnant women in KwaZulu-Natal, South Africa: prevalence and correlates. Drug Alcohol Depend. 2012;120(1):113–8.
26. Choi KW, Abler LA, Watt MH, Eaton LA, Kalichman SC, Skinner D, Pieterse D, Sikkema KJ. Drinking before and after pregnancy recognition among South African women: the moderating role of traumatic experiences. BMC Pregnancy Childbirth. 2014;14(1):1.
27. London L. The dop'system, alcohol abuse and social control amongst farm workers in South Africa: a public health challenge. Soc Sci Med. 1999;48(10):1407–14.
28. May PA, Blankenship J, Marais A, Gossage JP, Kalberg WO, Barnard R, De Vries M, Robinson LK, Adnams CM, Buckley D, Manning M, Jones KL, Parry C, Hoyme HE, Seedat S. Approaching the prevalence of the full spectrum of fetal alcohol spectrum disorders in a South African population-based study. Alcohol Clin Exp Res. 2013;37(5):818–30.
29. Stein DJ, Koen N, Donald KA, Adnams CM, Koopowitz S, Lund C, Marais A, Myers B, Roos A, Sorsdahl K, Stern M, Tomlinson M, van der Westhuizen C, Vythilingum B, Myer L, Barnett W, Brittain K, Zar H. Investigating the psychosocial determinants of child health in Africa: the Drakenstein Child Health Study. J Neuroscience methods. 2015;70(6):592–4.
30. Zar HJ, Barnett W, Myer L, Stein DJ, Nicol MP. Investigating the early-life determinants of illness in Africa: the Drakenstein Child Health Study. Thorax. 2015;70(6):592–4.
31. Western Cape Government. Regional development profile cape winelands district, 2013. Cape Town: Provincial Treasury. Accessed 21 Apr 2014.

32. World Health Organization. Guidelines on optimal feeding of low birth-weight infants in low-and middle-income countries. World Health Organization; 2011.
33. Mikolajczyk RT, Zhang J, Betran AP, Souza JP, Mori R, Gülmezoglu AM, Merialdi M. A global reference for fetal-weight and birthweight percentiles. Lancet. 2011;377(9780):1855–61.
34. Ali R, Awwad E, Babor T, Bradley F, Butau T, Farrell M, Formigoni M, Isralowitz R, de Lacerda BR, Marsden J. The alcohol, smoking and substance involvement screening test (ASSIST): development, reliability and feasibility. Addiction. 2002;97(9):1183–94.
35. Humeniuk R, Ali R, Babor T, Souza-Formigoni MLO, de Lacerda RB, Ling W, McRee B, Newcombe D, Pal H, Poznyak V. A randomized controlled trial of a brief intervention for illicit drugs linked to the alcohol, smoking and substance involvement screening test (ASSIST) in clients recruited from primary health-care settings in four countries. Addiction. 2012;107(5):957–66.
36. Humeniuk R, Ali R, Babor TF, Farrell M, Formigoni ML, Jittiwutikarn J, de Lacerda RB, Ling W, Marsden J, Monteiro M, Nhiwatiwa S, Pal H, Poznyak V, Simon S. Validation of the alcohol, smoking and substance involvement screening test (ASSIST). Addiction. 2008;103(6):1039–47.
37. Mertens JR, Flisher AJ, Ward CL, Bresick GF, Sterling SA, Weisner CM. Medical conditions of hazardous drinkers and drug users in primary care clinics in Cape Town, South Africa. J Drug Iss. 2009;39(4):989–1014.
38. Henry-Edwards S, Humeniuk R, Ali R, Poznyak V, Monteiro M. The alcohol, smoking and substance involvement screening test (ASSIST): guidelines for use in primary care (draft version 1.1 for field testing). Geneva: World Health Organization; 2003.
39. Siemens. Immulite 1000 nicotine metabolite testing phamplet. 2009.
40. Beck AT, Steer RA, Brown GK. Beck depression inventory-II. San Antonio: Psychological Corporation; 1996. pp. 78204–2498.
41. Bisconer SW, Gross DM. Assessment of suicide risk in a psychiatric hospital. Prof Psychol Res Pract. 2007;38(2):143.
42. Naragon-Gainey K, Watson D, Markon KE. Differential relations of depression and social anxiety symptoms to the facets of extraversion/positive emotionality. J Abnorm Psychol. 2009;118(2):299.
43. Landes M, van Lettow M, Chan AK, Mayuni I, Schouten EJ, Bedell RA. Mortality and health outcomes of HIV-exposed and unexposed children in a PMTCT cohort in Malawi. PLoS ONE. 2012;7(10):e47337.
44. Currivan D, Nyman AL, Turner CF, Biener L. Does telephone audio computer-assisted self-interviewing improve the accuracy of prevalence estimates of youth smoking? Evidence from the UMass tobacco study. Public Opin Q. 2004;68(4):542–64.
45. Morrison-Beedy D, Carey MP, Tu X. Accuracy of audio computer-assisted self-interviewing (ACASI) and self-administered questionnaires for the assessment of sexual behavior. AIDS Behav. 2006;10(5):541–52.
46. Litten RZ, Bradley AM, Moss HB. Alcohol biomarkers in applied settings: recent advances and future research opportunities. Alcohol Clin Exp Res. 2010;34(6):955–67.
47. Ford N, Mofenson L, Shubber Z, Calmy A, Andrieux-Meyer I, Vitoria M, Shaffer N, Renaud F. Safety of efavirenz in the first trimester of pregnancy: an updated systematic review and meta-analysis. AIDS. 2014;28(Suppl 2):S123–31.
48. Kourtis AP, Schmid CH, Jamieson DJ, Lau J. Use of antiretroviral therapy in pregnant HIV-infected women and the risk of premature delivery: a meta-analysis. AIDS. 2007;21(5):607–15.
49. Stein A, Desmond C, Garbarino J, Van IJzendoorn MH, Barbarin O, Black MM, Stein AD, Hillis SD, Kalichman SC, Mercy JA, BakermansKranenburg MJ, Rapa E, Saul JR, DobrovaKrol NA, Richter LM. Predicting long-term outcomes for children affected by HIV and AIDS: perspectives from the scientific study of children's development. AIDS. 2014;28(Supplement 3):S261–8.

5

Clinical characteristics, predictors of immune reconstitution inflammatory syndrome and long-term prognosis in patients with Kaposi sarcoma

Patricia Volkow[1*], Gabriela Cesarman-Maus[2], Pamela Garciadiego-Fossas[1], Enrique Rojas-Marin[3] and Patricia Cornejo-Juárez[1]

Abstract

Objective: To investigate the predictive factors for the development of Kaposi sarcoma-related immune reconstitution inflammatory syndrome (KS-IRIS) and long-term prognosis in patients starting combined antiretroviral therapy (cART).

Methods: We studied a retrospective-cohort of consecutive antiretroviral-naïve patients with KS initiating cART from January 2005 to December 2011 and followed through June 2013. KS-IRIS was defined as ≥2 of the following: abrupt increase in number of KS lesions, appearance or exacerbation of lung-opacities or lymphedema, concomitantly with an increase in CD4+ cell-count ≥50 cells/mm^3 and a decrease of >1 log in viral-load once started cART. We compared individuals who met KS-IRIS criteria with those that did not and described the long-term follow-up.

Results: We included 89 patients, 88 males; 35 (39%) developed KS-IRIS at a median of 10 weeks (IQR 4–16). KS-IRIS patients had more pulmonary-involvement (60% vs. 16.6% of patients; $p < 0.0001$), eight died attributed to pulmonary-KS. Thrombocytopenia <100,000/mm^3 at follow-up occurred in 36% of KS-IRIS vs. 4% in non-KS-IRIS patients ($p = 0.0002$), 45% KS-IRIS patients with thrombocytopenia died, non without KS-IRIS. Chemotherapy (bleomicyn–vincristine) was more frequently prescribed in KS-IRIS patients (88.6% vs. 29.6%) with no differences in outcome; 80% of all patients achieve KS complete remission, 52% of them never received chemotherapy. No difference between groups in the long-term follow-up (mean 52.4 ± 27.4 months) was found, only one patient developed a secondary malignancy (1.12%).

Conclusions: Lung-involvement was predictive of IRIS development. Thrombocytopenia in KS-IRIS patients at week 12 follow-up after cART initiation was associated with high mortality. Over a third of patients with KS achieve remission without chemotherapy. Individuals that survive the initial period of KS-IRIS adhere to cART had a good long-term prognosis.

Keywords: Kaposi sarcoma, Immune reconstitution inflammatory syndrome, Highly active antiretroviral therapy, Combined antiretroviral therapy, Thrombocytopenia, Pulmonary Kaposi sarcoma

*Correspondence: pvolkowf@gmail.com
[1] Infectious Diseases Department, Instituto Nacional de Cancerología (INCan), Av. San Fernando No. 22, Col. Sección XVI, Deleg. Tlalpan, 14080 Mexico City, Mexico
Full list of author information is available at the end of the article

Background

Kaposi sarcoma (KS) was first described in the nineteenth century. In 1981 it became one of the signs that marked the beginning of the AIDS epidemic. This enigmatic disease is now recognized as a cytokine-mediated angioproliferative disease [1, 2] caused by human herpesvirus 8 (HHV-8), also referred as Kaposi sarcoma-associated herpesvirus (KSHV) [3, 4] indeed HHV-8/KSHV fulfilled Koch principles for an infectious disease pathogen. KS course is unpredictable even in the combined antiretroviral therapy (cART) era, and it is still associated with significant mortality [5, 6].

The use of combined antiretroviral therapy (cART) has resulted in a dramatic reduction in opportunistic infections and mortality in patients with human immunodeficiency virus (HIV) infection [7, 8]. The major benefit of cART is the inhibition of viral replication that results in gradual restoration of the pathogen-specific immune response through partial recovery of the immune system [9, 10]. Initiation of cART, even in the presence of decreasing plasma HIV-1 RNA viral loads and rising CD4+ cell counts [9, 11], may lead to unexpected clinical deterioration which is known as immune reconstitution inflammatory syndrome (IRIS), [10, 12]. IRIS is attributed to "deregulation" of the reconstituting immune system and unmasking of pathogens or antigens that were previously present but clinically asymptomatic [9, 13–15]. IRIS has been reported to occur in 10–30% of antiretroviral-naïve patients with a 5–30% mortality rate [5, 16]. In Africa, it has become a significant cause of morbidity and mortality in HIV-infected patients with access to cART [5, 17, 18]. IRIS has been described in association with different infectious processes [10, 19–21]. It has also been described within the context of KS and is characterized by abrupt exacerbation of KS in patients on cART (KS-IRIS) [13].

In the present study, we describe the prevalence and risk factors associated with the development of IRIS: clinical characteristics, type of therapy, outcome, markers of poor prognosis and long-term prognosis in patients with KS from a cohort of patients in Mexico initiating cART. We also estimated the incidence of secondary malignancies in long-term survivors.

Methods

We performed a retrospective study of consecutive antiretroviral-naïve patients with KS who began cART between January 1, 2005 and December 31, 2011 at the National Cancer Institute of Mexico (INCan), a referral center for adult patients with AIDS-associated cancers. We included follow-up data up to June 30, 2013 provided the patients had >2 hospital-visits, and had not received systemic corticosteroids within the 2 months prior or concomitantly with the initiation of cART [22]. We obtained information on demographics, co-existence of other AIDS-defining events, cART regimen, CD4+ lymphocyte counts and viral load at HIV diagnosis and at 12 weeks follow-up.

We included the following clinical features related with KS: presence and extent of mucosal involvement, number of skin lesions (considered disseminated if there were > 20 lesions or affecting ≥ 2 regions of the body), the presence and extent of lymphedema, gastrointestinal involvement diagnosed by endoscopy and confirmed by biopsy, and lung involvement (lung opacities on chest X-ray and a negative gallium scan or typical lesions documented by bronchoscopy). We further classified patients accordingly to ACTG staging classification [23, 24], and compared each stage between the two groups and mortality.

IRIS criteria

KS-IRIS was diagnosed in patients receiving cART with a reduction of at least 1 log10 of HIV-1 RNA and/or an increase of ≥50 cells/mm^3 or ≥twofold rise in baseline CD4+ cell count associated with clinical abrupt worsening of previously existing KS ("paradoxical") or the development of KS ("unmasked") within the first 6 months after the initiation of cART [25].

KS exacerbation was defined with at least two of the following criteria: abrupt increase in the size or number of KS lesions, appearance or exacerbation of lymphedema, and the appearance or increase of otherwise unexplained, gallium-negative, lung opacities on chest X-rays after starting cART [5, 6, 16, 25, 26]. The agreement by two clinicians was necessary for the diagnosis of KS-IRIS. A radiologist blinded to the patients' diagnoses evaluated the chest roentgenograms.

We compared patients who met KS-IRIS criteria with those that did not. We evaluated clinical features, imaging studies, the use of chemotherapy, laboratory tests and patient outcomes.

The evolution of KS was classified at the last hospital visit as a complete response (CR) when patients had no clinically evident cutaneous or mucosal lesions; partial response (PR) when patients had >50% decrease in the number and/or size of the original lesions, with no new lesions; stable disease when patients had <50% decrease in lesions and no new lesions; disease progression when patients had an increase in size and/or number of KS lesions; and relapse when a patient who had been classified previously as PR or CR had new lesions or increased in lesion's size or number.

Survival and follow-up time was calculated from the date of HIV diagnosis to the date when the patient was last seen, or the date of the patient's death. The cause of death was attributed to KS in the presence of respiratory insufficiency, hemoptysis, gastrointestinal bleeding, and/or airway obstruction and the remainder as HIV-related, non-HIV-related, or unknown. Date and cause of death was corroborated at the Mexican National Death Certificate Registry. No autopsies were performed.

The chemotherapy regimen used in these patients was based on bleomycin (10 U/m^2) and vincristine (1.4 mg/m^2) [27], and was prescribed by the treating physician (usually for patients with extensive skin lesions and lymphedema and/or gastrointestinal or pulmonary involvement).

Statistical analysis

KS-IRIS and non-KS-IRIS groups were compared employing the Student t test for independent groups, the Fisher exact test, and the Mann–Whitney test or X^2 test as appropriate. Time to development of KS-IRIS was analyzed by Kaplan–Meier survival curves, whereas predictors of mortality and KS-IRIS were tested using Cox proportional hazard model, the variables with a $p \leq 0.1$ were included in this analysis. Independent risk factors were identified in multivariate analysis utilizing a forward step-wise procedure with the criterion, variable inclusion and $p > 0.10$ were removal from the model. p values $\leq$0.05 were considered statistically significant. Statistical analysis was performed utilizing STATA 14 software (STATA. Corp. College Station, TX, USA).

Results

A total of 394 new patients with HIV were seen at the INCan during the study period. One hundred sixty one (41%) presented with KS; 109 (68%) were antiretroviral-naïve or had initiated cART within 6 months of their first clinic appointment. Two patients were excluded from the analysis because they received systemic corticosteroids and 18 were excluded since they had two or less hospital visits.

Eighty-nine patients (88 males and 1 female) were included: 35 patients (39.3%) met the criteria for KS-IRIS and were compared with the 54 (60.6%) individuals who did not develop KS-IRIS. In the KS-IRIS group, there were four patients classified as "unmasked" and 31 classified as "paradoxical". The median time between the initiation of cART and KS-IRIS diagnosis was 10 weeks (IQR 4–16). For all male patients, the risk factor for HIV infection was men who have sex with men (MSM); the woman was infected through heterosexual intercourse.

Combined ART was based on Non-Nucleoside Reverse Transcriptase Inhibitors (NNRTI) in 45 patients (51%), protease inhibitors (PI) in 43 patients (48%), and there was one patient with three Nucleoside Reverse Transcriptase Inhibitors (NRTI), (p = 0.359). Clinical, ACTG staging and laboratory data are shown in Table 1. Mean age in the KS-IRIS group was 32 ± 7 years vs. 36 ± 8 years in the non-KS-IRIS group (p = 0.01). HIV was diagnosed at a median of 10 weeks (IQR 6–30 weeks) before the initiation of cART; median baseline CD4 count was 92 cells/mm^3 (IQR 33–214 cells/mm^3) and was 249 cells/mm^3 (IQR 144–387 cells/mm^3) at week 12 after starting cART. Median follow-up from the start of cART to the last hospital visit did not differ different between groups [20 months (IQR 6–46) in the KS-IRIS vs. 21.5 (IQR 11–33) in the non-KS-IRIS group, p = 0.9]. Seventy (81.5%) of the patients were in ACTG stage T1, with no difference among the stages between groups and in mortality (Table 1).

There was a significant difference between groups at baseline regarding the extension and number of KS lesions, as well as the presence of pulmonary involvement (Table 1) more common in the KS-IRIS group. Initial chest roentgenogram showed often disseminated reticular and nodular opacities, Gallium scans performed in 17 patients (14 with KS-IRIS and three with non-KS-IRIS) prompted by clinical symptoms and an abnormal chest X-ray were negative in nine and one respectively. Pleural effusion was also more frequent in patients in the KS-IRIS group compared to the non-KS-IRIS group (24% vs. 2%, p = 0.001).

The initial HIV viral load was significantly higher among patients with KS-IRIS (Table 1 include data and comparisons). By 12 weeks of cART, 73 patients (90%) had achieved a viral load <100 copies/ml (25/80.6% for KS-IRIS and 48/96% for non-KS-IRIS groups, respectively, p = 0.02). Thrombocytopenia (<100,000/mm^3), which did not differ at baseline between groups, developed in 11 of 35 patients with KS-IRIS at the 12-week follow-up visit and almost half of them (45.5%) died, including five of the seven individuals with platelet counts <50,000/mm^3. None of the patients in the non-KS-IRIS group had thrombocytopenia <50,000/mm^3 at follow-up and only two (4%) had platelet counts between 50,000 and 100,000/mm^3.

Chemotherapy was administered to 31 (88.5%) individuals in the KS-IRIS group and to 17 (31%) in the non-KS-IRIS group (p < 0.0001), with a mean number of chemotherapy cycles of 3.9 ± 2.3 and 3.8 ± 2 cycles respectively, (p = 0.8), (Table 2). Chemotherapy was well tolerated with no major adverse events recorded. Overall 80% of KS patients achieved CR, 23 patients (66%) of KS-IRIS group and 48 (89%) of non-KS-IRIS (p = 0.117); and PR in three (9%) and one (20%) patients respectively. One patient with PR abandoned cART after he had developed viral failure and relapsed 3 years later. In relation to complete remission there was no difference in

Table 1 Clinical and laboratory characteristics of patients with KS-IRIS- and non-KS-IRIS

Patient characteristics	IRIS-KS N = 35 (39%) (CI95% 29–50)	Non-IRIS-KS (N = 54) (60.6%) CI 95% 50–71)	All patients (N = 89)	p
Mean age ± 2 SD (years)	32 ± 7	36 ± 8	35 ± 8	0.01
Weeks from HIV diagnosis to cART (median, IQR)	10 (5–33)	10 (6–30)	10 (6–30)	0.24
Median baseline CD4+ cells/mm^3 (IQR)	82 (30–140)	110 (36–230)	91 (34–204)	0.43
Median CD4+ cells/mm^3 12 weeks after cART initiation (IQR)	212 (89–357)	308 (159–391)	249 (144–387)	0.28
ACTG staging				
S0T0	0	7 (13%)	7 (7.8%)	0.18
S1T0	1 (4.4%)	11 (20%)	12 (13.5%)	
S0T1	19 (54%)	18 (33%)	37 (41.5%)	
S1T1	15 (42.8%)	18 (33%)	33 (37%)	
Deaths ACTG staging				
S0T0	0	0	0	0.3
S1T0	0	0	0	
S0T1	5 (12.8%)	1 (1.1%)	6 (0%)	
S1T1	4 (10.2%)	4 (7.4%)	8 (9%)	
Median HIV-RNA copies/mm^3 at baseline. (IQR)	240,000 (106,000–612,000)	84,731 (31,300–250,000)	131,818 (57,200–361,124)	0.02
HIV-RNA at follow-up[a]: copies/mm^3				
Number of patients	31	50	81	0.02
<100	25 (80.6)	48 (96)	73 (90.1)	
101–1000	4 (12.91)	1 (2)	5 (6.2)	
1001–50,000	1 (3.2)	1 (2)	2 (2.5)	
>50,000	1 (3.2)	0	1 (1.2)	
Antiretroviral therapy—No (%)				
NNRTI	20 (57)	25 (46)	45 (50.6)	0.36
PI	15 (42)	28 (51.8)	43 (48.3)	
3 NRTI	0	1 (1.85)	1 (1)	
Mucosal involvement—No (%)	27 (77)	35 (65)	62 (70)	0.25
Confluent/disseminated skin lesions—No (%)	25 (71)	25 (46)	50 (56)	0.01
Lymphedema—No (%)	15 (43)	14 (26)	29 (32)	0.09
Deaths—No (%)	5 (33%)	2 (14)	7 (24)	0.39
Gastrointestinal involvement—No (%)[b]	14 (61)	10 (37)	24 (48)	0.16
Deaths %	6 (43%)	4 (40%)	10 (42%)	0.41
Pulmonary involvement—No (%)	22 (63)	9 (17)	31 (35)	<0.001
Deaths[c]	8 (38%)	2 (22%)	10 (30%)	0.45
Platelets at first visit[d]				
>100,000/mm^3	29 (85%)	46 (85)	75 (85%)	0.62
50–100,000	2 (6%)	4 (7%)	6 (7%)	
<50,000	3 (8.9%)	4 (7%)	7 ((8%)	
Platelets at follow-up[e]				
>100,000/mm^3	20 (64%)	48 (96%)	68 (84)	0.0003
50–100,000	4 (13%)	2 (4)	6 (7)	
<50,000	7 (23%)	0	7 (8.6)	

Table 1 continued

Patient characteristics	IRIS-KS N = 35 (39%) (CI95% 29–50)	Non-IRIS-KS (N = 54) (60.6%) CI 95% 50–71)	All patients (N = 89)	p
Deaths first year	9 (26%)	5 (9.3%)	14 (15.7)	0.07
KS attributable deaths	8 (89%)	0	8 (57%)	

IQR interquartile range, *cARTc* combined antiretroviral therapy, *HIV* Human immunodeficiency syndrome, *NS* not significant, *SD* standard deviation, *NNRTI* Non-nucleoside reverse transcriptase inhibitor, *PI* protease inhibitor, *NRTI* nucleoside reverse transcriptase inhibitor

[a] Viral load at follow-up was measured between weeks 12 and 16 after initiation of cART; four patients died before follow-up of viral load determination

[b] Endoscopy was performed in 50 patients (21 Immune reconstitution inflammatory syndrome-Kaposi's sarcoma [IRIS-KS] and in 29 with non-IRIS)

[c] Mortality for pulmonary involvement was evaluated in the first 48 weeks after cART initiation

[d] Complete blood counts (CBC) were not performed at the first visit in 2 patients

[e] In five patients, CBC was not performed at follow-up

Table 2 Outcome of Kaposi sarcoma patients with IRIS and non-IRIS; treated with chemotherapy or without it, at time of last follow-up

	IRIS-KS (*N* = 35)			Non-IRIS-KS (*N* = 54)			Total (*N* = 89)		
	CR	PR	Death	CR	PR	Death	CR	PR	Death
Chemotherapy—*N* (%)	19 (54)	3 (9)[a]	9 (26)	15 (28)	0	2 (4)	34 (38)	3 (3)	11 (12)
No-chemotherapy *N* (%)	4 (11)	0	0	33 (61)	1 (2)	3 (5)	37 (42)	1 (1)	3 (3)
Total, *N* (%)	23 (65)	3 (9)	9 (26)	48 (89)	1 (2)	5 (9)	71 (80)	4 (4)	14 (16)

IRIS-KS immune reconstitution inflammatory syndrome-Kaposi's sarcoma, *CR* complete response, *PR* partial response

[a] One patient abandoned treatment, had Kaposi's sarcoma progression and died with AIDS and related comorbidities

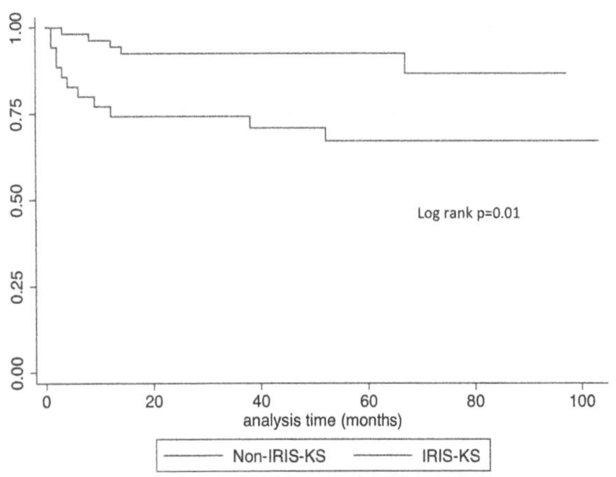

Fig. 1 Kaplan-Meier survival curve. Overall survival is shown in months from combined active antiretroviral therapy (cART) initiation for patients with and without Kaposi's sarcoma Immune Reconstruction Inflammatory Syndrome (KS-IRIS)

outcome whether patient received chemotherapy versus no chemotherapy.

Sixteen patients (18%) died; eleven in the KS-IRIS group, eight of them were attributed to KS lung disease; with a median survival of 16 weeks (IQR 9–50 weeks) after the initiation of cART. If patients survived the initial KS-IRIS phase and were adherent to cART, they had a good prognosis (p = 0.01). In the non- KS-IRIS group five patients died none related to KS, with a median survival time from cART initiation of 51 weeks (IQR 35–58) (Fig. 1).

Using Cox Proportional Hazard model the main predictor for the development of KS-IRIS was KS pulmonary involvement (HR 3.2, CI 95% 1.12–9.12, p = 0.02). Table 3 and only a platelet count bellow 100,000/mm^3 at 12 weeks at follow-up after cART initiation was associated with death (HR 7.79, CI 95% 1.22–49.43, p < 0.02). Table 4.

The mean follow up of 81 patients surviving at least 26 weeks after cART initiation was 52.4 ± 27.4 months, for a total of 4.3 person/years for the whole group. Except for one case of Hodgkin's lymphoma diagnosed 2 years after the diagnosis of KS, no other malignancies were diagnosed during follow-up. Incidence rate of secondary malignancy among patients with long-term follow up was 300 per 100,000 person-years.

Mean CD4 count at last visit was 400 ± 228 cells/mm^3, 75 patients (93%) had an undetectable HIV viral load. Five patients had viral replication (median 100,000 copies/ml, IQR 1660–801,682); two of them had abandoned cART and for one patient data was unavailable.

There were no differences between KS-IRIS and non-KS-IRIS patients in the prevalence of KS as a sole AIDS defining event or coexistence of other AIDS defining

Table 3 Cox regression model for IRIS development

Characteristics	IRIS-KS (n = 35)	Non-IRIS-KS (n = 54)	Unadjusted HR (95% CI)	p value	Adjusted HR (95% CI)	p value
IRIS						
HIV-RNA at follow-up[a]						
<100 copies/mm^3	25 (81)	48 (96)	1.00			
>100 copies/mm^3	6 (19)	2 (4)	5.76 (0.92–61)	0.04	2.26 (0.58–8.89)	0.239
Pulmonary involvement						
No	14 (40)	45 (83)	1.00			
Yes	21 (60)	9 (17)	7.5 (2.53–22.79)	<0.0001	3.20 (1.12-9.12)	0.02
Platelets at follow-up[b]						
>100,000/mm^3	20 (65)	48 (96)	1.00			
<100,000/mm^3	11 (35)	2 (4)	13.2 (2.46–128.61)	0.003	2.79 (0.92–8.43)	0.06

[a] Detectable viral load >1000 copies/mm^3 at 12-week follow up. Viral load was documented in 81 patients

[b] Platelets <100,000/mm^3 at 12-weeks follow-up. 81 patients had platelets count at follow-up

Table 4 Cox regression model for mortality

Characteristics	Death (n = 14)	Alive (n = 75)	Unadjusted HR (95% CI)	p value	Adjusted HR (95% CI)	p value
Mortality						
HIV-RNA at follow-up[a]						
<100 copies/mm^3	6 (67)	67 (93)				
>100 copies/mm^3	3 (33)	5 (7)	6.7 (0.81–44.41)	0.04	2.09 (0.33–13.23)	0.433
Platelets at follow-up[b]						
>100,000/mm^3	6 (46)	62 (91)	1.00		1.00	
<100,000/mm^3	7 (54)	6 (9)	10.16 (2.15–47.53)	0.001	7.79 (1.22–49.43)	0.02

[a] Detectable viral load >1000 copies/mm^3 at 12-week follow up. Viral load was documented in 81 patients

[b] Platelets <100,000/mm^3 at 12-weeks follow-up. 81 patients had platelets count at follow-up

illnesses. KS-related mortality was significantly higher among patients with KS-IRIS, but it was not different for patients with one or more defining AIDS events (Table 1).

Discussion

KS remains the most frequent AIDS associated malignancy in HIV-infected individuals seen at the National Institute of Cancer in Mexico, representing 41% of all initial visits to the AIDS Clinic during 2005–2011. In this study we describe the prevalence of KS-IRIS in a group of patients starting cART, Pulmonary involvement was associated to the risk of developing KS-IRIS, and thrombocytopenia at 12 week's follow-up after starting cART was associated to death. Over a third of patients with KS achieve remission without chemotherapy solely treated with cART.

The pathogenesis of KS is complex; it involves HHV-8/KSHV infection, cytokines and host-immune suppression [3, 28]. HHV-8 has oncogenic capacity, which mimics oncogenes that promote cell division, inhibit apoptosis, modulate inflammation and induce angiogenesis, but does not produce cell immortalization [29]; indeed spindle KS cells are not monoclonal. HHV-8 also induces viral and host cytokine production that promotes KS cell proliferation and differentiation (IL-6, oncostatin, alfa-TNF, PDGF, VEGF), and in HIV patients HIV-Tat protein also induces the expression of cytokines (N-kappa B activation, INF gamma, VEGF).

MSM with HIV or other active sexually transmitted diseases have the highest seropositive rates for HHV-8 [30]. At our hospital, only five women have been diagnosed with KS since 1990, and only one during the study period, consistent with the epidemiology reported in Mexico where KS is predominantly observed among MSM [31]. In our hospital we do not have HHV-8 serology.

In 1997, the first case of KS exacerbation in a patient who developed KS-induced airway obstruction 4 weeks after initiating cART was described [32]. To our knowledge, the rate of KS-IRIS found in our study is the highest reported to date (39% of patients) [33]. Our very high prevalence could be biased; since our institution is a tertiary-care center receiving patients with more extended KS disease [31]. The median time to development of KS-IRIS was 10 weeks, similar to the previously reported 6–14 week lapse after cART initiation [17, 19, 26, 33, 34].

IRIS associated to other pathogens (i.e., cytomegalovirus, MTB, MAC, and hepatitis B) has been reported to occur earlier within 2–5 weeks after cART initiation [33–35].

Higher HIV viral load was associated with the development of KS-IRIS by univariate analysis, which is a finding that had previously been reported though not consistently [33]. In two studies, an increase in CD4 count preceded KS progression in patients who had been severely immune-compromised before starting cART [4, 20, 35]. We also found an increase in CD4 counts at 12 weeks of follow-up, but this increase did not differ between the groups.

ACTG staging classification was not useful differentiating groups for IRIS-KS or mortality; we attribute this to the fact that most patients had extensive disease and low CD4.

cART has dramatically reduced opportunistic infections and mortality of HIV patients in established market-economy countries where early HIV diagnosis is promoted with extended access to HIV treatment [36, 37]. cART has also improved KS response and survival [38–42], it decreases HHV-8/KSHV viral load, and also produces complete regression of KS lesions with no additional therapy [8, 43]. However in countries such as Mexico with universal access to cART but where HIV diagnosis is delayed and patients arrive with severe immune suppression, [31] IRIS has increased the burden of mortality and morbidity of HIV-infected individuals [38].

Management of KS-IRIS has not been studied in controlled trials, but as opposed to some cases of *Mycobacterium* infection and cryptococcosis [9], corticosteroids are contraindicated in KS-IRIS, since it may further exacerbate KS lesions due to the synergy of cytokines with glucocorticoid receptors in KS spindle cells [22, 44, 45]. Herpes virus-specific immune reconstitution and the antiviral effect of combined cART plus chemotherapy has been recently documented with a trend toward better clinical outcome with cART plus chemotherapy compared with cART alone [46].

There are a wide variety of chemotherapy regimens published for KS [47–49]. In the present study chemotherapy was prescribed only for patients with more extended disease and outcome was not different between groups. It is important to note that 42% of patients achieving complete remission never received chemotherapy. The role of chemotherapy and its ultimate benefit in KS management remains a matter of debate and requires further research.

KS-IRIS is a time-limited phenomenon, but it can be a life-threatening one. Our experience shows that once the initial crisis is overcome, KS resolves in a high percentage of patients with limited or no chemotherapy and does not recur if patients maintain good adherence to cART.

The overall prevalence of pulmonary involvement in our series was higher (35%) compared to other studies (19–21%, respectively) [34, 50] likely reflecting sicker patients referred to our institution, and is one of the major risk for mortality described for KS-IRIS mortality [51, 52]. We found that pulmonary involvement was associated with the development of KS-IRIS, but not to death; only thrombocytopenia (<100,000 platelets/mm^3) at 12 weeks of follow-up was significantly associated with patient demise.

The overall incidence of secondary malignancies observed in this population is lower to what has been reported in patients receiving pegylated liposomal doxorubicin (PLD), 1.2% vs. 9.2% at a long-term follow-up, median time 48 months (IQR 33–80) for patient surviving >26 weeks, vs. 50 months (IQ-17–76) after last PLD dose, respectively [53]. It is important to consider that PLD treated patients were slightly older (35 vs. 40 years), and the number of chemotherapy cycles administered was more than twice for PLD KS treated patients compared with our patients (9 vs. 4). Decrease in CD4 count while on PLD has been described [54], this fact needs further research to understand the role of PLD in the development of secondary neoplasia and its ultimate benefit in Kaposi's therapy.

A limitation of the study that can contribute to the high prevalence of KS-IRIS we found, is that our institution is a referral tertiary care oncological center and only patients with more extensive disease are referred to our institution, while patients with few lesions and no organ involvement stay in primary care units for HIV patients. Other limitation is the analysis was retrospective and diagnosing a patient with KS-IRIS was based on published criteria [9, 13] with only two laboratory parameters and the rest mostly clinical. However, two experienced clinicians agreed on the diagnosis, and radiologic evaluation was blinded to clinical findings. Follow-up information was obtained from multiple sources such as the death certificates, pharmacy records, telephone calls and the National Program for Universal cART access, reducing uncertainty and biases.

Additional information on preventing and treating KS-IRIS is warranted including optimal timing of cART initiation for patients who present with extensive skin lesions and lung involvement, the impact of HIV and HHV-8/KSHV viral loads and CD4/CD8 counts as well as the production of inflammatory cytokines in diverse clinical scenarios as well as the role that other co-infections may have on the development of KS [55]. Anti-HHV-8/KSHV therapy should also be addressed, because both foscarnet and ganciclovir have proved activity in vitro [56] and epidemiological studies have shown that either antiviral given prophylactically for CMV infection diminishes the incidence of KS [57, 58].

It important to emphasize that abrupt clinical deterioration associated with IRIS does not represent cART failure; thus, a change of antiretroviral therapy is not warranted [26].

In summary KS patients with pulmonary involvement at diagnosis had higher risk of developing KS-IRIS. Thrombocytopenia at 12-week follow-up was significantly associated with mortality as determined by multivariate analysis. Over a third of patients with KS achieve remission without chemotherapy. Individuals that survive the initial period of KS-IRIS and adhere to cART had a good long-term prognosis. The information of the causes of death are available as Additional file 1: Table S1.

Authors' contributions

PVF, PCJ, PGF contributed collecting all the data, ERM evaluated and interpreted all the imagine studies, PVF, PCJ, PGF and GCM, analyzed and interpretied the data and PVF and PCJ drafted the first manuscript. All authors read and approved the final manuscript.

Author details

[1] Infectious Diseases Department, Instituto Nacional de Cancerología (INCan), Av. San Fernando No. 22, Col. Sección XVI, Deleg. Tlalpan, 14080 Mexico City, Mexico. [2] Hematology Department, Instituto Nacional de Cancerología (INCan), Mexico City, Mexico. [3] Radiology Department, Instituto Nacional de Cancerología (INCan), Mexico City, Mexico.

Acknowledgements

We thank Dr. Rogelio Pérez-Padilla for kindly reviewing the manuscript.

Competing interests

The authors declare that they have no competing interests.

References

1. Nakamura S, Salahuddin SZ, Biberfeld P, Ensoli B, Markham PD, Wong-Staal F, et al. Kaposi's sarcoma cells: long-term culture with growth factor from retrovirus-infected CD4+ T cells. Science. 1988;242:426–30.
2. Ensoli B, Nakamura S, Salahuddin SZ, Biberfeld P, Larsson L, Beaver B, et al. AIDS-Kaposi's sarcoma-derived cells express cytokines with autocrine and paracrine growth effects. Science. 1989;243:223–6.
3. Chang Y, Cesarman E, Pessin MS, et al. Identification of new herpesvirus like DNA sequences on AIDS-associated Kaposi's sarcoma. Science. 1994;266:1865–6.
4. Chang Y. KSHV, Kaposi's sarcoma, and related lymphoproliferative disorders. In: Parsonnet J, editor. Microbes and malignancy: infection as a cause of human cancers. New York: Oxford University Press; 1999. p. 207–31.
5. Letang E, Lewis JJ, Bower M, Mosam A, Borok M, Campbell TB, et al. Immune reconstitution inflammatory syndrome associated with Kaposi sarcoma: higher incidence and mortality in Africa than in the UK. AIDS. 2013;27(10):1603–13.
6. Maskew M, Fox MP, van Cutsem G, Chu K, Macphail P, Boulle A, Egger M, et al. Treatment response and mortality among patients starting antiretroviral therapy with and without Kaposi sarcoma: a cohort study. PLoS ONE. 2013;8(6):e64392.
7. Palella FJ Jr, Delaney KM, Moorman AC, Loveless MO, Fuhrer J, Satten GA, Aschman DJ, Holmberg SD. Declining morbidity and mortality among patients with advanced human immunodeficiency virus infection. HIV outpatient study investigators. N Engl J Med. 1998;338(13):853–60.
8. Ledergerber B, Egger M, Erard V, Weber R, Hirschel B, Furrer H, et al. AIDS-related opportunistic illnesses occurring after initiation of potent antiretroviral therapy. JAMA. 1999;282:2220–6.
9. Murdoch DM, Venter W, van Rie A, Feldman W. Immune reconstitution inflammatory syndrome (IRIS): review of common infectious manifestations and treatment options. (Abstract). AIDS Res Ther. 2007;4:9.
10. Lawn SD, Bekker LG, Miller RF. Immune reconstitution disease associated with mycobacterial infections in HIV-infected individuals receiving antiretrovirals. Lancet Infect. 2005;5:361–73.
11. Shelburne SA, Visnegarwala F, Harcourt J, Graviss EA, Giordano TP, White C Jr, et al. Incidence and risk factors for immune reconstitution inflammatory syndrome during highly active antiretroviral therapy. AIDS. 2005;19:399–406.
12. Cooney EL. Clinical indicators of immune restoration following highly active antiretroviral therapy. Clin Infect Dis. 2002;34:224–33.
13. Bower M, Nelson M, Young AM, Thirlwell C, Newsom-Davis T, Mandalia S, et al. Immune reconstitution inflammatory syndrome associated with Kaposi's sarcoma. J Clin Oncol. 2005;23:5224–8.
14. Shelburne SA 3rd, Hamill RJ, Rodríguez-Barradas MC, Greenberg SB, Atmar RL, Musher DW, et al. Immune reconstitution inflammatory syndrome: emergence of a unique syndrome during highly active antiretroviral therapy. Medicine. 2002;81:213–27.
15. Lipman M, Breen R. Immune reconstitution inflammatory syndrome in HIV. Curr Opin Infect Dis. 2006;19:20–5.
16. Murdoch DM, Venter WD, Feldman C, Van Rie A. Incidence and risk factors for the immune reconstitution inflammatory syndrome in HIV patients in South Africa: a prospective study. AIDS. 2008;22:601–10.
17. Klotz SA, Aziz Mohammed A, Girmai Woldemichael M, Worku Mitku M, Handrich M. Immune reconstitution inflammatory syndrome in a resource-poor setting. JIAPAC. 2009;8:122–7.
18. Kambugu A, Meya DB, Rhein J, O'Brien M, Janoff EN, Ronald AR, et al. Outcomes of cryptococcal meningitis in Uganda before and after the availability of highly active antiretroviral therapy. Clin Infect Dis. 2008;46:1694–701.
19. Ratnam I, Chiu C, Kandala NB, Easterbrook PJ. Incidence and risk factors for immune reconstitution inflammatory syndrome in an ethnically diverse HIV-1-infected cohort. Clin Infect Dis. 2006;42:418–27.
20. Race EM, Adelson-Mitty J, Kriegel GR, Barlam TF, Reimann KA, Letvin NL, et al. Focal mycobacterial lymphadenitis following initiation of protease-inhibitor therapy in patients with advanced HIV-1 disease. Lancet. 1998;351:252–5.
21. Park WB, Choe PG, Jo JH, Kim SH, Bang JH, Kim HB, et al. Tuberculosis manifested by immune reconstitution inflammatory syndrome during HAART. AIDS. 2007;21:875–7.
22. Volkow PF, Cornejo P, Zinser JW, Ormsby CE, Reyes-Terán G. Life-threatening exacerbation of Kaposi's sarcoma after prednisone treatment for immune reconstitution inflammatory syndrome. AIDS. 2008;22:663–5.
23. Chachoua A, Krigel R, Lafleur F, Ostreicher R, Speer M, Laubenstein L, Wernz J, Rubenstein P, Zang E, Friedman-Kien A. Prognostic factors and staging classification of patients with epidemic Kaposi's sarcoma. J Clin Oncol. 1989;7(6):774–80.
24. Krown SE, Testa MA, Huang J. AIDS-related Kaposi's sarcoma: prospective validation of the AIDS Clinical Trials Group staging classification. AIDS Clinical Trials Group Oncology Committee. J Clin Oncol. 1997;15(9):3085–92.
25. French MA, Price P, Stone SF. Immune restoration disease after antiretroviral therapy. AIDS. 2004;18(12):1615–27.
26. Nathan RV. Suspected immune reconstitution inflammatory syndrome associated with the proliferation of Kaposi's sarcoma during HAART. AIDS. 2007;21:775–6.
27. Gompels MM, Hill A, Jenkins P, Peters B, Tomlinson D, Harris JR, et al. Kaposi's sarcoma in HIV infection treated with vincristine and bleomycin. AIDS. 1992;6:1175–80.
28. Hengge UR, Ruzicka T, Tyrling SK, Stuschke M, Roggendorf M, Schwartz RA, et al. Update on Kaposi's syndrome and other HHV8 associated diseases. Part 1: epidemiology, Environmental predispositions, clinical manifestations, and therapy. Lancet Infect Dis. 2002;2:281–92.
29. Gantt S, Casper C. Human herpesvirus 8-associated neoplasms: the roles of viral replication and antiviral treatment. Curr Opin Infect Dis. 2011;24(4):295–301.
30. Hengge UR, Ruzicka T, Tyrling SK, Stuschke M, Roggendorf M, Schwartz RA, et al. Update on Kaposi's syndrome and other HHV8 associated diseases. Part 1: epidemiology. Environmental predispositions, clinical manifestations, and therapy. Lancet Infect Dis. 2001;2:281–92.
31. Crabtree-Ramírez B, Gómez-Palacio M, Rodríguez-Rivera V, Reyes-Terán G. Baseline characteristic of HIV-infected patients attending a National Institute of Health in Mexico City: evidence of late detection of HIV infection

and the urgent need for efficient voluntary counseling and testing (VCT) programs. AIDS 2008. THPEO244 International AIDS Conference; August 2008. p. 390.

32. Weir A, Wansbrough-Jones M. Mucosal Kaposi's sarcoma following protease inhibitor therapy in an HIV-infected patient. AIDS. 1997;11:1895–986.
33. Letang E, Almeida JM, Miró J, Ayala E, White I, Carrilho C, et al. Predictors of immune reconstitution inflammatory syndrome-associated with Kaposi sarcoma in Mozambique: a prospective study. J Acquir Immune Defic Syndr. 2010;53:589–97.
34. Leidner RS, Aboulafia DM. Recrudescent Kaposi's sarcoma after initiation of HAART: a manifestation of immune reconstitution syndrome. AIDS Patient Care ST. 2005;19:635–44.
35. Cheng VC, Yuen KY, Chan WM, Wong SS, Ma ES, Chan RM. Immunorestitution disease involving the innate and adaptive response. Clin Infect Dis. 2000;30:882–92.
36. Mocroft A, Kirk O, Clumeck N, Gargalianos-Kakolyris P, Trocha H, Chentsova N, et al. The changing pattern of Kaposi sarcoma in patients with HIV, 1994–2003: the EuroSIDA Study. Cancer. 2004;100:2644–54.
37. Eltom MA, Jemal A, Mbulaiteye SM, Devesa SS, Biggar RJ. Trends in Kaposi's sarcoma and non-Hodgkin's lymphoma incidence in the United States from 1973 through 1998. J Natl Cancer Inst. 2002;94(16):1204–10.
38. Tam HK, Zhang ZF, Jacobson LP, Margolick JB, Chmiel JS, Rinaldo C, et al. Effect of highly active antiretroviral therapy on survival among HIV-infected men with Kaposi sarcoma or non-Hodgkin lymphoma. Int J Cancer. 2002;98:916–22.
39. Paparizos VA, Kyriakis KP, Papastamopoulos V, Hadjivassiliou M, Stavrianeas WG. Response of AIDS-associated Kaposi sarcoma to highly active antiretroviral therapy alone. J Acquir Immune Syndr. 2002;30:257–8.
40. Nguyen HQ, Magaret AS, Kitahata MM, Van Rompaey SE, Wald A, Casper C. Persistant Kaposi sarcoma in the era of highly active antiretroviral therapy: characterizing the predictors of clinical response. AIDS. 2008;22:937–45.
41. Holkova B, Takeshita K, Cheng DM, Volm M, Wasserheit C, Dempoulos R, et al. Effect of highly active antiretroviral therapy on survival in patients with AIDS-associated pulmomary Kaposi's sarcoma treated with chemotherapy. J Clin Oncol. 2001;19:3848–51.
42. Bower M, Wein J, Francis N, Newsom-Davis T, Powles S, Crook T, et al. The effect of HAART in 254 patients with AIDS-related Kaposi's sarcoma. AIDS. 2009;23:1701–6.
43. Connick E, Kane MA, White IE, Ryder J, Campbell T. Immune reconstitution inflammatory syndrome associated with Kaposi sarcoma during potent antiretroviral therapy. Clin Infect Dis. 2004;39:1852–5.
44. Guo WX, Antakly T. AIDS-related Kaposi's sarcoma: evidence for direct stimulatory effect of glucocorticoids on cell proliferation. Am J Pathol.
45. Schulhafer EP, Grossman ME, Fagin G, Bell KE. Steroid-induced Kaposi's sarcoma in a patient with pre-AIDS. Am J Med. 1987;82:313–7.
46. Bihl F, Mosam A, Henry LN, Chisholm JV 3rd, Dollard S, Gubi P, et al. Kaposi's sarcoma-associated herpesvirus-specific immune reconstitution and antiviral effect of combined HAART/chemotherapy in HIV clade C-infected individuals with Kaposi's sarcoma. AIDS. 2007;21:1245–52.
47. Newell M, Milliken S, Goldstein D, Lewis C, Boyle M, Dolan G, et al. A phase II study of liposomal doxorubicin in the treatment of HIV-related Kaposi's sarcoma. Aust NZ J Med. 1998;28:777–83.
48. Tulpule A, Groopman J, Saville MW, Harrington W Jr, Friedman-Kien A, Espina BM, et al. Multicenter trial of low-dose paclitaxel in patients with advanced AIDS-related Kaposi sarcoma. Cancer. 2002;95:147–54.
49. Cooley T, Henry D, Tonda M, Sun S, O'Connell M, Rackoff W. A randomized, double-blind study of pegylated liposomal doxorubicin for the treatment of AIDS-related Kaposi's sarcoma. Oncologist. 2007;12:114–23.
50. Martin J, Laker M, Clutter D, Kambugu A, Janka D, Bennett J, et al. Kaposi's sarcoma-associated immune reconstitution syndrome in Africa: initial findings from prospective evaluation. 16th Conference on Retrovirus and Opportunistic Infections 2009. Abstract #31.
51. Crane HM, Deubner H, Huang JC, Swanson PE, Harrington RD. Fatal Kaposi's sarcoma-associated reconstitution following HAART initiation. Int J STD AIDS. 2005;16:80–3.
52. Palmieri C, Dhillon T, Thirlwell C, Newsom-Davis T, Young AM, Nelson M, et al. Pulmonary Kaposi sarcoma in the era of highly active antiretroviral therapy. HIV Med. 2006;7:291–3.
53. Martín-Carbonero L, Palacios R, Valencia E, Saballs P, Sirera G, Santos I, et al. Long-term prognosis of HIV-infected patients with Kaposi sarcoma treated with pegylated liposomal doxorubicin. Clin Infect Dis. 2008;47(3):410–7.
54. Volkow P, Lizano M, Carrillo-García A, Pérez-Montiel D, Garciadiego P. Triple secondary neoplasms: penis, lip and oral cavity in an AIDS patient treated with pegylated liposomal doxorubicin for cutaneous Kaposi's sarcoma. AIDS. 2014;28(15):2327–9.
55. Feller L, Lemmer J. Insights into pathogenic events of HIV-associated Kaposi sarcoma and immune reconstitution syndrome related Kaposi sarcoma. Infectious Agents Cancer. 2008;3:1. doi:10.1186/1750-9378-3-1.
56. Neyts J, Clerq E. Antiviral drug susceptibility of human herpesvirus. Antimicrob Agents Chemother. 1997;41:2754–6.
57. Mocroft A, Youle M, Gazzard B, Morcinek J, Halai R, Phillips A. Antiherpesvirus treatment and risk of Kaposi's sarcoma in HIV infection. AIDS. 1996;10:1101–5.
58. Glesby MJ, Hoover DR, Weng S, Graham NM, Phair JP, Detels R, et al. Use of antiherpes drugs and the risk of Kaposi's sarcoma: data from the Multicenter AIDS Cohort study. J Infect Dis. 1996;173:1477–80.

6

Barriers to uptake of early infant HIV testing in Zambia: the role of intimate partner violence and HIV status disclosure within couples

Karen M. Hampanda[1*], Abigail M. Nimz[2] and Lisa L. Abuogi[3,4]

Abstract

Background: Early detection of pediatric HIV through uptake of infant HIV testing is critical for access to treatment and child survival. While structural barriers have been well described, a greater understanding of social and behavioral factors that may relate to maternal uptake of early infant HIV testing services is urgently needed. The aim of this study was to explore how gender power dynamics within couples affect HIV-positive women's uptake of early infant HIV testing at a large health center in Lusaka, Zambia.

Methods: In 2014, 320 HIV-positive married postpartum women were recruited at a large public health facility in Lusaka to participate in a cross-sectional survey. Data on uptake of early infant HIV testing by 4–6 weeks of age was collected through medical records. Simple and multiple logistic regression models determined significant predictors of maternal uptake of early infant HIV testing.

Results: In the adjusted model, uptake of early infant HIV testing was associated with female-directed emotional intimate partner violence (aOR 0.41; 95% CI 0.21–0.79; $p < 0.01$), HIV status disclosure to the male partner (aOR 13.73, 95% CI 3.59–52.49, $p < 0.001$), and maternal postpartum ART adherence (aOR 2.28, 95% CI 1.15–4.55, $p < 0.05$).

Conclusions: Domestic relationship dynamics, including emotional violence and HIV status disclosure to the male partner, may play an important role in maternal uptake of early infant HIV testing. These findings provide additional evidence for the link between intimate partner violence against women and poor HIV-related health outcomes. Programs that adequately screen for and address various forms of intimate partner violence within the context of prevention of mother-to-child transmission are recommended.

Background

Despite commendable advances in prevention of mother-to-child transmission (PMTCT), pediatric HIV remains a significant public health challenge, particularly in sub-Saharan Africa. In 2015, 150,000 children under 15 years of age were newly infected with HIV and 1.8 million children were living with the virus—the majority residing in sub-Saharan Africa [1]. In the study setting, Zambia, an estimated 85,000 children were living with HIV in 2015 [2]. Early detection of HIV in infants through timely HIV testing is critical for their survival due to the increased risk of mortality without antiretroviral therapy (ART) compared to HIV-infected adults [3–5]. The World Health Organization (WHO) currently recommends testing of HIV-exposed infants in resource-limited settings using dry blood spot (DBS) polymerase chain reaction (PCR) technology at 4–6 weeks of life to optimize detection of intrauterine, intrapartum, and early postnatal mother-to-child HIV transmission [6]. Yet, most recent estimates indicate that less than half of the infants born to HIV-positive mothers in low- and middle-income

*Correspondence: karen.hampanda@ucdenver.edu
[1] Department of Community and Behavioral Health, Colorado School of Public Health, 13199 East Montview Boulevard, Suite 310, Mail Stop A090, Aurora, CO 80045, USA

countries receive an HIV test within the first two months of life [7].

Numerous healthcare system barriers to early diagnosis of HIV infection in infants in resource-limited settings have been identified. For example, DNA-PCR using DBS requires sophisticated and expensive nucleic acid testing, as well as highly trained staff and advanced laboratory infrastructure, which is generally only present in large, centralized laboratories [8–10]. Indeed, in Zambia, there are only three facilities with laboratories capable of processing PCR [11]. The situation is also exacerbated by restriction of sample collection sites to PMTCT clinics, stock outs of HIV testing commodities, poorly functioning sample transport networks, and limitations in supply chain management [8, 12, 13]. Current efforts are underway to address these acknowledged problems, including, for example, point-of-care technologies [12].

While healthcare system barriers related to infant HIV testing have been well described, less is known about the impact of social factors, including dynamics with the male partner, among HIV-positive mothers. The family—particularly the male partner—is arguably the most influential social unit affecting individual health behaviors [14]. In African settings in particular, male partners are known to play an essential role in household decision-making, including women's use of HIV-related services [15–17]. Moreover, dynamics with male partners, such as HIV status disclosure and fear of intimate partner violence (IPV), are known to effect women's uptake of some services in the PMTCT cascade of care [18, 19]. It is plausible that the same barriers related to dynamics within couples that exist for other PMTCT-related health behaviors may prevent HIV-positive mothers from accessing early infant HIV testing services. This study explores how gender power dynamics within couples, such as IPV against women and male controlling behaviors, women's participation in household decision-making, and women's relative earnings, as well as HIV status disclosure to male partners, affect HIV-positive mother's uptake of early infant HIV testing by the recommended 4–6 weeks postpartum in a large public health center in Lusaka, Zambia.

Methods

Study design

A cross-sectional survey was conducted with postpartum HIV-positive women who were currently married or cohabiting with a male partner. Recruitment occurred at a large public health center during routine pediatric immunizations from April to August of 2014. Quantitative data were collected through medical records (i.e., the child's Under-Five Card) and a face-to-face survey with closed-ended questions, including dynamics within the woman's current heterosexual relationship. The questionnaire was pretested during a pilot study in March of 2014. Trained Zambian research assistants verbally administered the survey in the local languages on paper forms in a private location at the health center after women completed their health care visit. The questionnaire was written in English, but translated into the two most commonly spoken dialects in Lusaka (Nynaja and Bemba). Participants received a small travel reimbursement for their time. Written informed consent or a thumbprint was obtained from all study participants. The study was designed and implemented in accordance with the WHO Ethical and Safety Recommendations for Research on Domestic Violence Against Women [20]. Research Assistants were trained in research ethics. Participants who reported IPV were offered referrals to a local organization for counseling and victim support services.

Study participants

Participants included 320 HIV-positive mothers who had brought their child for routine pediatric immunizations in the Maternal and Child Health Department of a large public health center in Lusaka, Zambia. The health center has a catchment population of over 160,000 individuals living in the surrounding low socioeconomic neighborhoods. Mothers who were diagnosed as HIV seropositive, over the age of 18 years, currently married or living with a man as if married, and whose youngest biological infant was between 3 and 9 months of age were invited to participate in the survey after completing their health care visit. Infant age criterion was selected based on the immunization schedule in Zambia and to limit recall bias. Immunization compliance in Zambia is high with 97% of all infants receiving at least some immunizations by 12 months of life [15–17].

Nurses determined eligibility for the study using the infant's "Under-Five Card," a mother's copy of her child's health record that she is required to bring to all pediatric health care visits and includes the child's birth date, height and weight, immunizations, medications, and PMTCT care. Nurses providing immunizations examined the Under-Five Card or other medical records if the card was not available and verbally invited eligible women to participate in the survey by proceeding to a designated private room (or waiting area outside if the room was occupied) in the clinic where research assistants conducted informed consent, asked additional screening questions, and verbally administered the survey questionnaire to consenting eligible participants. The response rate for eligible women was 85%.

Measures

The main outcome of interest, uptake of infant HIV testing by 4–6 weeks postpartum, was captured using the child's Under-Five Card or other available medical record. Research assistants indicated on the survey questionnaire whether the child had record of HIV testing at 4–6 weeks via PCR, and if available, the result of the test. Gender power dynamics within the couple, the independent variables of interest, were measured using the Revised Conflict Tactics Scale (CTS2). The CTS2 is one of the most widely used gender power measurement tools worldwide with strong reported psychometric properties [21]. The version of the CTS2 used in this study came directly from the Zambian Demographic and Health Survey (ZDHS) Domestic Violence Module [22, 23]. The DHS Domestic Violence Module was first developed and standardized in 2000 and has been continually used throughout sub-Saharan Africa [24]. The module includes questions regarding different forms of IPV against women, male partner controlling behaviors, women's participation in household decisions, and women's relative earnings. Participants were asked to report their experiences with specific emotional, physical, and sexual IPV events ever occurring in the course of their relationship with the current male partner. There were three possible specific events for emotional violence, seven possible events for physical violence, and two possible events for sexual violence. Participants also reported whether their male partner displays specific controlling behaviors from a set of six questions. In addition, the survey included four questions regarding women's participation in household decisions regarding daily household purchases, major household purchases, women's use of health care, and the final say over how money is spent. Women's relative earnings compared to the husband was measured by asking women if the they earn more money than the husband, about the same amount of money, or less money than the husband. We also added one additional question on women's HIV status disclosure to the husband.

Control variables included the woman's age, infant's age, parity, education, household wealth (a proxy for socioeconomic status), when the woman was diagnosed with HIV (before or during the most recent pregnancy), if the woman was taking lifelong triple ART or short course prophylaxis under WHO Option A, knowledge of PMTCT, the woman's postpartum ART adherence, and the male partner's HIV status (positive, negative, or unknown). Educational attainment was measured by asking women "what was the highest level of school you attended" (none, some primary, completed primary, some secondary, completed secondary, some college, completed college, or graduate level). We measured socioeconomic status by asking participants what household assets their home owned from a list of 21 possible items, including, for example, electricity, a car, and a refrigerator. Knowledge of PMTCT was measured by asking participants "are there any special drugs that a doctor or nurse can give to a woman infected with HIV to reduce the risk of transmission to the baby?." Lastly, postpartum ART adherence was measured using a visual analog scale (VAS) [25] that was verbally explained to women by the research assistants. Participants retrospectively reported on their estimate of ART adherence (doses taken at the appropriate time) since giving birth from 0 to 100%. Postpartum adherence rather than pregnancy adherence was included in our analysis because the time period more closely correlates with maternal uptake of infant HIV testing behaviors.

Data cleaning and statistical analysis

Survey data were double entered into CSPro and exported into Stata 12 for analysis. Surveys with more than 50% missing data were not included in the analyses (n = 4). Missing data (2.3%) were imputed using multivariate chained equations in Stata 12 [26, 27]. Data converged, indicating that the multivariate chained model was a good fit for the data set [28]. We created a binary dependent variable for uptake of early infant HIV testing based on whether or not a PCR test was specified on the child's health record/Under-Five Card by 4–6 weeks of age. For the independent variables regarding dynamics with the male partner, we created two binary variables to capture experiences with IPV: 1) if the woman reported any female-directed emotional IPV in the course of the relationship and 2) if the woman reported any female-directed physical/sexual IPV in the course of the relationship. We also created a binary variable to capture if the male partner displayed three or more controlling behaviors based on prior literature standards for analyzing this variable [24]. Additionally, we created a count variable to indicate the number of household decisions (0–4) women reported participating based on their responses to the individual household decision-making questions. Women were categorized as participating in a household decision if they made the decision alone or together with the male partner, compared to when the male partner alone makes the decision. For women's relative earnings, we created a binary variable to indicate whether women make more/about the same amount of money as the husband, compared to women who make less money than the husband. Lastly, a binary variable for status disclosure was created to capture whether women reported notifying their male partner of their HIV-positive status.

For the control variables, the woman's age and parity were treated as continuous variables in the analysis. Two variables based on reported educational attainment were created: if the woman completed primary education and if the woman completed secondary education. For socioeconomic status, we converted women's responses to the list of household assets into a linear index using principal-components analysis (PCA) to derive weights [29]. For example, if a household had electricity, it would move the participant 0.30 on the index; however, if a household owned a chair, it would only move the participant 0.17 on the index. The index was standardized prior to inclusion in the regression models. Additional binary control variables included: whether the woman was diagnosed with HIV during the most recent pregnancy, whether she was taking lifelong triple ART, and whether she had knowledge regarding PMTCT. Postpartum ART adherence was dichotomized into a variable indicating if the woman was at least 80% adherent to taking medication after giving birth based on recent studies suggesting this is the adequate doses needed to suppress the virus [30, 31]. Finally, three dummy variables were created to indicate the male partner's HIV status: (1) if the male partner was HIV-positive, (2) if the male partner had an unknown status or never tested for HIV, and (3) if the male partner was HIV-negative.

Descriptive statistics highlighted sample characteristics stratified by if the child had an early HIV test. Simple logistic regression models determined significant difference in the odds of early infant HIV testing by the independent variables of interest and control variables. We also ran a pairwise correlation to determine the correlation coefficients for experiencing any emotional IPV in the course of the relationship, the number of household decisions the woman participates, and if the male partner displays 3 or more controlling behaviors. These gender power variables were selected for the correlation analysis because they were significantly associated with early infant HIV testing in the bivariate model. Each measure in the correlation analysis was highly correlated with the other ($p < 0.001$), indicating a significant interaction between these variables.

Finally, a multiple logistic regression model determined significant differences in the odds of early infant HIV testing by the relevant independent variables (i.e., those associated with the dependent variable in the simple logistic regression models) after adjusting for control variables of age, parity, whether the woman completed secondary education, whether she was diagnosed with HIV during the most recent pregnancy, household wealth index, postpartum ART adherence, and the husband's HIV status. Secondary education, rather than primary education, was included in the multiple logistic regression models because it displayed greater variability in the sample. The variables capturing knowledge of PMTCT, if the woman was taking lifelong triple ART, any female-directed physical/sexual IPV, and if the woman had greater or equal earnings as male partner were not included in the multiple logistic regression model because they were not significantly associated with early infant HIV testing in the simple logistic regression models and have not previously been established in the literature as important covariates.

Results

Participant characteristics

Table 1 displays the participant characteristics, comparing infants who had an early HIV test and those who did not. Of the 320 HIV-positive female participants, the median age was 28 years (IQR 24, 34). Women had given birth to a median of 3 children (IQR 2, 4). Over 70% of women had completed primary education, but only 14% had completed secondary education. For the poorest 40% of the sample, the mean wealth index score was −1.97. For the mid-wealth participants (also 40% of the sample), the mean wealth index score was 0.88. For the wealthiest 20% of the sample, the mean wealth index score was 2.67. In terms of actual household assets, 75% of participants had electricity; 39% owned a refrigerator, and 5% owned a vehicle. Knowledge of PMTCT was nearly universal: 96% of women agreed that there are special drugs that can prevent mother-to-child HIV infection. The majority of participants (60%) reported being diagnosed with HIV during the most recent pregnancy while 40% knew their status prior to becoming pregnant. Fifty-six percent of participants were prescribed lifelong triple ART while 44% were not eligible for treatment and taking short-course prophylaxis under WHO programmatic Option A. Lastly, 81% of women reported being adherent to ART postpartum.

Disclosure of women's HIV status to the male partner was high with 92% of women reporting they had informed the current partner of their HIV-positive status. Approximately half (52%) of the participants' reported having a male partner who is also living with HIV (i.e., seroconcordant), 28% reported having a male partner who is HIV-negative (serodiscordant), and 21% reported having a male partner whose status was unknown or who had never tested for HIV. Experiences with IPV were common: 40% of women reported any female-directed emotional IPV in the course of the relationship and 50% of women reported any female-directed physical/sexual IPV in the course of the relationship. Male controlling behaviors were also common with 56% of women reporting their male partner displays three or more controlling behaviors. Women reported participating in a median of half (2.0 out of 4.0) of the household decisions. Twenty-five percent of women reported having equal or greater earnings as the male partner.

Uptake of early infant HIV testing and unadjusted associations

Seventy-three percent (n = 233) of infants had an HIV test by 4–6 weeks of age. Table 1 indicates which demographic and sexual relationship characteristics were associated with uptake of early infant HIV testing in the simple logistic regression models. Two demographic characteristics were associated with uptake of early infant HIV testing in the bivariate models: knowing one's HIV status prior to becoming pregnant ($p < 0.05$) and being adherent to postpartum ART ($p < 0.001$). Sexual relationship characteristics associated with uptake of early infant HIV testing included: HIV status disclosure to the male partner ($p < 0.001$), having an HIV-positive male partner ($p < 0.05$) and knowing the male partner's HIV status ($p < 0.05$), not experiencing any female-directed emotional IPV ($p < 0.001$), the male partner displaying <3 controlling behaviors ($p < 0.05$), and greater participation in household decision-making ($p < 0.01$).

Uptake of early infant HIV testing and adjusted associations

Table 2 displays the multiple logistic regression results for the adjusted odds of early infant HIV testing by dynamics within the couple and control variables. The only power dynamic that remained significantly associated with uptake of early infant HIV testing after including other gender power measures and control variables was female-directed emotional IPV: women who reported any female-directed emotional IPV in the course of their

Table 1 Participant Characteristics (n = 320)

Variable	Infant tested by 4–6 weeks (n = 233)	Infant not tested by 4–6 weeks (n = 87)	Total (n = 320)	
	Median (IQR)/N (%)	Median (IQR)/N (%)	Median (IQR)/N (%)	P
Demographic characteristics				
Age in years	29.0 (25.0, 34.0)	27.0 (24.0, 33.0)	28.0 (24.0, 34.0)	0.097
Parity	3.0 (2.0, 5.0)	3.0 (2.0, 4.0)	3.0 (2.0, 4.0)	0.161
Completed primary education	167 (72.8%)	63 (72.2%)	230 (71.9%)	0.572
Completed secondary education	35 (15.3%)	9 (11.4%)	44 (13.8%)	0.187
Standardized wealth Index	0.14 (−0.73, 0.89)	−0.08 (−0.83, 0.59)	0.06 (−0.78, 0.76)	0.106
Diagnosed with HIV during most recent pregnancy	130 (55.9%)	63 (72.0%)	192 (60.3%)	0.010
Prescribed lifelong triple ART[a]	138 (59.1%)	41 (47.7%)	179 (56.0%)	0.068
Knowledge of PMTCT	225 (96.5%)	81 (93.0%)	306 (95.6%)	0.183
Adherent to ART[b]	202 (86.8%)	57 (65.1%)	259 (80.9%)	0.000
Sexual relationship characteristics				
Disclosed HIV status to male partner	227 (97.6%)	66 (76.0%)	293 (91.8%)	0.000
Male partner HIV status				
Positive (seroconcordant)	128 (55.2%)	36 (41.9%)	164 (51.6%)	0.036
Negative (serodiscordant)	65 (27.8%)	24 (27.6%)	89 (27.8%)	0.980
Unknown/partner not tested	40 (17.0%)	26 (30.5%)	66 (20.6%)	0.010
Any female-directed emotional IPV in course of relationship	79 (33.9%)	50 (57.9%)	129 (40.3%)	0.000
Any female-directed physical/sexual IPV in course of relationship	113 (48.5%)	47 (54.4%)	160 (50.0%)	0.356
Male partner displays 3 + controlling behaviors[c]	131 (56.4%)	63 (72.0%)	194 (60.6%)	0.012
Number of household decisions the woman participates[d]	3.0 (2.0, 4.0)	2.0 (1.0, 3.0)	2.0 (1.0, 4.0)	0.007
Woman has greater or equal earnings as male partner	59 (25.3%)	17 (19.7%)	76 (23.8%)	0.294

[a] Comparison group: prescribed short-course prophylaxis under Option A

[b] Defined as the woman's self-report of taking >80% of medication doses postpartum (includes both short-course prophylaxis and lifelong triple ART)

[c] Out of six total behaviors

[d] Out of four total household decisions

Table 2 Multiple logistic regression results for the adjusted odds of early infant HIV testing

	Infant HIV testing by 4–6 weeks aOR (95% CI)
Dynamics with the male partner	
Any female-directed emotional IPV in course of relationship	0.41** (0.21–0.79)
Number of household decisions the woman participates	1.10 (0.86–1.39)
Male partner displays 3 + controlling behaviors	1.05 (0.53–2.06)
Disclosed HIV status to male partner	13.73*** (3.59–52.49)
Control variables	
Age in years	1.03 (0.96–1.11)
Parity	1.03 (0.80–1.32)
Completed secondary education	2.09 (0.81–5.40)
Standardized wealth Index	1.04 (0.76–1.40)
Diagnosed with HIV during most recent pregnancy	0.66 (0.36–1.22)
Maternal ART adherence postpartum	2.28* (1.15–4.55)
Male partner HIV status:	
HIV-Negative	ref.
Unknown	1.68 (0.67–4.19)
HIV-positive	1.13 (0.58–2.19)

* $p < 0.05$; ** $p < 0.01$; *** $p < 0.001$

relationship had 59% lower adjusted odds of early infant HIV testing (aOR 0.41; 95% CI 0.21–0.79; $p < 0.01$), compared to women who did not experience emotional IPV. Conversely, women's participation in household decisions was not significantly associated with early infant HIV testing, nor was the male partner displaying three or more controlling behaviors after adjusting for emotional IPV and other control variables. Women who reported disclosing their HIV status to the male partner, however, had 14 times higher adjusted odds of early infant HIV testing (aOR 13.73, 95% CI 3.59–52.49, $p < 0.001$), compared to women who did not disclosure their status. Finally, women who reported >80% adherence to ART after birth had 2 times higher adjusted odds of early infant HIV testing (aOR 2.28, 95% CI 1.15–4.55, $p < 0.05$), compared to women who reported <80% ART adherence and after adjusting for dynamics with the male partner and other control variables.

Discussion

Over one-quarter of the HIV-exposed infants in this study failed to receive early PCR testing by the recommended 4–6 weeks—hindering early diagnosis and treatment, and the odds of survival [3–5]. This study demonstrates that dynamics with the male partner may have a significant affect on the odds of maternal uptake of early infant HIV testing. In this study, female-directed emotional IPV was strongly associated with reduced adjusted odds of early infant HIV testing. Notably, there was a significant interaction between female-directed emotional IPV, women's participation in household decisions, and male partner controlling behaviors—with emotional IPV driving the relationship with uptake of infant HIV testing. Our findings add to the growing body of literature linking different forms of IPV to poor medical outcomes across the continuum of care for HIV-infected mothers and their children [19, 32–34]. Our findings also underscore the importance of examining IPV as a multidimensional phenomenon [35] and including emotional/psychological forms of abuse as potential predictors for poor health outcomes.

We hypothesize several potential explanations for the relationship between emotional IPV and reduced odds of early infant HIV testing, which warrant further exploration. First, partners in emotionally violent relationships may have poor communication, which is known to be important for other PMTCT-related health behaviors [36–38]. In addition, male partners who are emotionally violent may be less willing to participate in PMTCT-related care, which, again, is a known facilitator for uptake of other PMTCT protocols [39–41]. Lastly, women experiencing emotional IPV may be afraid of finding out the infant is HIV-positive and enduring additional potential emotional abuse from their male partner. We recommend that future qualitative research with peripartum HIV-positive women explore the mechanisms within emotionally violent relationships that are different than those in physically/sexually violent relationships, which may impede the uptake of HIV-related health behaviors differentially.

Another dynamic within sexual relationships related to early infant HIV testing is women's HIV status disclosure to male partners. This study supports prior research from sub-Saharan Africa indicating women's HIV status disclose to male partners improves participation in PMTCT programs [42, 43]. In this study, we document a direct quantitative relationship between non-disclosure of women's HIV status to male partners and lower uptake of early infant HIV testing. Recent qualitative work also indicates that women's fear of stigma and involuntary HIV status disclosure to family members or the community are barriers to early infant diagnosis and the continuation of HIV care for mothers and their children [44, 45].

Outside of dynamics with the male partner, maternal HIV-related health behaviors also affect the odds of early infant HIV testing. Our findings indicate that women who reported better postpartum ART adherence were more likely to have their child tested for HIV by 4–6 weeks. Importantly, this finding suggests that the HIV-exposed children who are at the greatest risk of contracting HIV (due to maternal non-adherence to PMTCT) may be least likely to be diagnosed through early infant HIV testing. It is therefore critical for PMTCT programs to promote maternal adherence early in the cascade of care and prioritize outreach and counseling with women who are non-adherent to ART—both for their own health and to ensure that they are not lost to follow-up and miss opportunities for early infant HIV testing.

Our prior research indicates that IPV against HIV-positive women, including emotional IPV, negatively affects adherence to several steps in the PMTCT cascade, including maternal ART adherence during and after pregnancy [32]. The present study adds that early infant HIV testing, a critical step in the cascade of care for HIV-exposed infants, is also affected by emotional IPV. Thus, programs within the context of PMTCT that adequately screen for and address various forms of IPV are urgently needed. Counseling within PMTCT programs should attempt to evaluate women's home circumstances and determine who may be at risk for low compliance because of IPV, including emotional abuse. An appropriate referral system between PMTCT programs and IPV services should also be prioritized.

The results of this study should be interpreted within several limitations. First, it is cross-sectional and cannot establish causality or the timing of events. Second, status disclosure and gender power dynamics are based on self-report, which can be vulnerable to recall and social desirability biases. The sample is also non-representative and clinic-based, limiting the generalizability of findings. This study may also have selection bias because all participants were bringing their children for pediatric immunizations, which may not be representative of all mother-baby pairs needing infant HIV testing. We did not measure communication within the couple or male partner support for health behaviors, which may be mediating factors in the relationship between emotional IPV and uptake of early infant HIV testing. We were also unable to test the relationship between dynamics within couples and the odds of the infant being diagnosed with HIV because only one-third of children had any available test results due to the slow turn-around time for PCR in Zambia at the time of the study.

Conclusion

This study highlights the role of dynamics within heterosexual couples and uptake of early infant HIV testing. Emotional IPV and non-disclosure of an HIV-positive status to male partners are strongly associated with reduced odds of early infant HIV testing. Given the high prevalence of IPV in the region, including emotional IPV, these findings have far-reaching implications for early infant HIV diagnosis and treatment. Programs that adequately screen for and address various forms of IPV within the context of PMTCT are recommended.

Authors' contributions

KH conceived of the research study; designed the research methods; led the acquisition, analysis, and interpretation of data; and participated in the drafting and revising of this article. LA contributed to the analysis and interpretation of data and the writing and revising of this article. AN participated in the interpretation of data and in the drafting and revising of the article. All authors read and approved the final manuscript.

Author details

[1] Department of Community and Behavioral Health, Colorado School of Public Health, 13199 East Montview Boulevard, Suite 310, Mail Stop A090, Aurora, CO 80045, USA. [2] University of Colorado School of Medicine, 13001 E 17th Place, Aurora, CO 80045, USA. [3] Department of Pediatrics, University of Colorado School of Medicine and Children's Hospital Colorado, Aurora, CO, USA. [4] Center for Global Health, University of Colorado School of Medicine School of Public Health, 13199 East Montview Boulevard, Suite 310, Mail Stop A090, Aurora, CO 80045, USA.

Acknowledgements

The authors would like to thank Dr. Sara Yeatman, Dr. Patrick Krueger, Dr. Karen Spencer, Dr. Sheana Bull, Dr. Yusuf Ahmed, Christine Chewe Sakala, Grace Lungeani Phiri, Franklin Munsanje, and Bibi Lambert Manda for their support of the study.

Competing interests

The authors declare that they have no competing interests.

Funding

Research reported in this publication was supported by the Center for Global Health at the University of Colorado Denver and the National Institute of Mental Health of the National Institutes of Health under Award Number F31MH107348. The content is solely the responsibility of the authors and does not necessarily represent the official views of the National Institutes of Health.

References

1. UNAIDS. Children and HIV: fact sheet July 2016. Geneva: Joint United Nations Programme on HIV/AIDS; 2016.
2. HIV and AIDS estimates. Zambia. 2015. http://www.unaids.org/en/regionscountries/countries/zambia.

3. Becquet R, Mofenson LM. Early antiretroviral therapy of HIV-infected infants in resource-limited countries: possible, feasible, effective and challenging. AIDS. 2008;22:1365–8.
4. Prendergast A, Mphatswe W, Tudor-Williams G, Rakgotho M, Pillay V, Thobakgale C, McCarthy N, Morris L, Walker BD, Goulder P. Early virological suppression with three-class antiretroviral therapy in HIV-infected African infants. AIDS. 2008;22:1333–43.
5. Edmonds A, Yotebieng M, Lusiama J, Matumona Y, Kitetele F, Napravnik S, Cole SR, Van Rie A, Behets F. The effect of highly active antiretroviral therapy on the survival of HIV-infected children in a resource-deprived setting: a cohort study. PLoS Med. 2011;8:e1001044.
6. WHO. WHO recommendations on the diagnosis of HIV infection in infants and children. In: WHO, editor. WHO Library Cataloguing-in-Publication Data. Geneva: World Health Organization; 2010.
7. The gap report. http://www.unaids.org/en/resources/documents/2014/20140716_UNAIDS_gap_report.
8. Ciaranello AL, Park JE, Ramirez-Avila L, Freedberg KA, Walensky RP, Leroy V. Early infant HIV-1 diagnosis programs in resource-limited settings: opportunities for improved outcomes and more cost-effective interventions. BMC Med. 2011;9:59.
9. Creek TL, Sherman GG, Nkengasong J, Lu L, Finkbeiner T, Fowler MG, Rivadeneira E, Shaffer N. Infant human immunodeficiency virus diagnosis in resource-limited settings: issues, technologies, and country experiences. Am J Obstet Gynecol. 2007;197:S64–71.
10. Stevens W, Sherman G, Downing R, Parsons LM, Ou CY, Crowley S, Gershy-Damet GM, Fransen K, Bulterys M, Lu L, et al. Role of the laboratory in ensuring global access to ARV treatment for HIV-infected children: consensus statement on the performance of laboratory assays for early infant diagnosis. Open AIDS J. 2008;2:17–25.
11. ZMOH. PMTCT 2010 National Protocol Guidelines. Integrated prevention of mother-to-child transmission of HIV. In: Bweupe M, Chitembo L, Maswenyeho S, Murless E, Mwale J, Tambatamba B, Vwalika C, Mbewe R, editors. Zambia: Ministry of Health; 2010. Available at: https://aidsfree.usaid.gov/sites/default/files/tx_zambia_pmtct_2010.pdf.
12. Diallo K, Modi S, Hurlston M, Beard RS, Nkengasong JN. A proposed framework for the implementation of early infant diagnosis point-of-care. AIDS Res Hum Retrovir. 2017;33(3):203–10. doi:10.1089/AID.2016.0021.
13. Penazzato M, Revill P, Prendergast AJ, Collins IJ, Walker S, Elyanu PJ, Sculpher M, Gibb DM. Early infant diagnosis of HIV infection in low-income and middle-income countries: does one size fit all? Lancet Infect Dis. 2014;14:650–5.
14. Simons-Morton BG, Hayne D, Noelcke E. Social Influences: the effects of socialization, selection, and social normative processes on health behavior. In: DiClemente RJ, Crosby RA, Kegler MC, editors. Emerging theories in health promotion practice and research. San Francisco: Wiley; 2009.
15. Albrecht S, Semrau K, Kasonde P, Sinkala M, Kankasa C, Vwalika C, Aldrovandi GM, Thea DM, Kuhn L. Predictors of nonadherence to single-dose nevirapine therapy for the prevention of mother-to-child HIV transmission. J Acquir Immune Defic Syndr. 2006;41:114–8.
16. Aluisio A, Richardson BA, Bosire R, John-Stewart G, Mbori-Ngacha D, Farquhar C. Male antenatal attendance and HIV testing are associated with decreased infant HIV infection and increased HIV-free survival. J Acquir Immune Defic Syndr. 2011;56:76–82.
17. CSO. Zambia Demographic and Health Survey 2013–14. Rockville: Central Statistical Office, Ministry of Health, and ICF International; 2014.
18. Maman S, Mbwambo J, Hogan NM, Kilonzo GP, Sweat M. Women's barriers to HIV-1 testing and disclosure: challenges for HIV-1 voluntary counselling and testing. AIDS Care. 2001;13:595–603.
19. Hatcher AM, Stöckl H, Christofides N, Woollett N, Pallitto CC, Garcia-Moreno C, Turan JM. Mechanisms linking intimate partner violence and prevention of mother-to-child transmission of HIV: a qualitative study in South Africa. Soc Sci Med. 2016;168:130–9.
20. WHO. Putting women first: ethical and safety recommendations for research on domestic violence against women. In: WHO, editor. Department of Gender and Women's Health: Family and Community Health. Geneva: World Health Organization; 2001.
21. Straus MA, Hamby SL, BoneyMcCoy S, Sugarman DB. The revised conflict tactics scales (CTS2)—development and preliminary psychometric data. J Fam Issues. 1996;17:283–316.
22. Hindin MJ, Kishor S, Ansara DL: Intimate partner violence among couples in 10 DHS countries: predictors and health outcomes. In: DHS analytical studies, vol. No. 18. Calverton: Macro International Inc.; 2008.
23. CSO: Zambia Demographic and Health Survey 2007. Calverton, Maryland, USA: Central Statistical Office (CSO), Ministry of Health (MOH), Tropical Diseases Research Centre (TDRC), University of Zambia, & Macro International Inc.; 2009.
24. MacQuarrie KL, Winter R, Kishor S: Spousal violence in Sub-Saharan Africa: structure, forms, and levels. In: Session 177: methodological innovations in intimate partner violence research population association ofamerica annual meeting, May 1-3, Boston, MA; 2014
25. Simoni JM, Kurth AE, Pearson CR, Pantalone DW, Merrill JO, Frick PA. Self-report measures of antiretroviral therapy adherence: a review with recommendations for HIV research and clinical management. AIDS Behav. 2006;10:227–45.
26. van Buuren S, Brand JPL, Groothuis-Oudshoorn CGM, Rubin DB. Fully conditional specification in multivariate imputation. J Stat Comput Simul. 2006;76:1049–64.
27. Raghunathan TE, Lepkowski JM, Hoewyk JV, Solenberger P. A multivariate technique for multiply imputing missing values using a sequence of regression models. Surv Methodol. 2001;27:85–95.
28. StataCorp. Stata 11 multiple-imputation reference manual. College Station: Stata Press; 2009.
29. Filmer D, Pritchett L. Estimating wealth effect without expenditure data or tears: an application to educational enrollments in States of India. Demography. 2001;38:115–32.
30. Kobin AB, Sheth NU. Levels of adherence required for virologic suppression among newer antiretroviral medications. Ann Pharmacother. 2011;45:372–9.
31. Gordon LL, Gharibian D, Chong K, Chun H. Comparison of HIV virologic failure rates between patients with variable adherence to three antiretroviral regimen types. AIDS Patient Care STDS. 2015;29:384–8.
32. Hampanda K. Intimate partner violence and HIV-positive women's non-adherence to antiretroviral medication for the purpose of prevention of mother-to-child transmission in Lusaka, Zambia. Soc Sci Med. 2016;153:123–30.
33. Hatcher AM, Woollett N, Pallitto CC, Mokoatle K, Stockl H, MacPhail C, Delany-Moretlwe S, Garcia-Moreno C. Bidirectional links between HIV and intimate partner violence in pregnancy: implications for prevention of mother-to-child transmission. J Int AIDS Soc. 2014;17:19233.
34. Hampanda K. Intimate Partner violence against HIV-positive women is associated with sub-optimal infant feeding practices in Lusaka, Zambia. Matern Child Health J. 2016;20(12):2599–606.
35. Johnson MP. A typology of domestic violence: intimate terrorism, violent resistance, and situational couple violence. Boston, MA; Hanover, NH: Northeastern University Press; Published by University Press of New England; 2008.
36. Dahl V, Mellhammar L, Bajunirwe F, Bjorkman P. Acceptance of HIV testing among women attending antenatal care in south-western Uganda: risk factors and reasons for test refusal. AIDS Care. 2008;20:746–52.
37. Sarker M, Sanou A, Snow R, Ganame J, Gondos A. Determinants of HIV counselling and testing participation in a prevention of mother-to-child transmission programme in rural Burkina Faso. Trop Med Int Health. 2007;12:1475–83.
38. Msuya SE, Mbizvo EM, Hussain A, Uriyo J, Sam NE, Stray-Pedersen B. Low male partner participation in antenatal HIV counselling and testing in northern Tanzania: implications for preventive programs. AIDS Care. 2008;20:700–9.
39. Kiarie JN, Farquhar C, Richardson BA, Kabura MN, John FN, Nduati RW, John-Stewart GC. Domestic violence and prevention of mother-to-child transmission of HIV-1. AIDS. 2006;20:1763–9.
40. Wettstein C, Mugglin C, Egger M, Blaser N, Salazar L, Estill J, Bender N, Davies MA, Wandeler G, Keiser O. Missed opportunities to prevent mother-to-child-transmission in sub-Saharan Africa: systematic review and meta-analysis. AIDS. 2012;26(18):2361.
41. Auvinen J, Suominen T, Valimaki M. Male participation and prevention of human immunodeficiency virus (HIV) mother-to-child transmission in Africa. Psychol Health Med. 2010;15:288–313.

42. Jasseron C, Mandelbrot L, Dollfus C, Trocme N, Tubiana R, Teglas JP, Faye A, Rouzioux C, Blanche S, Warszawski J. Non-disclosure of a pregnant woman's HIV status to her partner is associated with non-optimal prevention of mother-to-child transmission. AIDS Behav. 2011;17(2):488–97.
43. Spangler SA, Onono M, Bukusi EA, Cohen CR, Turan JM. HIV-positive status disclosure and use of essential PMTCT and maternal health services in rural Kenya. J Acquir Immune Defic Syndr. 2014;67(Suppl 4):S235–42.
44. Donahue MC, Dube Q, Dow A, Umar E, Van Rie A. "They have already thrown away their chicken": barriers affecting participation by HIV-infected women in care and treatment programs for their infants in Blantyre, Malawi. AIDS Care. 2012;24:1233–9.
45. Braitstein P, Songok J, Vreeman RC, Wools-Kaloustian KK, Koskei P, Walusuna L, Ayaya S, Nyandiko W, Yiannoutsos C. "Wamepotea" (they have become lost): outcomes of HIV-positive and HIV-exposed children lost to follow-up from a large HIV treatment program in western Kenya. J Acquir Immune Defic Syndr. 2011;57:e40–6.

7

High level of HIV-1 drug resistance mutations in patients with unsuppressed viral loads in rural northern South Africa

Elizabeth M. Etta[1], Lufuno Mavhandu[1], Cecile Manhaeve[2], Keanan McGonigle[3], Patrick Jackson[3], David Rekosh[1,3], Marie-Louise Hammarskjold[1,3], Pascal O. Bessong[1*] and Denis M. Tebit[1,3*]

Abstract

Background: Combination antiretroviral therapy (cART) has significantly reduced HIV morbidity and mortality in both developed and developing countries. However, the sustainability of cART may be compromised by the emergence of viral drug resistance mutations (DRM) and the cellular persistence of proviruses carrying these DRM. This is potentially a more serious problem in resource limited settings.

Methods: DRM were evaluated in individuals with unsuppressed viral loads after first or multiple lines of cART at two sites in rural Limpopo, South Africa. Seventy-two patients with viral loads of >1000 copies/ml were recruited between March 2014 and December 2015. Complete protease (PR) and partial Reverse Transcriptase (RT) sequences were amplified from both plasma RNA and paired proviral DNA from 35 of these subjects. Amplicons were directly sequenced to determine subtype and DRM using the Stanford HIV Drug Resistance Interpretation algorithm.

Results: Among the 72 samples, 69 could be PCR amplified from RNA and 35 from both RNA and DNA. Sixty-five (94.2%) viruses were subtype C, while one was subtype B (1.4%), one recombinant K/C, one recombinant C/B and one unclassified. Fifty-eight (84%) sequences carried at least one DRM, while 11 (15.9%) displayed no DRM. DRM prevalence according to drug class was: NRTI 60.8% NNRTI 65.2%, and PI 5.8%. The most common DRMs were; M184V (51.7%), K103N (50%), V106M (20.6%), D67N (13.3%), K65R (12%). The frequency of the DRM tracked well with the frequency of use of medications to which the mutations were predicted to confer resistance. Interestingly, a significant number of subjects showed predicted resistance to the newer NNRTIs, etravirine (33%) and rilpivirine (42%), both of which are not yet available in this setting. The proportion of DRM in RNA and DNA were mostly similar with the exception of the thymidine analogue mutations (TAMs) D67N, K70R, K219QE; and K103N which were slightly more prevalent in DNA than RNA. Subjects who had received cART for at least 5 years were more likely to harbour >2 DRM ($p < 0.05$) compared to those treated for a shorter period. DRM were more prevalent in this rural setting compared to a neighbouring urban setting.

Conclusion: We found a very high prevalence of NRTI and NNRTI DRM in patients from rural Limpopo settings with different durations of treatment. The prevalence was significantly higher than those reported in urban settings in South Africa. The dominance of NNRTI based mutations late in treatment supports the use of PI based regimens for second line treatment in this setting. The slight dominance of TAMs in DNA from infected PBMCs compared to plasma

*Correspondence: pascal.bessong@univen.ac.za; dmt6u@virginia.edu
[1] HIV/AIDS & Global Health Research Program, Department of Microbiology, University of Venda, Thohoyandou 0950, South Africa
[3] Department of Microbiology, Immunology and Cancer Biology, Myles H. Thaler Center for AIDS and Human Retrovirus Research, University of Virginia, Charlottesville, VA 22908, USA

virus requires further studies that should include cART subjects with suppressed virus. Such studies will improve our understanding of the pattern of drug resistance and dynamics of viral persistence in these rural settings.

Keywords: HIV drug resistance, Antiretroviral therapy, Peripheral blood mononuclear cells, Plasma, Rural South Africa

Background

HIV drug resistance remains a major threat to the success of scaling up of combination antiretroviral therapy (cART) in developing countries, especially in Africa where about 60% of HIV-infected individuals were on cART in 2012 [1]. The increased availability of cART has led to remarkable treatment results in most programs in sub-Saharan Africa (SSA), leading to a significant reduction of new infections [2]. Despite this success, some patients with incomplete adherence to treatment protocols might fail therapy and develop resistant viruses [3]. One challenge of cART in SSA has been the inability to routinely monitor virological parameters such as viral load (VL) and drug resistance, which are important to guide patient management and choose the right salvage treatments [4, 5]. Recent WHO recommendations stipulate that VL monitoring be utilized as the preferred method to determine treatment failure in SSA [6]. Within the past years, VL monitoring has in fact been successfully implemented as part of care in South Africa [6].

Sequencing is the most accurate method to track the emergence of DRM and is typically done by Sanger sequencing. However, cost and availability of infrastructure to perform these assays still remain major obstacles [7]. As a consequence, most patients failing therapy remain on first-line therapy for long periods causing an accumulation of mutations, which might lead to the emergence of high-level resistance [8, 9]. This is particularly true for patients who started treatment long before VL was more widely available. Samples from such long term cART patients provide a good source to track previous DRM which can be found only in the cellular compartment.

Genotypic drug resistance studies of subjects with unsuppressed VL have been performed in several SSA countries including South Africa and suggest a high level of DRM as well as some subtype specific mutations [10–16]. For example, previous studies among South Africans reported that infections with HIV-1 subtype C may lead to a rapid emergence of certain non-nucleoside reverse transcriptase (NNRTI) or nucleotide reverse transcriptase inhibitor (NRTI) DRM, which are less common among other subtypes. Specifically, V106M (NNRTI), K65R (NRTI) and N348I are more common among subtype C strains compared to other group M strains [17–19].

The South African treatment protocols are consistent with the 2016 WHO guidelines, which recommend a combination of two NRTIs and one NNRTIs as a first-line regimen and two-NRTI and one protease inhibitor (PI) as second line. According to the April 2014 South African revised guidelines, a preferred first-line regimen could be: tenofovir (TDF)/lamivudine (3TC) + efavirenz (EFV)/nevirapine (NVP), or alternatively abacavir (ABC) + 3TC + EFV; or stavudine (d4T) + 3TC + EFV. For second line treatment, TDF + 3TC + lopinavir/ritonavir (LPV/r); or 3TC + AZT + LPV/r could be used.

Despite the benefits of cART, a significant number of patients still experience treatment failure, associated with the development of DRM due to incomplete adherence to therapy or the presence of transmitted DRM [20, 21]. Given the changing treatment strategies and options, genotypic and phenotypic drug resistance patterns will continue to evolve. Although considerable data on virologic failure in patients with unsuppressed VL on first or second line treatment from South Africa are available, these studies have been mostly done in urban settings [15, 22, 23]. On the contrary, rural settings (making up almost 40% of the South African population) still remain largely understudied. Such rural populations often face significant challenges such as distance to treatment sites and access to virological monitoring. In addition, cultural beliefs often increase stigma and could impact adherence and prevalence of DRM [24, 25]. Two recent studies in Uganda and South Africa reported that the intensity of virological monitoring, frequency and pattern of DRM is influenced by the location (urban or rural) of the treatment site [26, 27]. Such results illustrate that inadequate infrastructure and low per capita income common in rural settings might influence the successful implementation of cART. It is therefore imperative that frequent monitoring of DRM is implemented in order to better understand the relationship between drug resistance development and therapy failures in these rural settings.

The use of integrated proviral DNA rather than RNA isolated from circulating virus to monitor HIV drug resistance in patients failing treatment has been considered as an alternative method for drug resistance genotyping [28]. Sequencing of DNA is also an efficient method to study the archived and persistent viral reservoirs in patients with low or suppressed viral loads [29]. With the current focus on HIV persistence, it is important that studies investigating persisting viral populations during suppression are performed to better understand the viral dynamics and alternative future treatment options.

In this study, we describe the drug resistance profile of HIV-1 infected individuals experiencing unsuppressed VL attending two rural HIV treatment centres; the HIV/AIDS Prevention Group Wellness Clinic (HAPG) in Bela-Bela and the Donald Frazer Hope Clinic (DFHC) in Vhufhuli, both located in the Limpopo Province of northern South Africa. Our findings show a high prevalence of NNRTI and NRTI, but low level PI mutations. DRM were more prevalent in this rural setting than reported for a nearby urban setting in Pretoria. Furthermore, by comparing the DRM (NRTI and NNRTI) in viral RNA as well as proviral DNA among circulating viruses in plasma and peripheral blood compartments in 35 subjects, we found that the DRM in these two compartments were mostly similar with a slight dominance of thymidine analogue mutations (TAMs) in DNA, a result that necessitates further studies with a larger cohort.

Methods

Subjects and specimen collection

From July 2013 to December 2015, blood specimens were collected from participating subjects who comprised a random selection of those with unsuppressed viremia at the HIV/AIDS Prevention Group Wellness Clinic (HAPG) in Bela-Bela and the Donald Frazer Hope Clinic (DFHC) in Vhufhuli, in Limpopo Province of rural northern South Africa. All recruited patients met the study criteria of plasma VL > 1000 copies/ml in one of the following ways: (i) two consecutive VL greater than 1000 copies/ml after previous suppression (ii) one VL > 1000 copies/ml after previous suppression followed by a change in treatment (iii) one VL > 1000 copies/ml after 6 months on ART without suppression.

CD4 count, viral load determination and sample processing

VL and $CD4^+$ T cell counts were all performed by the National Health Laboratory Services (NLS) of South Africa. VL were done annually as stipulated by the 2015 South African Treatment Guideline and involved clinic staff usually calling to remind patients of their next VL testing. For drug resistance determination, 5 ml of whole blood was collected from each study participant and transported to the HIV/AIDS and Global Health Research and Training Laboratory at the Department of Microbiology, University of Venda for processing and analyses. On arrival in the laboratory, plasma was separated from cells by centrifuging at 3000 rpm for 5 min and stored at −80 °C in several aliquots. Total cells comprising mostly buffy coats were stored at 4 °C until further processing.

DNA and RNA extractions

Plasma RNA and proviral DNA from total cells were extracted using Qiagen Viral RNA Mini Kit and Qiagen blood DNA Midi Kit (Qiagen, Valencia, CA, USA), respectively, according to the manufacturers' protocols. Extracted DNA and RNA from these samples were then used for PCR and RT-PCR, respectively.

Polymerase chain reaction and sequencing

A fragment of the pol gene approximately 1.5 kb in size (comprising the complete PR and the first 1200 bp of RT) was amplified using a nested PCR protocol described previously [10, 30]. Briefly, cDNA was prepared from viral RNA and used for a nested PCR [30]. Cycling conditions for cDNA and PCRs are available upon request. Amplicons were purified using the Qiaquick PCR purification kit (Qiagen, Valencia, CA, USA) according to the manufacturers' protocol.

Direct population based Sanger sequencing was performed on an ABI 3730XL platform using the ABI Prism® BigDye™ Terminator v3.1 ready reaction sequencing kit (Applied Biosystems, Warrington, UK). The resulting forward and reverse nucleotide sequence electro-pherograms were assembled, manually edited and translated into predicted amino acids with SeqMan Pro II software, version 8.0 (DNASTAR, Lasergene, USA). Primer sequences used for amplification and sequencing are available upon request.

Phylogenetic analysis

Phylogenetic analyses were performed to determine the viral subtypes in relation to reference subtypes from the Los Alamos National Laboratory. Sequence alignment of the gene fragments was performed using MUSCLE in MEGA 6 software [31]. The phylogenetic trees were derived using the Maximum Likelihood Model, which calculates the difference in transition and transversion rates. The reliability of the tree was assessed by bootstrapping of 1000 replicates.

Drug resistance genotyping

For drug resistance genotyping, the newly derived sequences were submitted to the Stanford HIV Drug Resistance Database (http://hivdb.stanford.edu) for examination of drug resistance mutations. Observed predicted DRM were confirmed using the International AIDS Society-USA (IAS) Panel for drug resistance guideline [32]. All sequences associated with high level resistance according to Stanford and IAS algorithms were considered to be resistant.

Statistical analyses

The Wilcoxon rank sum test was used to compare groups. P-value <0.05 was considered to be significant. Correlation between the rural and urban settings was performed using the Pearson Correlation.

Results

Study participants, clinical data and study sites

Subjects for this study comprised patients attending either the HAPG clinic in Bela-Bela or the Donald Fraser Clinic in Vhufhuli, both in the Limpopo Province of northern South Africa. Participation was purely voluntary and included patients who had been on ART for periods ranging from 2 to 10 years. The HAPG in Bela-Bela Clinic currently enrolls almost 1200 patients, while the Donald Fraser Clinic has about 1500 subjects on ART. Sample collection covered a period of 2.5 years; from July 2013 to December 2015. Blood specimens were collected from a total of 72 HIV-1 ART experienced patients who had an unsuppressed viral load >1000 copies/ml (median VL 15,548 copies/ml). The median age of the participants was 37 years (range 5–64), 41 (56.9%) of whom were females (Table 1). The median $CD4^+$ cell count was 293 cells/mm^3. More than 80% of the subjects were classified as CDC (Centers for Disease Control) stage B or C ($CD4^+$ T-cell count less than 500 cells/mm^3). VL and $CD4^+$ cell counts were available for all study participants (Table 1). The most common regimens in use were TDF/FTC/EFV (n = 22; 29.3%), TDF/3TC/EFV (n = 13; 18.1%) and TDF/3TC/LPV/r (n = 9; 12.5%; Table 1).

Table 1 Demographic, clinical and virological characteristics of 72 patients on ART experiencing an unsuppressed viral load

Parameter	Value
Number of patients	72
Female	41 (56.9)
Male	31 (43.1)
Median age (range) in years	37 (5–64)
Median CD4 count (range) in cells/mm^3	293 (6–196)
Median plasma viral load (range) in copies/ml	15,548 (50–73,389)
ART regimen at time of genotyping	
TDF/FTC/EFV	22 (29.3)
TDF/3TC/EFV	13 (18.1)
TDF/3TC/LPV/r	9 (12.5)
ABC/3TC/EFV	7 (9.7)
AZT/3TC/LPV/r	5 (6.9)
TDF/3TC/NVP	3 (4.2)
Others[a]	13 (18.1)
Time on ART (months)	
<24	20 (27.8)
25–60	25 (34.7)
>60	27 (37.5)
Clinical stage (CDC) (%)	
A: >500	14 (19.4)
B: 200–500	36 (50)
C: <200	22 (30.6)
Amplified Genotypes (%)	
Subtype C	65 (94.2)
Subtype B	1 (1.4)
Others (K/C, C/B and unclassified)	3 (4.4)

[a] Other regimen combinations included AZT/DDI/EFV, TDF/DDI/3TC, AZT/DDI/LPV/r, AZT/3TC/EFV, ABC/3TC/LPV/r, AZT/3TC/NVP

HIV genotyping and drug resistance prediction

PR and RT nucleotide sequences were obtained for 69 plasma samples. The majority of these sequences (n = 65; 94.2%) were subtype C while one each (1.4%) of subtype B, recombinant K/C, recombinant C/B and unclassified were also found (Table 1). Using the Stanford Drug Resistance Database algorithm, 11 (15.9%) sequences did not carry any DRM while 58 (84.1%) had at least one PI, NRTI or NNRTI DRM. Based on drug class, the most common DRM were against NRTI 60.8%; NNRTI 65.2%, and PI 5.8%. The most dominant DRM against the reverse transcriptase inhibitors (RTI), were M184V (51.7%), K103N (50%), V106AM (20.6%), G190A (13.8%), D67N (13.8%), K65R (12.1%) and K219Q/E (12.1%; Fig. 1). The Q151M multi-drug resistant mutation was found in one subject while the transitional mutation (Q151L) which precedes the emergence of Q151M was observed in 2 patients. M230L which causes high level resistance to the entire NNRTI class, occurred in a single case (Fig. 1). E138A/K/Q, a mutation related to the NNRTIs etravirine (ETR) and rilpivirine (RPV) was found in 8.6% of subjects, although these drugs are not currently available and not part of the standard treatment regimen in South Africa. Excluding E138A/K/Q among NNRTI mutations reduced the NNRTI resistance prevalence from 65.2 to 62.5%. Among EFV exposed patients, a relatively high prevalence of P225H (12.1%), was found in combination with K103N, confirming previous observations that this mutation rarely occurs independently. Four cases of the H221Y (7%; Fig. 1) DRM were present, always in combination with Y181C. Although H221Y has minimal detectable effect on NNRTI susceptibility, it has been found to frequently occur in combination with Y181C in RPV exposed patients [33]. However, in the present study H221Y was identified only in patients with EFV exposure.

Three subjects carried the accessory mutation A62V that has been reported to be widespread among subtype A viruses from countries of the former Soviet Union [34]. A62V often occurs in combination with multi-resistance NRTI mutations K65R and Q151M. In this study, all the A62V mutations described were linked to K65R, but not

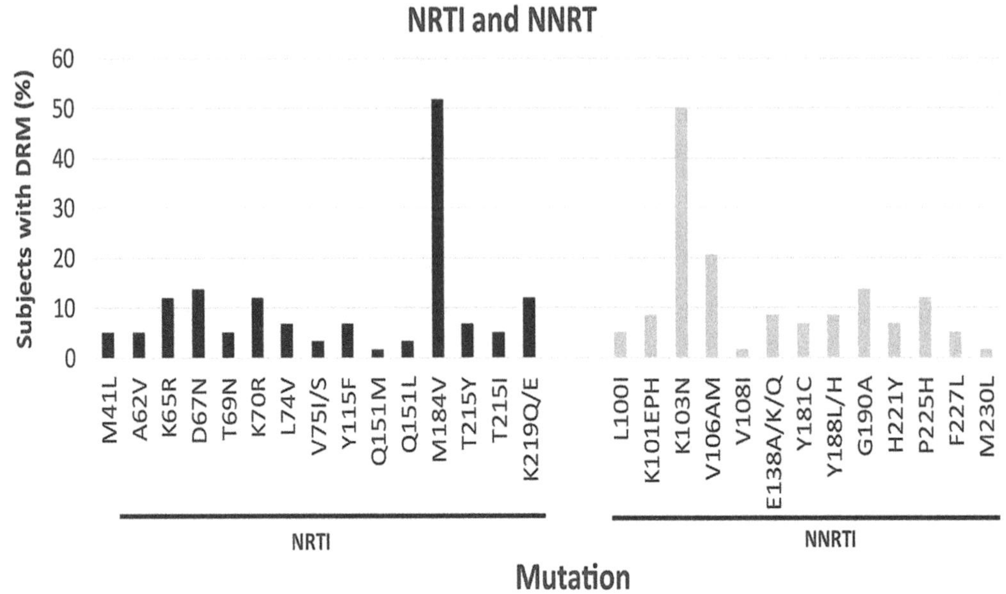

Fig. 1 Prevalence and pattern of HIV drug resistance mutations from two treatment centers in rural Limpopo Province. *NRTI* nucleoside reverse transcriptase inhibitor; *NNRTI* non-nucleoside reverse transcriptase inhibitor

to Q151M [35]. Out of the five patients who carried multiple thymidine analogue mutations (TAMs) only one had the K65R mutation, suggesting that these TAMs likely resulted from previous AZT or d4T treatment and not exposure to TDF. TAMs were dominated by D67N (13.8%), followed by K219Q/E (12.1%) and K70R (12.1%) with a low occurrence of T215Y/F (6.9%). The T215Y/F mutation seem to be subtype specific as it was recently found as the dominant TAM in 33.6% of non-subtype C infected study subjects in five Central African countries [36]. Interestingly, among the viruses with mutations at this position, tyrosine (Y) was the dominant amino acid (6.9%; T215Y) compared to the complete absence of phenylalanine (F) (0%; T215F; Fig. 1). Five percent of viruses carried an isoleucine (I, encoded by ATT, ATC) mutation at position 215 (215I) which resulted from a single nucleotide changing threonine (ACT, ACC) to isoleucine. The 215I mutation seems to be transitional (intermediate) to T215F (phenylalanine-TTT, TTC).

Considering that the history of ART influences circulating DRM, we grouped these DRM using the Stanford Drug Resistance algorithm into high, intermediate and low level resistance mutations and compared them to the antiretroviral drugs that these patients were receiving at the time of testing (Fig. 2). The prevalence of the RTIs administered to patients at the time of this study were in the following order: TDF > EFV > 3TC > FTC > AZT > ABC > NVP > ddI (Fig. 2). Lopinavir boosted ritonavir (LPV/r) was the most commonly used PI 20/69 (29%) of study participants (Table 1). However, when we compared the prevalence of the predicted high and medium level DRM to the drugs in use, the highest level of resistance was to NNRTIs, (NVP and EFV) in accordance with their low barrier to resistance. The rank order of the predicted frequency of resistance to the cART in use were as follows: NVP > EFV > ABC > 3TC > FTC > ddI > d4T > TDF > AZT. It is interesting to note that although TDF was the most frequently used drug, it had one of the lowest number of DRM frequencies (high resistance barrier; Fig. 2). Abacavir (ABC) is a recommended component of the first line therapy provided to children and adolescents who made up 25% of the study participants. A relatively high level (>60%) of ABC DRM was observed among study subjects, clearly higher than the number of subjects on ABC. Some of the ABC resistance could also be attributed to its cross resistance to ddI, which shares a similar DRM pattern. Predicted resistance was highest among patients whose regimen included NVP and EFV, two NNRTIs which are also components of first line treatment. Two (3.0%) subjects harbored major PI DRM (D30N, M46I and V32I). T74S, a minor PR mutation, was detected in 45 (65.2%) of the 69 participants. LPV/r was administered as part of the first line treatment to children and adolescents or as second line to adults.

More than two-thirds of subjects had been on ART for at least 24 months, the majority (62%) of these had been exposed to more than one drug regimen. We therefore assessed the frequency of current NRTI and NNRTI DRM in correlation with the length of time of cART exposure (Fig. 3). Subjects were categorized

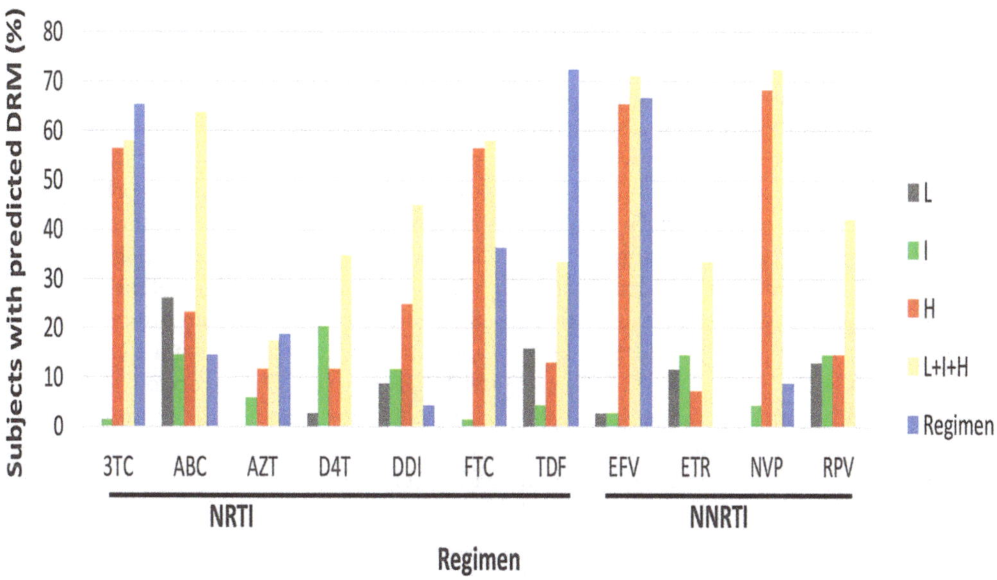

Fig. 2 Prevalence of genotypic drug resistance to various antiretroviral drugs. NRTI, nucleoside reverse transcriptase inhibitor; *NNRTI* non-nucleoside reverse transcriptase inhibitor, *3TC* Lamivudine, *ABC* Abacavir, *AZT* Zidovudine, *d4T* Stavudine, *ddI* didanosine, *FTC*, Emtricitabine, *TDF* Tenofovir, *EFV* Efavirenz, *ETR* Etravirine, *NVP* Nevirapine, *RPV* Rilpivirine, *L* Low, *I* Intermediate, *H* High level resistance

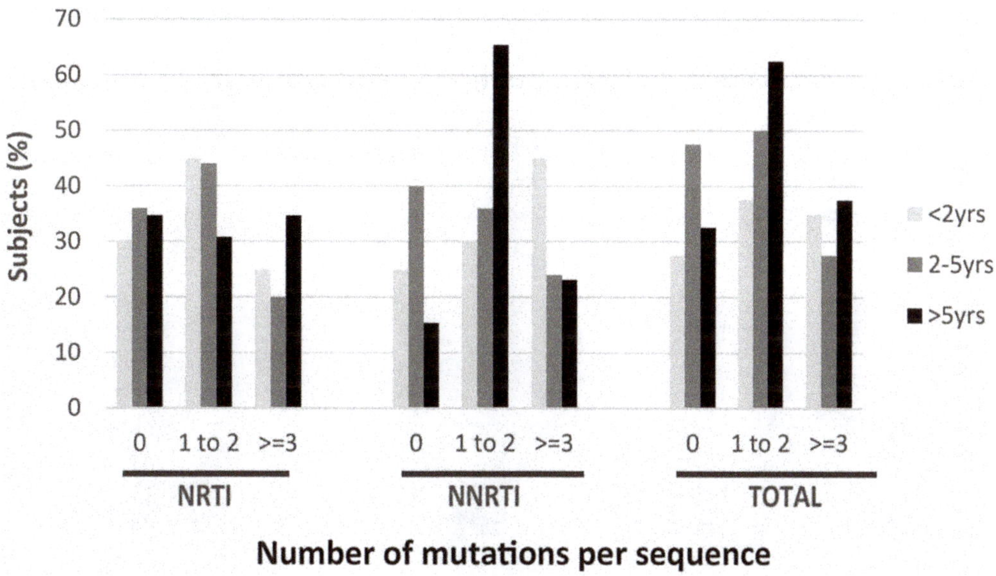

Fig. 3 Comparing the frequency of NRTI versus NNRTI drug resistance mutations over time. *NRTI* nucleoside reverse transcriptase inhibitor, *NNRTI* non-nucleoside reverse transcriptase inhibitor

based on the number of DRM (0, 1–2, and ≤3) and the length of time on cART (<2, 2–5 and >5 years; Fig. 3). The distribution of NRTI DRM was mostly similar over time (<5 years) for subjects harbouring less than 3 mutations (Fig. 3). After 5 years of treatment, the number of subjects carrying >3 NRTI mutations were higher (but not significantly) than those with <2 mutations suggesting an accumulation of DRM overtime. For the NNRTIs, one or two DRM (either K103N, V106M or G190A) were the most common and were more prevalent in subjects that had been on treatment for >5 years ($p < 0.05$; Fig. 3).

Healthcare facilities and living standards differ greatly between urban and rural settings in SSA countries including South Africa. Recently, a higher level of DRM was observed in a rural area of KwaZulu-Natal compared to an urban cohort in Pretoria [26]. As the rural settings of Limpopo and KwaZulu-Natal differ somewhat especially in population density, we compared the DRM data from the Pretoria study to those from our study (Table 2). Twenty NRTI and NNRTI DRM positions were considered and the frequency of these mutations in rural versus urban settings were compared. More than half of these mutations (K65R, D67N, K70R, L74V, V75I/S, Y115F, K219Q/E, K101E/P/H, K103N, V106AM, Y181C and Y188L/H) were significantly more prevalent ($p < 0.05$) in the rural settings of Limpopo than in urban Pretoria (Table 2). The prevalence of these DRM in the two rural sites of Limpopo and KwaZulu-Natal correlated well ($r^2 = 0.93$). Exceptionally, the M184V mutation prevalence in rural Limpopo was more closely related to urban Pretoria (51.7% vs. 53.4%) than rural Kwazulu-Natal (79.8%; Table 2).

In order to assess if integrated proviral DNA can be used to analyze drug resistance in patients failing therapy, we amplified and sequenced the PR and RT genes of 35 subjects from proviral DNA (PBMC). DNA sequences generated were compared to corresponding paired RNA sequences (Fig. 4a, b). Of the 13 different NRTI DRM that were detected by any method in this study, nine DRM were found in the same or greater proportion of the population using the viral RNA assay as compared with the proviral DNA assay (Fig. 4a, b). Interestingly, four DRM were detected in a greater proportion of the population using the DNA assay, of which three were TAMs; namely D67N, K70R and K219Q/R/E (Fig. 4a). A similar observation was made among the NNRTI mutations in which 8/13 of the DRM were found to be either identical to or more prevalent using the viral RNA assay than the proviral DNA assay. The exception was the K103N mutation which was significantly more prevalent ($p < 0.05$) in assays of proviral DNA compared to assays using viral RNA (Fig. 4b).

Discussion

This study was performed among patients failing treatment in two treatment centres in rural South Africa: the HAPG Wellness Clinic which started cART administration in 2000, 4 years before the roll-out of antiretroviral therapy in the public health sector in South Africa; and the Donald Fraser Clinic which started providing treatment in 2004. Although both sites have been

Table 2 Comparison of the NRTI and NNRTI DRM prevalence from Limpopo (rural), KwaZulu-Natal (rural) and urban (Pretoria)

Mutation	Limpopo	Kwazulu-Natal (rural)[a]	Pretoria (urban)[a]	p-value (Limpopo vs. Pretoria)[b]
M41L	5.2	7.1	5.8	1
A62V	5.2	2.6	1	0.89
K65R	12.1	13.1	1.9	*<0.01*
D67N	13.8	16.8	5.8	*0.014*
K70R	12.1	14.3	7.8	*0.039*
L74V	6.9	2.6	1	*0.023*
V75I/S	3.4	3.8	0	0.089
Y115F	6.9	5.3	0	*0.014*
Q151M	1.7	1.8	1.9	0.91
M184V	51.7	79.8	51.7	1
T215Y	6.9	12.5	8.7	0.5
K219Q/E	12.1	13.3	5.8	*<0.01*
L100I	5.2	3	2.9	0.09
K101EPH	8.6	1.8	1	*<0.01*
K103N	50.0	44.5	34	*<0.01*
V106AM	20.7	28.9	34	*<0.01*
V108I	1.7	10.5	3.9	0.17
Y181C	6.9	12.5	11.7	*0.03*
Y188L/H	8.6	10.1	2.9	*0.01*
G190A	13.8	15.8	9.7	0.05

[a] Data obtained from study by Rossouw et al. [26]

[b] The p-values represent significance (in itatlics) of comparisons between the rural sites from this study (Limpopo) and the urban site (Pretoria) from the study by Rossouw et al. [26]

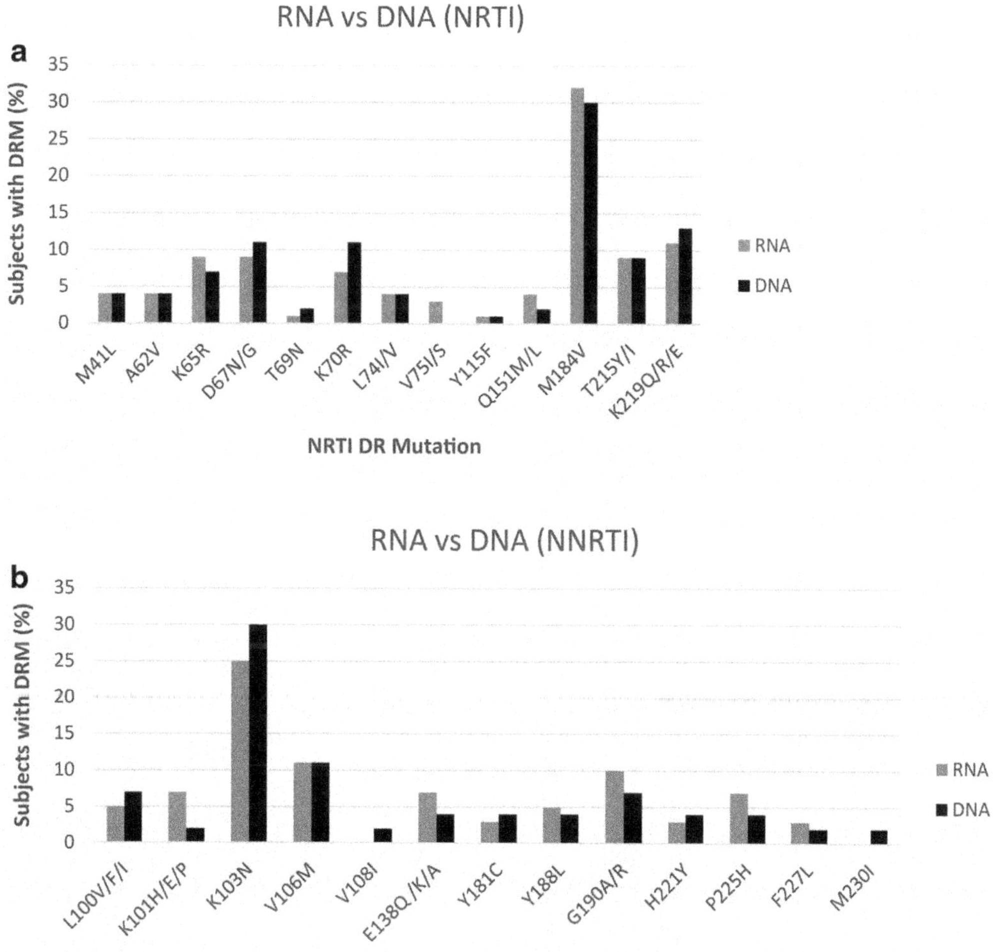

Fig. 4 Comparing the DRM in RNA (plasma) and DNA (peripheral blood mononuclear cells). **a** NRTI. **b** NNRTI

implementing VL and $CD4^+$ T-cell count monitoring, according to national guidelines, and as part of HIV management for several years, the prevalence of DRM was still high. The M184V mutation was the most prevalent DRM, observed in 52% of study subjects. This coincided with the extensive use of 3TC, surpassed only by the use of TDF and EFV in the population. Interestingly, TDF mutations were one of the least common DRM in the study despite its frequent usage, supporting its inclusion as the main backbone during first line treatment.

Although currently used cART is effective for all group M subtypes, the pattern of drug resistance differs between subtypes [10, 36]. Our study confirmed the dominance of K65R and V106M, two mutations which are most common among subtype C strains [36, 37]. In fact, very recently in a cohort of more than 3700 subjects failing cART in several West and Central Africa countries, these two DRM were found to be more prevalent among subtypes C strains compared to CRF02_AG, CRF06cpx, and subtypes A and G [17, 18, 36]. This dominance has been attributed to the genomic sequence of subtype C, which requires only a single nucleotide change at these codon positions to transition to a drug resistant amino acid residue [37]. Similarly, we speculate that the occurrence of the E138A/K/Q mutation could be due to the codon usage of subtype C RT at this position which is GAA versus GAG in other group M strains. In fact, in the Stanford Drug Resistance database, subtype C strains from drug exposed patients have a higher prevalence of the E138A/K/Q mutation compared to other group M strains (8–9.5% vs. 2–5%). Further verification of such subtype-specific differences in the pattern of resistance mutations would clearly be of great significance for treatment management and also for a better understanding of the overall resistance mechanism.

The high occurrence of both K103N and V106M could be a reflection of the wide use of EFV and NVP as part of the first line therapy. In addition, the high levels of

V106M mutations could also be attributed to subtype-specificity, since this mutation had been found most frequently among subtype C [17, 36]. It seems quite clear that NNRTIs should not be used for second line treatment in rural South African populations. This conclusion is supported by the fact that a significant number of the patients we studied already show resistance to newer NNRTIs (ETR and RPV), which have not even been introduced in South Africa.

The selection of TAMs such as D67N, M41L and T215Y could be attributed to treatment with the thymidine analogues AZT and d4T, which also cause cross resistance to other NRTIs [8]. Similarly, patients harbouring TAMs also had high level resistance to NNRTIs (EFV and NVP) and 3TC supporting the point that they were likely failing thymidine containing ART at the point when TDF replaced AZT in the national guidelines [38]. TAMs have been reported to be more common among CRF06cpx strains than other HIV-1 subtypes or CRFs [10, 36]. In this study, there was a noticeable absence among subjects of the L210W and very low occurrence of the M41L DRM, both components of the Type 1 TAMs pathway (M41L, L210W and T215Y). Although, this could likely be related to the reduced usage of d4T, recent reports suggest that compared to other dominant HIV-1 genotypes (subtypes A, CRF02_AG and CRF06cpx), subtype C show the lowest prevalence of M41L DRM [36]. The absence of M41L and L210W was initially reported from a subtype C cohort in Botswana where the most common TAM pathway was D67N, K70R and T215Y [39]. In our study, we observed that the four TAMs (D67N, K70R, T215Y and K219Q/E) which make up the Type 2 TAM pathway, occurred more frequently and correlated well with the usage of AZT. Although we could not state categorically the order of emergence of these mutations as this was a cross sectional study, the mutations D67N and K70R were the most frequent single occurring TAMs. Both AZT and d4T have been reported to cause TAMs at an equal rate [40].

The majority of participants in this study were adults >18 years old. This is not surprising given that treatment of children and adolescents with cART has not been vigorously pursued in SSA until recently. Out of the 13 subjects <18 years old with unsuppressed virus, DRM could be detected in 70% (6 were TAMs and 3 were either NNRTI or other NRTI). DRM has been reported to be highly prevalent among African children with unsuppressed VL [41]. In Uganda and South Africa, DRMs were higher in children from rural compared to urban clinics indicating a better management and/or easier adherence in urban clinics [26, 27]. Due to the low number of children and adolescents in this study, we could not independently confirm this. With the increasing usage of cART in children and adolescents in SSA, more longitudinal studies are required to better understand the pattern of DRM among this group.

The observed high levels of DRM in these rural settings could be linked to several factors. First, the availability of transportation to treatment centers is generally significantly reduced in rural areas compared to urban settings. Secondly, shortage of cART supplies are common occurrences in rural areas. Finally, cultural differences or stigma might affect the open administration of cART especially among women, a phenomenon that is more strongly present in rural areas. Another factor that likely influenced the high rates of DRM in one of the study sites (HAPG) was the inadequate planning and poor follow-up by health authorities. In 2009, at the HAPG privately run facility in Bela-Bela, patients' healthcare providers were switched as patients were transferred from HAPG to a newly opened nearby Public Health Clinic (PHC). Records dating from the beginning of cART therapy at HAPG in 2004 showed good patient follow-up and less treatment failure. However, after the massive patient transfer in 2009 to the PHC and their return to the HAPG private clinic in 2012, the rate of virologic failure increased significantly among returning patients. Despite the high prevalence of DRM observed in this study, the number of patients with detectable VL, but no DRM was similar to previous reports (16% vs. 19–36% respectively) in some urban centres in South Africa [22, 36, 42, 43].

There are few reports on the prevalence and pattern of DRM in rural South Africa [26, 30, 44]. A recent study compared the frequency of DRM from rural KwaZulu-Natal and urban Pretoria, and found a clear difference between these two sites [26]. In our current study, we confirmed the findings of Rossouw et al. Notably, the number of DRMs at the two sites in rural Limpopo were generally higher than in neighboring urban Pretoria (Table 2). Only two DRMs were substantially more common in Pretoria as compared with the Limpopo population. The mutations V106A/M and Y181C were 13.3 and 4.8% more common in Pretoria than in Limpopo, respectively. Both mutations are associated with exposure to NVP [45]. At the time of sequencing, the Pretoria subjects were much more likely to be exposed to NVP than were the subjects in Limpopo (32.4% vs. 5%). Although subjects in these rural settings would be predicted to respond to the ART regimens that are currently in use, we suggest that the WHO recommendation that includes a PI in the second line treatment and close monitoring be strictly observed in order to reduce the transmission of DRM. This recommendation is supported by the very low level of PI DRMs observed in this study.

We compared DRM from both plasma (RNA) and cellular (proviral DNA) compartments from patients experiencing unsuppressed viral load who had received treatment for varying periods, ranging from 1 to 10 years. Plasma is routinely used for drug resistance testing, because viral RNA reflects the current replicating virus in blood. The prevalence of DRM in RNA and DNA was mostly similar with the exception of the TAMs, which were more prevalent in DNA than RNA. The persistence of some TAMs in DNA could be explained by the formerly common administration of NRTI (AZT and d4T) regimens. Of note is the fact that d4T is gradually being phased out and was not included in any of the current treatment regimens received by the study subjects. Three viral RNA and two proviral DNA derived sequences from patients who had never been treated with ddI, ABC, or TDF harboured a K65R mutation.

It is important to point out that our analyses were done using routine population-based Sanger sequencing that does not allow the detection of minority viral variants which comprise less than 20% of the viral population in a patient sample [46, 47]. Recent methods such as next generation sequencing would most likely detect minor drug resistant variants at levels as low as 1% [47, 48]. Considering the fact that undetected drug resistant minority variants may persist when cART is discontinued or changed, it will be worthwhile to perform comparative RNA/DNA drug resistance studies using more sensitive next generation sequencing [47]. Although advances in cART has improved the lives of HIV infected patients, current regimens have failed to eliminate latent reservoirs, and it is acknowledged that eradication of the virus is not possible with current cART regimens alone [49]. Furthermore, the efficacy of switching drugs for patients experiencing a rebound in VL will depend mainly on the number of DRM persisting in the proviral reservoir, following previous therapeutic failures [50, 51].

Overall, these results clearly show that patients receiving cART, but experiencing therapeutic failure, harbour diverse drug-resistant variants, which in some cases persisted in the cellular blood compartment. Detection of this persisting variants can be improved by using more sensitive methods such as next generation sequencing. The proviral variants observed in this study closely resemble the population found in the plasma compartment (viral RNA) with the exception of some persistent TAMs; confirming the known fact that proviral DNA constitutes a reservoir for drug-resistant variants which might replenish plasma pool during suboptimal therapy.

Two limitations should be noted in our investigation: first, this was a cross-sectional study in which data on adherence to treatment was not available; as a result, it was not possible to associate the observed virologic failure to poor adherence. Second, information on prior exposure to NVP in the early days of mother-to-children transmission (MTCT) prevention efforts was also not available. The use of nevirapine monotherapy could have potentially impacted on the observed level of NNRTI mutations particularly K103N.

In conclusion, this study suggests that there is a high level of DRM in rural South Africa and confirms recent observations from KwaZulu-Natal that DRMs are more prevalent in rural than urban areas. It also confirms that long term ART with no virological monitoring could lead to an accumulation of DRMs especially of the NRTI class. Although plasma and PBMCs presented largely identical DRMs, the later compartment may act as an archive of drug resistant variants, especially TAMs, an observation that needs further studies with a larger sample size including subjects with suppressed virus. Such studies could shed more light on the persistence of DRMs and their impact on HIV treatment and cure.

Authors' contributions

DMT, PB, DR and MLH designed the study; EME, CM, LM, KMG were involved in sampling and performing experiments; PJ interpreted the data and participated in writing the manuscript. All authors read and approved the manuscript.

Author details

[1] HIV/AIDS & Global Health Research Program, Department of Microbiology, University of Venda, Thohoyandou 0950, South Africa. [2] Bela-Bela HIV/AIDS Prevention Group Wellness Clinic (HAPG), Bela-Bela, South Africa. [3] Department of Microbiology, Immunology and Cancer Biology, Myles H. Thaler Center for AIDS and Human Retrovirus Research, University of Virginia, Charlottesville, VA 22908, USA.

Acknowledgements

We are grateful to all members of the HIV/AIDS & Global Health Research laboratory, Department of Microbiology, University of Venda for their help with sample processing.

Competing interests

The authors declare that they have no competing interests.

Funding

KMG was supported by a stipend from the Division of Global Health, Department of Infectious Diseases, University of Virginia for a Summer Internship Program at the University of Venda, South Africa. DMT was supported by Funds from the Myles H. Thaler Center for AIDS and Human Retrovirus Research. DMT also received partial support through a Carnegie African Diaspora Fellowship Award. EME was supported by the Research and Publications Committee of the University of Venda. POB received grant support from the South African Medical Research Council and the National Research Foundation (GUN 76684). The contents expressed here do not necessarily represent the views of the South African Medical Research Council or the National Research Foundation.

References

1. WHO U, UNAIDS: Global update on HIV treatment 2013: results, impact and opportunities. 2014.
2. Tanser F, de Oliveira T, Maheu-Giroux M, Barnighausen T. Concentrated HIV subepidemics in generalized epidemic settings. Curr Opin HIV AIDS. 2014;9(2):115–25.
3. Bangsberg DR. Preventing HIV antiretroviral resistance through better monitoring of treatment adherence. J Infect Dis. 2008;197:S272–8.
4. Gupta RK, Jordan MR, Sultan BJ, Hill A, Davis DH, Gregson J, Sawyer AW, Hamers RL, Ndembi N, Pillay D, et al. Global trends in antiretroviral resistance in treatment-naive individuals with HIV after rollout of antiretroviral treatment in resource-limited settings: a global collaborative study and meta-regression analysis. Lancet. 2012;380(9849):1250–8.
5. Richman DD, Margolis DM, Delaney M, Greene WC, Hazuda D, Pomerantz RJ. The challenge of finding a cure for HIV infection. Science. 2009;323(5919):1304–7.
6. Peter T, Ellenberger D, Kim AA, Boeras D, Messele T, Roberts T, Stevens W, Jani I, Abimiku A, Ford N, et al. Early antiretroviral therapy initiation: access and equity of viral load testing for HIV treatment monitoring. Lancet Infect Dis. 2017;17(1):e26–9.
7. Roberts T, Cohn J, Bonner K, Hargreaves S. Scale-up of routine viral load testing in resource-poor settings: current and future implementation challenges. Clin Infect Dis. 2016;62(8):1043–8.
8. Goodall RL, Dunn DT, Nkurunziza P, Mugarura L, Pattery T, Munderi P, Kityo C, Gilks C, Kaleebu P, Pillay D, et al. Rapid accumulation of HIV-1 thymidine analogue mutations and phenotypic impact following prolonged viral failure on zidovudine-based first-line ART in sub-Saharan Africa. J Antimicrob Chemother. 2017;72(5):1450–5.
9. Boender TS, Kityo CM, Boerma RS, Hamers RL, Ondoa P, Wellington M, Siwale M, Nankya I, Kaudha E, Akanmu AS, et al. Accumulation of HIV-1 drug resistance after continued virological failure on first-line ART in adults and children in sub-Saharan Africa. J Antimicrob Chemother. 2016;71(10):2918–27.
10. Tebit DM, Sangare L, Makamtse A, Yameogo S, Somlare H, Bado G, Kouldiaty BG, Sathiandee K, Tiba F, Sanou I, et al. HIV drug resistance pattern among HAART-exposed patients with suboptimal virological response in Ouagadougou, Burkina Faso. J Acquir Immune Defic Syndr. 2008;49(1):17–25.
11. Delaugerre C, Braun J, Charreau I, Delarue S, Nere ML, de Castro N, May T, Marchou B, Simon F, Molina JM, et al. Comparison of resistance mutation patterns in historical plasma HIV RNA genotypes with those in current proviral HIV DNA genotypes among extensively treated patients with suppressed replication. HIV Med. 2012;13(9):517–25.
12. Aghokeng AF, Kouanfack C, Eymard-Duvernay S, Butel C, Edoul GE, Laurent C, Koulla-Shiro S, Delaporte E, Mpoudi-Ngole E, Peeters M. Virological outcome and patterns of HIV-1 drug resistance in patients with 36 months' antiretroviral therapy experience in Cameroon. J Int AIDS Soc. 2013;16:18004.
13. Dolling DI, Dunn DT, Geretti AM, Sabin CA, Database UHDR. Study UKCHC: HIV-1 subtype and virological response to antiretroviral therapy: a confirmatory analysis. Clin Infect Dis. 2013;56(1):162–3.
14. El-Khatib Z, Delong AK, Katzenstein D, Ekstrom AM, Ledwaba J, Mohapi L, Laher F, Petzold M, Morris L, Kantor R. Drug resistance patterns and virus re-suppression among HIV-1 subtype C infected patients receiving non-nucleoside reverse transcriptase inhibitors in South Africa. J AIDS Clin Res. 2011;2(117). doi:10.4172/2155-6113.1000117
15. Wallis CL, Aga E, Ribaudo H, Saravanan S, Norton M, Stevens W, Kumarasamy N, Bartlett J, Katzenstein D. Drug susceptibility and resistance mutations after first-line failure in resource limited settings. Clin Infect Dis. 2014;59(5):706–15.
16. TenoRes Study G. Global epidemiology of drug resistance after failure of WHO recommended first-line regimens for adult HIV-1 infection: a multicentre retrospective cohort study. Lancet Infect Dis. 2016;16(5):565–75.
17. Brenner B, Turner D, Oliveira M, Moisi D, Detorio M, Carobene M, Marlink RG, Schapiro J, Roger M, Wainberg MA. A V106M mutation in HIV-1 clade C viruses exposed to efavirenz confers cross-resistance to non-nucleoside reverse transcriptase inhibitors. AIDS. 2003;17(1):F1–5.
18. Li JZ, Paredes R, Ribaudo HJ, Kozal MJ, Svarovskaia ES, Johnson JA, Geretti AM, Metzner KJ, Jakobsen MR, Hullsiek KH, et al. Impact of minority nonnucleoside reverse transcriptase inhibitor resistance mutations on resistance genotype after virologic failure. J Infect Dis. 2013;207(6):893–7.
19. Brehm JH, Koontz DL, Wallis CL, Shutt KA, Sanne I, Wood R, McIntyre JA, Stevens WS, Sluis-Cremer N, Mellors JW, et al. Frequent emergence of N348I in HIV-1 subtype C reverse transcriptase with failure of initial therapy reduces susceptibility to reverse-transcriptase inhibitors. Clin Infect Dis. 2012;55(5):737–45.
20. Nachega JB, Hislop M, Nguyen H, Dowdy DW, Chaisson RE, Regensberg L, Cotton M, Maartens G. Antiretroviral therapy adherence, virologic and immunologic outcomes in adolescents compared with adults in southern Africa. J Acquir Immune Defic Syndr 1999. 2009;51(1):65–71.
21. Tang MW, Shafer RW. HIV-1 antiretroviral resistance: scientific principles and clinical applications. Drugs. 2012;72(9):e1–25.
22. Orrell C, Walensky RP, Losina E, Pitt J, Freedberg KA, Wood R. HIV type-1 clade C resistance genotypes in treatment-naive patients and after first virological failure in a large community antiretroviral therapy programme. Antivir Ther. 2009;14(4):523–31.
23. Hoffmann CJ, Charalambous S, Sim J, Ledwaba J, Schwikkard G, Chaisson RE, Fielding KL, Churchyard GJ, Morris L, Grant AD. Viremia, resuppression, and time to resistance in human immunodeficiency virus (HIV) subtype C during first-line antiretroviral therapy in South Africa. Clin Infect Dis. 2009;49(12):1928–35.
24. Heckman TG, Somlai AM, Peters J, Walker J, Otto-Salaj L, Galdabini CA, Kelly JA. Barriers to care among persons living with HIV/AIDS in urban and rural areas. AIDS Care. 1998;10(3):365–75.
25. Wilson DP, Kahn J, Blower SM. Predicting the epidemiological impact of antiretroviral allocation strategies in KwaZulu-Natal: the effect of the urban–rural divide. Proc Natl Acad Sci USA. 2006;103(38):14228–33.
26. Rossouw TM, Nieuwoudt M, Manasa J, Malherbe G, Lessells RJ, Pillay S, Danaviah S, Mahasha P, van Dyk G, de Oliveira T. HIV drug resistance levels in adults failing first-line antiretroviral therapy in an urban and a rural setting in South Africa. HIV Med. 2017;18(2):104–14.
27. Musiime V, Kayiwa J, Kiconco M, Tamale W, Alima H, Mugerwa H, Abwola M, Apilli E, Ahimbisibwe F, Kizito H, et al. Response to antiretroviral therapy of HIV type 1-infected children in urban and rural settings of Uganda. AIDS Res Hum Retrovir. 2012;28(12):1647–57.
28. Kabamba-Mukadi B, Duquenne A, Henrivaux P, Musuamba F, Ruelle J, Yombi JC, Bodeus M, Vandercam B, Goubau P. HIV-1 proviral resistance mutations: usefulness in clinical practice. HIV Med. 2010;11(8):483–92.
29. Gallien S, Charreau I, Nere ML, Mahjoub N, Simon F, de Castro N, Aboulker JP, Molina JM, Delaugerre C. Archived HIV-1 DNA resistance mutations to rilpivirine and etravirine in successfully treated HIV-1-infected individuals pre-exposed to efavirenz or nevirapine. J Antimicrob Chemother. 2015;70(2):562–5.
30. Bessong PO, Mphahlele J, Choge IA, Obi LC, Morris L, Hammarskjold ML, Rekosh DM. Resistance mutational analysis of HIV type 1 subtype C among rural South African drug-naive patients prior to large-scale availability of antiretrovirals. AIDS Res Hum Retrovir. 2006;22(12):1306–12.
31. Tamura K, Stecher G, Peterson D, Filipski A, Kumar S. MEGA6: molecular evolutionary genetics analysis version 6.0. Mol Biol Evol. 2013;30(12):2725–9.
32. Thompson MA, Aberg JA, Hoy JF, Telenti A, Benson C, Cahn P, Eron JJ, Gunthard HF, Hammer SM, Reiss P, et al. Antiretroviral treatment of adult HIV infection: 2012 recommendations of the International Antiviral Society-USA panel. JAMA. 2012;308(4):387–402.
33. Rimsky L, Vingerhoets J, Van Eygen V, Eron J, Clotet B, Hoogstoel A, Boven K, Picchio G. Genotypic and phenotypic characterization of HIV-1 isolates obtained from patients on rilpivirine therapy experiencing virologic failure in the phase 3 ECHO and THRIVE studies: 48-week analysis. J Acquir Immune Defic Syndr (1999). 2012;59(1):39–46.
34. Kolomeets AN, Varghese V, Lemey P, Bobkova MR, Shafer RW. A uniquely prevalent nonnucleoside reverse transcriptase inhibitor resistance mutation in Russian subtype A HIV-1 viruses. AIDS. 2014;28(17):F1–8.
35. Rhee SY, Varghese V, Holmes SP, Van Zyl GU, Steegen K, Boyd MA, Cooper DA, Nsanzimana S, Saravanan S, Charpentier C, et al. Mutational correlates of virological failure in individuals receiving a WHO-recommended tenofovir-containing first-line regimen: an international collaboration. EBioMedicine. 2017;18:225–35.
36. Villabona-Arenas CJ, Vidal N, Guichet E, Serrano L, Delaporte E, Gascuel O, Peeters M. In-depth analysis of HIV-1 drug resistance mutations in HIV-infected individuals failing first-line regimens in West and Central Africa. AIDS. 2016;30(17):2577–89.
37. Brenner BG, Oliveira M, Doualla-Bell F, Moisi DD, Ntemgwa M, Frankel F, Essex M, Wainberg MA. HIV-1 subtype C viruses rapidly develop K65R resistance to tenofovir in cell culture. AIDS. 2006;20(9):F9–13.

38. Gregson J, Kaleebu P, Marconi VC, van Vuuren C, Ndembi N, Hamers RL, Kanki P, Hoffmann CJ, Lockman S, Pillay D, et al. Occult HIV-1 drug resistance to thymidine analogues following failure of first-line tenofovir combined with a cytosine analogue and nevirapine or efavirenz in sub Saharan Africa: a retrospective multi-centre cohort study. Lancet Infect Dis. 2017;17(3):296–304.
39. Novitsky V, Wester CW, DeGruttola V, Bussmann H, Gaseitsiwe S, Thomas A, Moyo S, Musonda R, Van WE, Marlink RG, et al. The reverse transcriptase 67N 70R 215Y genotype is the predominant TAM pathway associated with virologic failure among HIV type 1C-infected adults treated with ZDV/ddI-containing HAART in southern Africa. AIDS Res Hum Retrovir. 2007;23(7):868–78.
40. Sarmati L, Nicastri E, Parisi SG, D'Ettorre G, Narciso P, Mancino G, Gallo I, Abbadessa V, Dalle NE, Traina C, et al. Failure of stavudine–lamivudine combination therapy in antiretroviral-naive patients with AZT-like HIV-1 resistance mutations. J Med Virol. 2001;65(4):631–6.
41. Boerma RS, Sigaloff KC, Akanmu AS, Inzaule S, van Boele Hensbroek M, de Rinke Wit TF, Calis JC. Alarming increase in pretreatment HIV drug resistance in children living in sub-Saharan Africa: a systematic review and meta-analysis. J Antimicrob Chemother. 2017;72(2):365–71.
42. Wallis CL, Papathanasopolous MA, Fox M, Conradie F, Ive P, Orrell C, Zeinecker J, Sanne I, Wood R, McIntyre J, et al. Low rates of nucleoside reverse transcriptase inhibitor resistance in a well-monitored cohort in South Africa on antiretroviral therapy. Antivir Ther. 2012;17(2):313–20.
43. Hamers RL, Sigaloff KC, Kityo C, Mugyenyi P, de Wit TF. HIV-1 drug resistance in antiretroviral-naive patients in sub-Saharan Africa. Lancet Infect Dis. 2013;13(3):196–7.
44. Hamers RL, Derdelinckx I, van VM, Stevens W, de Wit TFR, Schuurman R. The status of HIV-1 resistance to antiretroviral drugs in sub-Saharan Africa. Antivir Ther. 2008;13(5):625–39 **[Erratum in: Antivir Ther. 2008;13(8):1129]**.
45. Rhee SY, Gonzales MJ, Kantor R, Betts BJ, Ravela J, Shafer RW. Human immunodeficiency virus reverse transcriptase and protease sequence database. Nucleic Acids Res. 2003;31(1):298–303.
46. Gibson RM, Meyer AM, Winner D, Archer J, Feyertag F, Ruiz-Mateos E, Leal M, Robertson DL, Schmotzer CL, Quinones-Mateu ME. Sensitive deep-sequencing-based HIV-1 genotyping assay to simultaneously determine susceptibility to protease, reverse transcriptase, integrase, and maturation inhibitors, as well as HIV-1 coreceptor tropism. Antimicrob Agents Chemother. 2014;58(4):2167–85.
47. Kyeyune F, Gibson RM, Nankya I, Venner C, Metha S, Akao J, Ndashimye E, Kityo CM, Salata RA, Mugyenyi P, et al. Low frequency drug resistance in HIV-infected Ugandans on antiretroviral treatment is associated with regimen failure. Antimicrob Agents Chemother. 2016;60(6):3380–97.
48. Palmer S, Boltz V, Martinson N, Maldarelli F, Gray G, McIntyre J, Mellors J, Morris L, Coffin J. Persistence of nevirapine-resistant HIV-1 in women after single-dose nevirapine therapy for prevention of maternal-to-fetal HIV-1 transmission. Proc Natl Acad Sci USA. 2006;103(18):7094–9.
49. Kimata JT, Rice AP, Wang J. Challenges and strategies for the eradication of the HIV reservoir. Curr Opin Immunol. 2016;42:65–70.
50. Devereux HL, Loveday C, Youle M, Sabin CA, Burke A, Johnson MA. Reduction in human immunodeficiency virus type 1 mutations associated with drug resistance after initiating new therapeutic regimens in pretreated patients. J Infect Dis. 2000;181(5):1804–7.
51. Turriziani O, Boni A, Falasca F, Graziano F, Bucci M, D'Ettorre G, Fantauzzi A, Paoletti F, Massetti AP, Mezzaroma I, et al. Mutational resistance pattern of HIV type 1 in $CD14^{+}$ monocytes, $CD4^{+}$ T cells, and plasma from treated patients. AIDS Res Hum Retrovir. 2010;26(6):625–34.

8

COHORT PROFILE: The Complications of Long-Term Antiretroviral Therapy study in Uganda (CoLTART)

Billy Nsubuga Mayanja[1*], Ivan Kasamba[1,2], Jonathan Levin[1], Ivan Namakoola[1], Patrick Kazooba[1], Jackson Were[1], Pontiano Kaleebu[1,3], Paula Munderi[1] and on behalf of the CoLTART study team

Abstract

Background: Antiretroviral therapy (ART) improves the survival and quality of life of HIV-positive individuals, but the effects of long-term ART use do eventually manifest. The Complications of Long-Term Antiretroviral Therapy cohort study in Uganda (CoLTART) was established to investigate the metabolic and renal complications of long-term ART use among Ugandan adults. We describe the CoLTART study set-up, aims, objectives, study methods, and also report some preliminary cross–sectional study enrolment metabolic and renal complications data analysis results.

Methods: HIV-positive ART naïve and experienced adults (18 years and above) in Uganda were enrolled. Data on demographic, dietary, medical, social economic and behaviour was obtained; and biophysical measurements and a clinical examination were undertaken. We measured: fasting glucose and lipid profiles, renal and liver function tests, full blood counts, immunology, virology and HIV drug resistance testing. Plasma samples were stored for future studies.

Results: Between July 2013 and October 2014, we enrolled 1095 individuals, of whom 964 (88.0%) were ART experienced (6 months or more), with a median of 9.4 years (IQR 7.0–9.9) on ART. Overall, 968 (88.4%) were aged 35 years and above, 711 (64.9%) were females, 608 (59.6%) were or had ever been on a Tenofovir ART regimen and 236 (23.1%) on a Protease Inhibitor (PI) regimen. There were no differences in renal dysfunction between patients on Tenofovir and Non-Tenofovir containing ART regimens. Patients on PI regimens had higher total cholesterol, lower high density lipoprotein, higher low density lipoprotein, higher triglycerides, and a high atherogenic index for plasma than the non-PI regimen, $p = 0.001$ or < 0.001. Patients on Non-PI regimens had higher mean diastolic hypertension than patients on PI regimens, $p < 0.001$.

Conclusions: Our finding of no differences in renal dysfunction between patients on Tenofovir and those on Non-Tenofovir containing ART regimens means that Tenofovir based first line ART can safely be initiated even in settings without routine renal function monitoring. However, integration of cardiovascular risk assessment, preventive and curative measures against cardiovascular disease are required. The CoLTART cohort is a good platform to investigate the complications of long-term ART use in Uganda.

Keywords: Cohort profile, Antiretroviral therapy, Metabolic abnormalities, Renal complications, HIV, Uganda

*Correspondence: billy.mayanja@mrcuganda.org; billymayanja@yahoo.com
[1] MRC/UVRI Uganda Research Unit on AIDS, P.O. Box 49, Entebbe, Uganda
Full list of author information is available at the end of the article

Background

Since the Universal roll-out of antiretroviral therapy (ART) in 2004, access to and availability of ART has improved. By June 2016, globally 18.2 million HIV-positive people were receiving ART, up from 15.8 million in June 2015 and 7.5 million in 2010 [1]. In Uganda, 750,896 (50%) HIV-positive people were receiving ART by December 2014 [2]. Although in industrialised countries ART has been used for over 20 years, in sub-Sahara, ART availability in public health facilities only began around 2004. In Uganda, reports suggest that the prevalence of non-infectious diseases like diabetes mellitus, and cardiovascular morbidity and mortality are increasing [3, 4].

Long-term ART use is associated with metabolic, cardiovascular, hepatic, renal, bone, bone marrow and other complications or toxicities [5–9]. These complications of ART are variably associated with all major classes of ARVs. The three most common metabolic abnormalities that are related to ART are dyslipidaemia, lipodystrophy and dysregulation of glucose metabolism [5–9]. Renal impairment among HIV-positive individuals may be due to HIV associated nephropathy, co-infections and co-morbidities, or renal toxicity from ART and concurrent medications [10, 11]. Due to its cost, in resource limited settings Tenofovir had been reserved for use with Protease inhibitors in second line ART regimens. The WHO recommendation to use Tenofovir in first line ART regimens has been widely adopted by ART programmes in Africa including Uganda, Kenya and Tanzania [12–15]. However, Tenofovir is often associated with renal toxicity, manifesting as a decline in estimated glomerular filtration rate (eGFR), proximal renal tubular dysfunction and acute renal failure especially among patients with risk factors for kidney disease [16–23]. It has been suggested, that patients of African origin are at higher risk for HIV associated kidney disease [24], a suggestion that remains to be clarified by studies conducted in Africa. Therefore, for long-term HIV care in Africa, health workers need research-based evidence on renal function beyond 5 years of Tenofovir containing ART, and how these patients should be monitored.

In sub-Saharan Africa, there is scarce literature on the long-term impact of ARVs toxicities among African populations. Current ART guidelines in sub-Saharan Africa are therefore based on evidence from industrialised country settings. However, there are differences between industrialised countries and sub-Saharan Africa in terms of patient profiles, background risk factors for co-infections, co-morbidities, ART regimen choices and drug toxicities. In 2013, the Complications of Long-Term Antiretroviral Therapy (CoLTART) cohort was therefore established by the MRC/UVRI Uganda Research Unit on AIDS (MRC/UVRI Uganda Unit) as a platform for studying the complications of long-term ART among Ugandan HIV-positive adults. The study aimed at examining the metabolic and renal complications of long-term ART use among Ugandan HIV-positive adults aged 18 years and above. In this paper, we describe the CoLTART study set-up, aims, objectives, study methods, and also report some preliminary cross-sectional study enrolment renal and metabolic complications data analysis results.

Methods

The CoLTART study design and settings

The CoLTART study was a prospective clinical cohort conducted at two study clinics; (a) the former Development of Antiretroviral therapy in Africa (DART) Trial study clinic in Entebbe [25], and (b) the former Rural Clinical Cohort (RCC) study clinic in Kyamulibwa, approximately 120 kilometres from Entebbe [26]. The MRC/UVRI Uganda Unit's Head offices and central Clinical Diagnostic Laboratory Services (CDLS) are located in Entebbe.

CoLTART study aims and objectives

The CoLTART study aims were to study the metabolic and renal complications of long-term ART, and the long-term treatment outcomes of a triple nucleoside first ART regimen. The primary objectives were to compare the: (a) mean values for cardio-metabolic markers among patients on a Protease Inhibitor (PI)-containing ART regimen and those on a non PI-containing regimen. (b) Mean values of proximal renal tubular function and eGFR among patients on a Tenofovir (TDF) containing regimen and those on a non-TDF containing regimen.

CoLTART study participants

Between July 2013 and October 2014, CoLTART study participants (Fig. 1) who were HIV-positive adults (aged 18 and above) on ART were recruited from; (a) the former DART Trial Cohort, which was a randomised clinical trial of monitoring strategy for the management of ART in adults with HIV infection in Africa established in 2003 [25]. (b) The former RCC which was an open clinical cohort established in 1990 to study the natural history of HIV infection [26] and later the impact of ART after its introduction in 2004 [27–30]. ART naïve HIV-positive study participants, but who were eligible to initiate ART were enrolled from: (a) the RCC, (b) the General Population Cohort that was established in 1989 in rural southwest Uganda to examine the dynamics of the HIV epidemic [31] and (c) the Entebbe Pre-ART cohort that was established in 1995 as a double blind, randomised and placebo controlled trial of a 23-valent pneumococcal polysaccharide vaccine in HIV-positive adult Ugandans

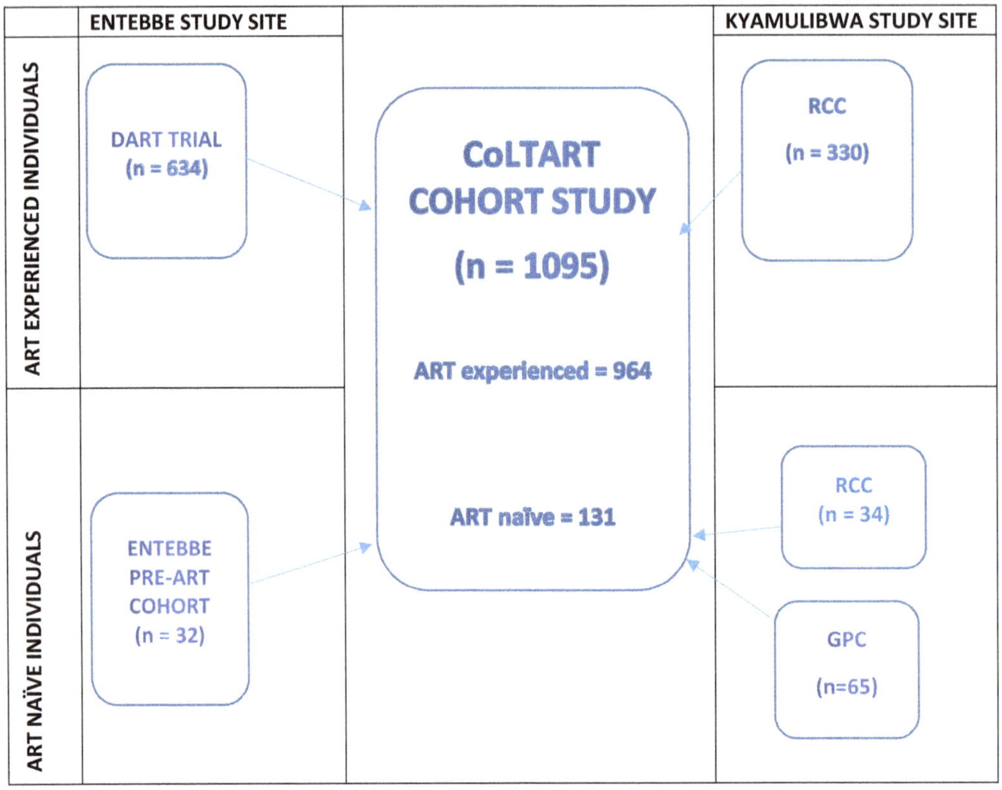

Fig. 1 Sources of enrolled CoLTART cohort study participants

[32]. ART was provided according to existing National ART guidelines [13, 33]. The study included HIV-positive adults (aged 18 years and above), who were on ART or eligible to initiate ART, not participating in another study, who were willing to undergo regular clinical, biophysical and laboratory evaluation and to complete a study questionnaire. Individuals who were too sick to undergo study procedures, unable or unwilling to give informed consent were excluded from the study.

Participants' enrolment and follow-up

Consenting eligible individuals were enrolled, and requested to fast from midnight of the day prior enrolment, and they received a drink and snack after the blood draw and biophysical measurements. We measured the body weight using the Seca digital measuring scale, height using a portable Seca 213 Leicester stadiometer and body circumferences using a non-stretchable Seca 201 Ergonomic Circumference Measuring tape (Table 1). Details of the methods for taking biophysical measurements and calibrating the equipment used have been described elsewhere [34]. Blood pressure and pulse rate were measured using the Omron M6 comfort automatic blood pressure monitor. At enrolment and six monthly follow-up visits, a modified WHO STEPS cardiovascular risk data surveillance questionnaire was administered to collect the relevant data [35]. Every three months, participants renewed their prescriptions for ART and/or cotrimoxazole or Dapsone prophylaxis and adherence data was collected using self-report and pill count. Every 6 months (Table 1), participants attended for scheduled follow-up visits, and they fasted as done at enrolment, and the data collected were recorded on a follow-up questionnaire and clinical examination form. At these 6 monthly visits, participants also renewed their medicines prescriptions and adherence data was collected. Participants who fell sick in between the scheduled visits attended the study clinics to receive medical care.

Laboratory procedures

Specimen collection and storage

At enrolment and follow-up visits, about 10–15 ml of venous blood were collected in three tubes as follows: (a) 4 ml of whole blood in an EDTA tube for haematology, immunology and viral loads measurements. (b) 5 ml plain serum tube blood to measure fasting serum lipids; renal and liver function tests. (c) 4 ml Sodium fluoride tube blood to measure fasting blood glucose. At enrolment only, serum for hepatitis B serology and two aliquots of plasma were stored at −80 °C for future testing.

Table 1 Measurements and data collected in the CoLTART cohort

Phase	Data collected at enrolment
Baseline	Demographic data and self-reported social economic status
July 2013	Medical, dietary and socio-economic and behavioural risk factors
	Biophysical measurements: weight, height, blood pressure, pulse rate; waist, hip and mid-upper arm circumferences
	Clinical examination
	Antiretroviral therapy and cotrimoxazole/dapsone adherence
	Laboratory measurements data
	Biochemistry
	(i) Fasting blood lipid profiles: total cholesterol, triglycerides, low density lipoproteins, high density lipoproteins
	(ii) Fasting blood glucose
	(iii) Renal function tests: urine strip testing, phosphates and creatinine
	Serum phosphates, creatinine and urea
	(vi) Liver function tests: alanine transaminase, aspartate transaminase, alkaline phosphatase and bilirubin
	Haematology and immunology
	(i) Full blood counts
	(ii) CD3, CD4 and CD8 cell counts
	Virology
	(i) HIV viral loads
	(ii) HIV drug resistance testing—when indicated
	Serology (for future testing)
	Serum for Hepatitis B virus serology and plasma aliquots stored at −80 °C
6 monthly	*Data collected at follow up*
Follow-up	Biophysical measurements
January 2014	Medical, dietary and socio-economic and behavioural risk factors
	Clinical examination
	Antiretroviral therapy and cotrimoxazole/dapsone adherence
	Laboratory measurements
	Fasting blood glucose and lipid profiles
	Renal and liver function tests
	Full blood counts and immunology—CD3, CD4 and CD8
	HIV viral loads
	HIV drug resistance testing—when indicated
	Whole blood for genomics studies stored at −80 °C (once)

Blood tubes were labelled with a unique individual study and laboratory number and transferred under appropriate conditions to the CDLS laboratory for analysis. At one follow-up visit, a 4 ml of whole blood sample in an EDTA tube was stored at −80 °C for future genomics testing. Participants with viral loads of 1000 copies/ml or higher had antiretroviral drug resistance testing done. Participants (excluding women in their menses) provided a fresh midstream urine specimen in a plain sterile container, that was later portioned in two plastic centrifuge tubes (one plain for urine creatinine and the other acidified for urine phosphates measurements), and a dipstick strip test was done on the urine remaining in the container.

Laboratory testing

All samples were analysed in the MRC/UVRI Uganda Unit's CDLS laboratories. The Clinical chemistry analyser, COBAS Integra 400 *plus* (Roche Diagnostics) was used to measure fasting serum lipids and blood glucose, and renal and liver function test parameters. Full blood counts were measured using the Coulter AcT5 Diff CP Analyser (Beckman Coulter, USA). CD4 cell counts were measured using either the FACSCount or FACSCalibur machine (Becton–Dickinson, USA). Plasma HIV-1 RNA was quantified using the COBAS Ampliprep/Taqman V2.0 HIV-1 viral load assay (Roche Molecular Diagnostics [RMD], NJ, USA) with a lower detection limit of 20 copies/ml. For urine strip testing, we used the Siemens Multistix 10SG and read with Clinitek Status Analyzer (Siemens Healthcare Diagnostics). For ARV drug resistance, PCR and sequencing reactions were conducted and the sequences submitted to the Stanford University HIV Drug Resistance database. The surveillance drug resistance mutations were identified using the 2009 WHO list for surveillance of transmitted drug resistances [36], using the Stanford calibrated population resistance analysis tool version 5.0 beta [37]. Sequences with genetic mixtures of wild-type and mutant sequences at amino acid sites that code for SDRMs were considered to be drug-resistant.

Laboratory data quality assurance

Standard operating procedures and internal quality measurements ensured internal quality control. The United Kingdom National External Quality Assurance Service, College of American Pathologists and the Royal College of Pathologists of Australasia were used for

External quality Assurance for both haematological and biochemistry assays. Virology Quality Assurance Scheme (Rush University, Chicago, IL) was used for External Quality Assurance for virological assays.

Data management and statistical methods

Data was collected on the case report forms which together with the Laboratory result forms were sorted, batched and submitted to the Statistics section for data entry. Data was managed in accordance with the ICH-GCP data management principles using a single Ms. Access study database using common identifiers to incorporate relevant retrospective data from the DART Trial Cohort and RCC databases. All the data was backed up on a central Unit server with a password restricted access. Enrolment statistical analyses were done in STATA 13 (Stata Corporation, College Station, USA). Participants' socio-demographic and economic characteristics, lifestyle and anthropometric as well as clinical, history of diseases and ART exposure were examined across study sites and by sex. Renal function outcomes were determined using measured renal function tests, and calculated Fractional Tubular reabsorption of phosphates and estimated glomerular filtration rate (eGFR). Different formulae were used to calculate eGFR; (a) the Cockcroft-Gault formulae with and without body surface area adjustment, (b) the Modified Diet in Renal Disease formulae with race adjustment and (c) the Chronic Kidney Disease Epidemiology.

Abnormal renal function outcomes were defined as: serum urea of more than 11.9 mmol/l, serum creatinine of more than 109 μmol/l, Fractional Tubular phosphates reabsorption of less than 82% and eGFR less than 60 ml/min/1.73 m^2, Diabetis mellitus as a measured fasting blood glucose more than or equal to 6.4 mmol/l or history of and or being on medications for diabetis mellitus. Hypertension was a measured systolic blood pressure (SBP) of more than or equal to 140 mmHg or diastolic blood pressure (DBP) more than or equal to 90 mmHg or any history of and or being on medications for hypertension. The renal function outcomes were compared across the Tenofovir exposure groups: (i) non-Tenofovir containing ART regimen (Non-TDF), (ii) Tenofovir containing ART regimen (TDF-ART) and (iii) previously on Tenofovir containing ART regimen but stopped (TDF-stopped). Mean values of renal function outcomes were compared by Tenofovir exposure using general linear models. General linear regression models adjusted for several factors were used to compare mean values of renal function outcomes across groups of Tenofovir exposure categories. The mean values of SBP, DBP, total serum cholesterol, high density lipoprotein, low density lipoprotein, triglyceride, atherogenic index of plasma and fasting blood glucose and Framingham risk score were compared between PI-based and non-PI based ART regimens using general linear regression models, adjusted for duration on ART and other factors.

Results

Between July 2013 and October 2014, we assessed 1108 HIV-positive individuals for study eligibility, of whom 1095 (98.8%) were enrolled into the study. At the Entebbe site, 673 individuals were assessed for study eligibility and 666 (99.0%) were enrolled and 7 (1.0%) were not enrolled because; 3 (0.4%) were participating in another study, 3 (0.4%) did not return for enrolment while 1 (0.1%) died before enrolment. At the Kyamulibwa site, 436 individuals were assessed for study eligibility and 429 (98.4%) were enrolled, 7 (1.6%) were not enrolled because 3 (0.7%) requested for transfer to other ART care centres, 1 (0.2%) had mental illness, 1 (0.2%) declined consent for participation, 1 (0.2%) defaulted and 1 (0.2%) died before enrolment. Of the 1095 individuals enrolled, 964 (88.0%) were ART experienced (6 months or more) with a median of 9.4 years (IQR 7.0–9.9) on ART. Overall, 968 (88.4%) were aged 35 years and above, 711 (64.9%) were females, 608 (59.6%) were or had ever been on a Tenofovir containing ART regimen and 236 (23.1%) on a Protease Inhibitor containing ART regimen. Participants at the urban (Entebbe) site were older, mean age (SD); 46.1 (8.1) vs 42.7 (10.6) years and had a higher education level; 54.3% vs 15.4% had attained secondary level education and above. Whereas most of rural participant were peasants (69.5%), those from the urban site were mainly in gainful employment or self-employed—80.3% (Table 2).

Among our study population, the overall prevalence of hypertension was 14.5%, Diabetes mellitus—2.1% and renal disease—0.6%. Participants from the urban site had been on ART for a longer duration, with 90.7% on ART for 9 years and over compared to 11.7% at the rural site. Overall, 236 (23.1%) of our participants were on a PI containing ART regimen with a higher proportion of patients being at the urban Entebbe site; 32.4% compared to 7.6% among those at the rural Kyamulibwa site and 608 (59.6%) were or had ever been on a Tenofovir containing ART regimen; 78.3% of those at the urban site and 28.3% at the rural site (Table 3). We found that among individuals on long-term ART; (a) there were no differences in renal dysfunction (glomerular function and renal tubular function) between patients on Tenofovir containing and Non-Tenofovir containing ART regimens (Table 4). (b) Patients on PI containing ART regimens had higher total cholesterol, lower high density lipoprotein, higher low density lipoprotein, higher triglycerides, and a high atherogenic index for plasma than patients on non-PI containing ART regimen, $p = 0.001$ or < 0.001. (c)

Table 2 Characteristics of participants at enrolment into the CoLTART study by sex and study site

Characteristic	All combined	Entebbe site			Kyamulibwa site		
	n (%)	All, n (%)	Sex		All, n (%)	Sex	
			Females, n (%)	Males, n (%)		Females, n (%)	Males, n (%)
All by site	1095	666	459 (68.9)	207 (31.1)	429	252 (58.7)	177 (41.3)
Age, years							
18–34	127 (11.6)	34 (5.1)	29 (6.3)	5 (2.4)	93 (21.8)	65 (26.0)	28 (15.8)
35–49	649 (59.3)	426 (64.0)	295 (64.3)	131 (63.3)	222 (52.0)	126 (50.4)	96 (54.2)
50+	319 (29.1)	206 (30.9)	135 (29.4)	71 (34.3)	112 (26.2)	59 (23.6)	53 (30.0)
Mean age, years (SD)	44.8 (9.3)	46.1 (8.1)	45.5 (8.1)	47.3 (7.9)	42.7 (10.6)	41.6 (10.4)	44.3 (10.8)
Marital status							
Never married	87 (8.0)	28 (4.2)	24 (5.2)	4 (1.9)	59 (13.8)	40 (15.9)	19 (10.7)
Married/cohabiting	469 (42.8)	263 (39.5)	105 (22.9)	158 (76.3)	206 (48.0)	93 (36.9)	113 (63.8)
Separated/divorced	265 (24.2)	150 (22.5)	126 (27.5)	24 (11.6)	115 (26.8)	78 (31.0)	37 (20.9)
Widowed	274 (25.0)	225 (33.8)	204 (44.4)	21 (10.1)	49 (11.4)	41 (16.2)	8 (4.5)
Education level							
Incomplete primary	498 (45.5)	185 (27.8)	133 (29.0)	52 (25.1)	313 (73.0)	181 (71.8)	132 (74.6)
Complete primary	169 (15.4)	119 (17.9)	85 (18.5)	34 (16.4)	50 (11.6)	27 (10.7)	23 (13.0)
Secondary+	428 (39.1)	362 (54.3)	241 (52.5)	121 (58.5)	66 (15.4)	44 (17.5)	22 (12.4)
Employment[a]							
Peasant/farmer	362 (33.1)	64 (9.6)	45 (9.8)	19 (9.2)	298 (69.5)	179 (71.0)	119 (67.2)
Gainful employment	221 (20.2)	174 (26.2)	113 (24.7)	61 (29.5)	47 (11.0)	26 (10.3)	21 (11.9)
Self-employed/business	427 (39.0)	360 (54.1)	242 (52.8)	118 (57.0)	67 (15.6)	36 (14.3)	31 (17.5)
Unemployed	84 (7.7)	67 (10.1)	58 (12.7)	9 (4.3)	17 (3.9)	11 (4.4)	6 (3.4)
SES score tertile[b]							
Low	458 (42.0)	277 (41.9)	222 (48.9)	55 (26.6)	181 (42.2)	111 (44.0)	70 (39.5)
Middle	413 (37.9)	245 (37.1)	159 (35.0)	86 (41.5)	168 (39.2)	104 (41.3)	64 (36.2)
High	219 (20.1)	139 (21.0)	73 (16.1)	66 (31.9)	80 (18.6)	37 (14.7)	43 (24.3)
Tobacco consumption[c]							
Never	898 (82.1)	575 (86.4)	430 (93.8)	145 (70.0)	323 (75.2)	234 (92.8)	89 (50.3)
Ex-smoker	105 (9.6)	61 (9.2)	14 (3.1)	47 (22.7)	44 (10.3)	4 (1.6)	40 (22.6)
Current	91 (8.3)	29 (4.4)	14 (3.1)	15 (7.2)	62 (14.5)	14 (5.6)	48 (27.1)
Alcohol consumption[d]							
Never	408 (37.6)	248 (37.7)	186 (41.1)	62 (30.4)	160 (37.4)	112 (44.4)	48 (27.1)
Ever >1 month	383 (35.3)	255 (38.9)	183 (40.4)	72 (35.3)	128 (29.7)	80 (31.7)	48 (27.1)
Within <1 month	295 (27.1)	154 (23.4)	84 (18.5)	70 (34.3)	141 (32.9)	60 (23.9)	81 (45.8)
Work involves moderate/vigorous activity[e]							
No	494 (45.2)	433 (65.1)	333 (72.7)	100 (48.3)	61 (14.3)	48 (19.0)	13 (7.4)
Yes	599 (54.8)	232 (34.9)	125 (27.3)	107 (51.7)	367 (85.7)	204 (81.0)	163 (92.6)
Days/week-animal proteins[f]							
0	300 (27.6)	127 (19.3)	98 (21.6)	29 (14.1)	173 (40.3)	123 (48.8)	50 (28.2)
1 or 2	487 (44.8)	298 (45.3)	210 (46.4)	88 (42.9)	189 (44.1)	98 (38.9)	91 (51.4)
3+	300 (27.6)	233 (35.4)	145 (32.0)	88 (42.9)	67 (15.6)	31 (12.3)	36 (20.4)
Adds salt to food[g]							
No	625 (57.8)	399 (61.0)	283 (63.0)	116 (56.6)	226 (52.8)	148 (58.7)	78 (44.3)
Yes	457 (42.2)	255 (39.0)	166 (37.0)	89 (43.4)	202 (47.2)	104 (41.3)	98 (55.7)
Type of oil/fat used in cooking[h]							
None	146 (13.6)	68 (10.5)	43 (9.6)	25 (12.3)	78 (18.3)	54 (21.4)	24 (13.7)
Vegetable oil	793 (73.6)	488 (75.1)	334 (74.9)	154 (75.5)	305 (71.4)	183 (72.6)	122 (69.7)
Animal fat	111 (10.3)	73 (11.2)	53 (11.9)	20 (9.8)	38 (8.9)	13 (5.2)	25 (14.3)
Others/none in particular	27 (2.5)	21 (3.2)	16 (3.6)	5 (2.5)	6 (1.4)	2 (0.8)	4 (2.3)

Table 2 continued

Characteristic	All combined	Entebbe site			Kyamulibwa site		
	n (%)	All, n (%)	Sex		All, n (%)	Sex	
			Females, n (%)	Males, n (%)		Females, n (%)	Males, n (%)
Total teaspoons of sugar added to drink/day[i]							
<3	337 (31.5)	247 (38.4)	149 (33.7)	98 (48.8)	90 (21.0)	46 (18.3)	44 (25.0)
4/7	428 (39.9)	279 (43.4)	202 (45.7)	77 (38.3)	149 (34.8)	84 (33.3)	65 (36.9)
8+	306 (28.6)	117 (18.2)	91 (20.6)	26 (12.9)	189 (44.2)	122 (48.4)	67 (38.1)

All combined combines both Entebbe and Kyamulibwa sites. SES score tertile—Social Economic Status score computed from asset index based on household ownership of items

Number of participants with missing data: [a]Employment—1, [b]SES score tertile—5, [c]Tobacco consumption—1, [d]Alcohol consumption—9, [e]Work involves moderate/vigorous activity—2, [f]Days/week-animal proteins—8, [g]Adds salt to food—13, [h]Type of oil/fat used in cooking—18, [i]Total teaspoons of sugar added to drink/day—24

Patients on non-PI containing ART regimen had higher diastolic hypertension than patients on PI containing ART regimen, $p < 0.001$ (Table 5).

Discussion

In sub Saharan Africa, there is paucity of data on the complications of long-term ART use generated from the region. The CoLTART cohort therefore provides a good platform to investigate the complications of long-term ART in a Ugandan population. In this cross-sectional analysis of data collected at enrolment of patients who had been on ART for a median of 9.4 years, we found no differences in renal function (eGFR and fractional tubular phosphate reabsorption) between patients on Tenofovir and Non-Tenofovir containing ART regimens. However, we found that patients on PI containing ART regimens had higher cardiometabolic risk factors including higher total cholesterol, lower high density lipoprotein, higher low density lipoprotein, higher triglycerides, and a high atherogenic index for plasma compared to the non-PI regimen.

These findings are reassuring against concerns about Tenofovir induced renal toxicity, especially as it is now recommended by WHO for initiating ART, and has been widely adopted by ART programmes in many resource limited countries including Uganda [12–15]. Short to medium follow up studies have reported an association between Tenofovir and renal dysfunction, leading to glomerular and proximal renal tubular damage and acute renal failure [17–20]. Our failure to find differences in renal dysfunction by Tenofovir use might be due to the fact that most of our patients had been on ART for more than 9 years. Similarly, other previous studies have reported that the loss in eGFR attributable to Tenofovir seemed to occur during the early years of exposure between 0.5 and 31.2 months and stabilized after that [38–41].

As HIV infected individuals live longer due to improved survival on ART, cardiometabolic co-morbidity will manifest, and the association of HIV infection and cardiovascular disease will be compounded by ART use. The association of PI containing ART regimen and cardiometabolic risk is important since PIs are the backbone of second line ART regimens in resource limited settings. With the advocacy and availability of virological monitoring of patients on ART, more patients with virological failure will be identified and switched to PI containing second line ART regimens. HIV care programmes in resource limited settings therefore need to integrate CVD risk assessment and preventive measures, including routine biochemical and biophysical monitoring as well as stocking of lipid lowering drugs, increasing physical exercises, dietary adjustments.

Study strengths

The CoLTART cohort study participants have been on ART for close to a decade and thus enables assessment of the temporal relationship between ART and ART complications. The DART and RCC cohorts have systematically collected data on clinical, immunological and virological treatment outcomes, ARV toxicities, with regular haematology, liver and kidney function biochemical test results that can be used retrospectively. Stored serum and plasma samples that can be used for various analyses for the status during the early ART period (DART) and during the Pre-ART and early ART periods (RCC) are also available. The MRC/UVRI Uganda Unit's CDLS has the capacity for analysing and storing research samples.

Study weakness

Study participants of the former cohorts may not be representative of the general HIV-positive population, and those who were available for enrolment may be a biased sample due to their longer survival. The study included limited outcomes, other long-term ART complications, such as reduced bone mineral density and osteoporosis were not studied due to the costs of the non-invasive DXA (DECK-sa) scan, a procedure used to measure bone

Table 3 Medical history of participants at enrolment into the CoLTART study by sex and site

Medical condition	All combined	Entebbe site			Kyamulibwa site		
	n (%)	All, n (%)	Sex		All, n (%)	Sex	
			Females, n (%)	Males, n (%)		Females, n (%)	Males, n (%)
All	1095	666	459 (68.9)	207 (31.1)	429	252 (58.7)	177 (41.3)
Hypertension history							
Never had hypertension	936 (85.5)	556 (83.5)	378 (82.4)	178 (86.0)	380 (88.6)	222 (88.1)	158 (89.3)
Ever had hypertension	159 (14.5)	110 (16.5)	81 (17.6)	29 (14.0)	49 (11.4)	30 (11.9)	19 (10.7)
Diabetes mellitus history[a]							
No known diabetes mellitus	1067 (97.9)	645 (97.3)	445 (97.4)	200 (97.1)	422 (98.8)	248 (98.8)	174 (98.9)
Known diabetes mellitus	23 (2.1)	18 (2.7)	12 (2.6)	6 (2.9)	5 (1.2)	3 (1.2)	2 (1.1)
Renal disease history[b]							
No renal disease	1087 (99.4)	659 (99.1)	456 (99.3)	203 (98.5)	428 (99.8)	252 (100.0)	176 (99.4)
Known renal disease	7 (0.6)	6 (0.9)	3 (0.7)	3 (1.5)	1 (0.2)	0 (0.0)	1 (0.6)
ART exposure, years							
ART naïve	74 (6.8)	27 (4.1)	21 (4.6)	6 (2.9)	47 (11.0)	22 (8.7)	25 (14.1)
<1 years	79 (7.2)	13 (2.0)	11 (2.4)	2 (1.0)	66 (15.4)	35 (13.9)	31 (17.5)
1 to <5 years	164 (15.0)	7 (1.1)	6 (1.3)	1 (0.5)	157 (36.6)	98 (38.9)	59 (33.3)
5 to <9 years	124 (11.3)	15 (2.3)	9 (2.0)	6 (2.9)	109 (25.4)	65 (25.8)	44 (24.9)
9+ years	654 (59.7)	604 (90.7)	412 (89.8)	192 (92.8)	50 (11.7)	32 (12.7)	18 (10.2)
Metabolic abnormalities study groups[c]							
Non-protease Inhibitor based ART	785 (76.9)	432 (67.6)	306 (69.9)	126 (62.7)	353 (92.4)	212 (92.2)	141 (92.8)
Protease Inhibitor based ART	236 (23.1)	207 (32.4)	132 (30.1)	75 (37.3)	29 (7.6)	18 (7.8)	11 (7.2)
Renal dysfunction study groups[d]							
Tenofovir containing ART	608 (59.6)	500 (78.3)	337 (76.9)	163 (81.1)	108 (28.3)	64 (27.8)	44 (29.0)
Non-Tenofovir containing ART	413 (40.5)	139 (21.8)	101 (23.1)	38 (18.9)	274 (71.7)	166 (72.2)	108 (71.1)
Body mass index (kg/m^2)[e]							
<18.5	114 (10.6)	48 (7.4)	29 (6.5)	19 (9.4)	66 (15.4)	29 (11.5)	37 (21.0)
18.5–24.9	674 (62.8)	365 (56.6)	217 (49.0)	148 (73.3)	309 (72.2)	175 (69.4)	134 (76.1)
25.0–29.9	218 (20.3)	172 (26.7)	140 (31.6)	32 (15.8)	46 (10.8)	41 (16.3)	5 (2.8)
≥30	67 (6.3)	60 (9.3)	57 (12.9)	3 (1.5)	7 (1.6)	7 (2.8)	0 (0.0)
Haemoglobin (g/dl)[f]							
Normal	908 (83.3)	570 (86.2)	387 (85.1)	183 (88.8)	338 (78.8)	199 (79.0)	139 (78.5)
Abnormal	182 (16.7)	91 (13.8)	68 (14.9)	23 (11.2)	91 (21.2)	53 (21.0)	38 (21.5)
CD4 cell counts at enrolment (cells/μl)[g]							
≤350	307 (30.1)	182 (30.6)	102 (25.2)	80 (42.3)	125 (29.3)	65 (26.1)	60 (33.9)
351–500	327 (32.1)	171 (28.8)	118 (29.1)	53 (28.0)	156 (36.6)	89 (35.7)	67 (37.9)
501+	386 (37.8)	241 (40.6)	185 (45.7)	56 (29.6)	145 (34.0)	95 (38.2)	50 (28.2)
Viral loads at enrolment (cells/ml)[h]							
≤1000 copies/ml	823 (77.7)	528 (81.6)	363 (81.2)	165 (82.5)	295 (71.6)	180 (75.3)	115 (66.5)
>1000 copies/ml	236 (22.3)	119 (18.4)	84 (18.8)	35 (17.5)	117 (28.4)	59 (24.7)	58 (33.5)

Number of participants with missing data: [a]Diabetes mellitus history—5, [b]Renal disease history—1, [c]Metabolic abnormalities study groups—74 patients who were ART naïve at enrolment, [d]Renal dysfunction study groups—74 patients who were ART naïve at enrolment, [e]Body Mass Index—22, [f]Haemoglobin—5, [g]CD4 cell counts at enrolment—75, [h]Viral loads at enrolment-36; the 1059 included the 74 ART naïve individuals pending ART initiation

NNRTI nucleoside reverse transcriptase inhibitor, *NNRTI* non-nucleoside reverse transcriptase inhibitor

density, as well as mineral content in the body. In our study, a small number of patients; 50 (8.9%) had discontinued Tenofovir but we did not consider the period since Tenofovir was discontinued and the reasons why it was discontinued. If Tenofovir was stopped due to Tenofovir induced renal dysfunction, this might have biased our results. Due to the low prevalence of antibody seropositivity and confirmed Hepatitis C virus (HCV) RNA infection in Uganda [42, 43], we did not screen for HCV in this study. Other potential sources of bias included the

Table 4 Proportion of renal dysfunction/failure, and adjusted mean differences in renal function measures by TDF exposure among 964 adults on ART for more than 6 months

Renal function assessment parameter	Renal dysfunction/failure, n (%)	Adjusted mean differences (95% CI), non-TDF as reference	p value
eGFR (Cockcroft-Gault, adj for BSA)			
Non-TDF	99/378 (26.2%)	Ref	0.797
TDF	142/501 (28.3%)	−2.15 (−8.53 to 4.22)	
TDF-stopped	14/50 (28.0%)	−0.62 (−12.74 to 11.50)	
eGFR (Cockcroft-Gault, without BSA adj)			
Non-TDF	141/379 (37.2%)	Ref	0.914
TDF	196/502 (39.0%)	−2.42 (−14.45 to 9.62)	
TDF-stopped	19/50 (38.0%)	−3.01 (−25.90 to 19.89)	
eGFR (CKD-Epi)			
Non-TDF	60/383 (15.7%)	Ref	0.837
TDF	109/514 (21.2%)	−0.88 (−3.84 to 2.08)	
TDF-stopped	9/50 (18.0%)	−0.78 (−6.42 to 4.87)	
eGFR (MDRD with race)			
Non-TDF	28/383 (7.3%)	Ref	0.872
TDF	57/514 (11.1%)	−0.61 (−8.09 to 6.87)	
TDF-stopped	4/50 (8.0%)	3.11 (−11.14 to 17.36)	
Fractional tubular PO4 reabsorption			
Non-TDF	16/339 (4.7%)	Ref	0.131
TDF	16/386 (4.1%)	−0.74 (−1.84 to 0.36)	
TDF-stopped	1/42 (2.4%)	1.12 (−0.92 to 3.15)	
Serum urea			
Non-TDF	0/382 (0.0%)	Ref	0.252
TDF	2/514 (0.4%)	0.03 (−0.19 to 0.25)	
TDF-stopped	0/50 (0.0%)	0.35 (−0.07 to 0.77)	
Serum creatinine (μmol/l)			
Non-TDF	4/383 (1.0%)	Ref	0.336
TDF	10/514 (1.9%)	2.03 (−1.40 to 5.46)	
TDF-stopped	3/50 (6.0%)	3.98 (−2.55 to 10.51)	
Serum phosphates (mmol/l)			
Non-TDF	64/383 (16.7%)	Ref	0.575
TDF	50/503 (9.9%)	0.01 (−0.04 to 0.06)	
TDF-stopped	8/48 (16.7%)	−0.04 (−0.13 to 0.05)	

Mean difference adjusted for site, duration on ART, smoking status, social-economic status, log viral load, CD4 cell count, hypertension and Glucose; Renal dysfunction/failure defined as <90 for estimated Glomerular Filtration Rates, >11.9 mmol/l for serum Urea, >109 μmol/l for serum creatinine and <0.81 mmol/l for serum phosphates (Hypophosphataemia)

eGFR estimated glomerular filtration rate, *BSA* body surface area adjustment, *CKD-Epi* Chronic Kidney Disease Epidemiology formula, *MDRD* Modified Diet in Renal Disease formulae with race adjustment

self-reported thus subjectively measured individual level exposures especially dietary, socio-economic and behavioural factors. There might have been some inaccuracies in tracking time on particular regimens of ART e.g. the exact dates of ART switches or substitutions.

Conclusions

Our findings allay fears of Tenofovir renal toxicity and the WHO recommendation to use Tenofovir in first line ART can safely be implemented even in resource limited settings with limited renal function monitoring. However, further evaluation of renal function among patients on Tenofovir beyond 10 years is advised. Integration of cardiovascular risk assessment, institution of preventive and curative or control remedies against cardiovascular disease are recommended.

Data available

Data available includes demographic, social economic status, medical, dietary and lifestyle risk factors. Biophysical measurements data available includes weight, height, blood pressure and pulse rate; waist, hip and mid-upper

Table 5 Proportion of abnormal values for CVD risk factors and differences in mean values of CVD risk measures by PI exposure among the 964 adults on ART for more than 6 months

CVD risk measure	Abnormal values for CVD risk, n (%)	ADJUSTED mean differences (95% CI), non-PI as reference	p value
Total cholesterol ≥5.2 μmol/l			
Non-PI regimen	176/714 (24.6%)	Ref	<0.001
PI regimen	121/230 (52.6%)	0.78 (0.57 to 0.98)	
HDL <1 mmol/l (males), <1.3 mmol/l (females)			
Non-PI regimen	265/714 (37.1%)	Ref	0.001
PI regimen	67/230 (29.1%)	0.12 (0.05 to 0.20)	
LDL ≥3.4 mmol/l			
Non-PI regimen	144/714 (18.6%)	Ref	<0.001
PI regimen	93/230 (40.3%)	0.45 (0.29 to 0.62)	
Total cholesterol/HDL ratio (>5.1)			
Non-PI regimen	90/714 (12.6%)	Ref	0.420
PI regimen	42/230 (18.3%)	0.10 (−0.15 to 0.35)	
Triglycerides ≥1.69 mmol/l			
Non-PI regimen	109/713 (15.3%)	Ref	<0.001
PI regimen	99/230 (43.0%)	0.52 (0.24 to 0.80)	
Glucose (>6.4 mmol/l)			
Non-PI regimen	26/714 (3.6%)	Ref	0.814
PI regimen	7/231 (3.0%)	0.00 (−0.03 to 0.04)	
Systolic blood pressure (≥140 mmHg)			
Non-PI regimen	110/707 (15.6%)	Ref	0.060
PI regimen	19/234 (8.1%)	−3.120 (−6.413 to 0.174)	
Diastolic blood pressure (≥90 mmHg)			
Non-PI regimen	112/707 (15.8%)	Ref	<0.001
PI regimen	13/234 (5.6%)	−3.931 (−5.967 to 1.895)	
AIP $\log_{10}$ (Triglycerides/HDL) ≥0.1			
Non-PI regimen	183/713 (25.7%)	Ref	<0.001
PI regimen	102/230 (44.3%)	0.12 (0.07 to 0.17)	
Abnormal BMI (≥30 kg/m^2)			
Non-PI regimen	44/703 (6.3%)	Ref	0.074
PI regimen	17/231 (7.3%)	−2.370 (−5.005 to 0.264)	
Abnormal waist circumference [≥94 cm (men)/≥80 (women)]			
Non-PI regimen	287/706 (40.6%)	Ref	0.805
PI regimen	94/234 (40.2%)	−0.202 (−1.829 to 1.425)	
Abnormal waist/hips ratio [>0.95 (men)/>85 (women)]			
Non-PI regimen	369/706 (52.3%)	Ref	0.118
PI regimen	133/234 (56.8%)	0.008 (−0.002 to 0.019)	
Abnormal Framingham score (>10%)			
Non-PI regimen	130/703 (18.5%)	Ref	0.434
PI regimen	28/229 (12.2%)	−0.344 (−1.218 to 0.530)	

Mean differences adjusted for site, duration on ART, sex, age-groups, smoking status, alcohol consumption, days/week-animal proteins, salt and sugar intake, physical activity, social-economic status, log viral load, CD4 cell count

HDL high density lipoprotein, *LDL Low Density Lipoprotein*, *AIP* atherogenic index for plasma, *BMI* body mass index

arm circumferences. Clinical examination and ART and cotrimoxazole/dapsone adherence data is also available. Available laboratory data includes: fasting blood glucose and lipid profiles (total cholesterol, triglycerides, low density lipoproteins, high density lipoproteins); renal function tests (Urine strip test, phosphates and creatinine and serum phosphates, creatinine and urea). Full blood counts, immunology (CD3, CD4 and CD8), viral loads and HIV drug resistance test results for blood samples with viral loads ≥1000 copies/ml. Liver function tests (alanine transaminase, aspartate transaminase, alkaline phosphatase and bilirubin). Stored samples are also available for Hepatitis B virus serology, genomic studies and other studies.

Data resource access

The CoLTART database has data on the participants biophysical measurements, clinical examination findings and laboratory measurements. All data from the cohort are managed by the Statistics Section of the MRC/UVRI Uganda Research Unit on AIDS. Data access inquiries can be made to the Director, MRC/UVRI, Uganda Research Unit on AIDS by email to: mrc@mrcuganda.org or the corresponding author.

Abbreviations

AIDS: Acquired Immune Deficiency Syndrome; ART: antiretroviral therapy; ARVs: antiretroviral drugs; CAP: College of American Pathologists; CDLS: Clinical Diagnostics Laboratory Services; CRFs: case report forms; CoLTART: Complications of Long-Term Antiretroviral Therapy; CPR: calibrated population resistance tool; CVD: cardiovascular disease; DART: Development of Antiretroviral therapy in Africa; DXA: dual-energy X-ray absorptiometry; EDTA: ethylenediaminetetraacetic acid; eGFR: estimated glomerular filtration rate; GCP: Good Clinical Practice; HIV: human immunodeficiency virus; ICH: International Council for Harmonisation; MRC: Medical Research Council; NRTI: Nucleoside Reverse Transcriptase Inhibitors; NNRTI: Non Nucleoside Reverse Transcriptase Inhibitors; PCR: Polymerase Chain Reaction; PI: protease inhibitor; RCC: Rural Clinical Cohort; RCPA: Royal College of Pathologists of Australasia; RMD: Roche Molecular Diagnostics; RNA: ribonucleic acid; SDRMs: surveillance drug resistance mutations; STEPS: STEPwise approach to surveillance; TDF: Tenofovir Disoproxil Fumarate; TDR: transmitted drug resistance; UKNEQAS: United Kingdom National External Quality Assurance Service; UVRI: Uganda Virus Research Institute; WHO: World Health Organisation.

Authors' contributions

BNM, JL, PM, PK conceived and designed the study; BNM, IN, PK, JW participated in data collection; JW participated in the laboratory analyses; IK, JL compiled and analysed data; BNM, IK, drafted the initial manuscript; BNM, IK, PM, PK interpreted the analysis; all authors contributed to manuscript revising. All authors read and approved the final manuscript.

Author details

[1] MRC/UVRI Uganda Research Unit on AIDS, P.O. Box 49, Entebbe, Uganda. [2] MRC Tropical Epidemiology Group, London School of Hygiene and Tropical Medicine, Keppel Street, London WC1E 7HT, United Kingdom. [3] Department of Clinical Research, London School of Hygiene and Tropical Medicine, Keppel Street, London WC1E 7HT, United Kingdom.

Acknowledgements

We acknowledge the contribution of CoLTART study participants, the CoLTART study team, and staff of the Clinical Diagnostic Laboratory Services, Basic Science and Statistics section. We also acknowledge the contribution of the MRC/UVRI Uganda Unit's Scientific Advisory Committee.

The CoLTART study team

Kyamulibwa study site: Billy N. Mayanja, Judith Nalwadda, Gladys Nakibuuka, Harriet Namugenyi, Patrick Kazooba, Rosemary Lubega. ***Entebbe study site:*** Annet Mugisha, Apophia Tereka, Apuuli Kalyebara, Arthur Namara, Diana Nakitto, Deus Wangi, Fred Nume, George Ssemwanga, Gertrude Nabulime, Gladys Nassuna, Gloria Lubega, Ivan Namakoola, Joseph Lutaakome, Lillian Generous, Lydia Matama, Rosemary Massa, Salome Tino, William Nakahima. ***Basic Science Virology:*** Anne A. Kapaata, Brian Magambo, Chris Parry, Frederick Lyagoba, Jamirah Nazziwa, Maria Nannyonjo. ***Clinical Diagnostic Laboratory Services:*** Edward Muhigirwa, Faith Wamalugu, Florence Kabajuma, Hope Grania Nakazibwe, Jackson Were, Joan Bwandinga, Juliet Bukenya, Member Zephyrian Kamushaaga, Peter Hughes, Peter Nkurunziza, Priscilla Agatha Balungi, Simon Mukasa, Sureyah Nassimbwa, Tobias Vudriko, William Senyonga, Wilfred Ochola. ***Statistics:*** Annet Nakimbugwe, Catherine Nampewo, Doreen Nambuba, Erima Naphtali, Grace Barigye, Irene Nakamanya, Ivan Kasamba, Jonathan Levin, Joseph Kahwa, Joy Namutebi Matovu, Lillian Namayirira, Ruth Namulindwa Lubega, Sandra Nabalayo, Solomon Kaddu. ***Principal Investigator:*** Paula Munderi.

Competing interests

The authors declare that they have no competing interests.

Funding

This research was jointly funded by the UK Medical Research Council (MRC) and the UK Department for International Development (DFID) under the MRC/DFID Concordant agreement.

References

1. UNAIDS. Fact sheet November 2016. http://www.unaids.org/en/resources/fact-sheet. Accessed 3 Dec 2016.
2. UNAIDS. The HIV and AIDS Uganda Country Progress Report 2014. http://www.unaids.org/sites/default/files/country/documents/UGA_narrative_report_2015.pdf. Accessed 6 Oct 2015.
3. Maher D, Waswa L, Baisley K, Karabarinde A, Unwin N. Epidemiology of hypertension in low-income countries: a cross-sectional population-based survey in rural Uganda. J Hypertens. 2011;29:1061–8.
4. Bimenya G, Okot J, Nangosa H, Anguma S, Byarugaba W. Plasma cholesterol and related lipid levels of seemingly healthy public service employees in Kampala, Uganda. Afr Health Sci. 2006;6:139–44.
5. Haugaard SB. Toxic metabolic syndrome associated with HAART. Expert Opin Drug Metab Toxicol. 2006;2:429–45.
6. Hofman P, Nelson AM. The pathology induced by highly active antiretroviral therapy against human immunodeficiency virus: an update. Curr Med Chem. 2006;13:3121–32.
7. Bradbury RA, Samaras K. Antiretroviral therapy and the human immunodeficiency virus—improved survival but at what cost? Diabetes Obes Metab. 2008;10:441–50.
8. Montessori V, Press N, Harris M, Akagi L, Montaner JS. Adverse effects of antiretroviral therapy for HIV infection. CMAJ. 2004;170:229–38.
9. Herman JS, Easterbrook PJ. PJ E. The metabolic toxicities of antiretroviral therapy. Int J STD AIDS. 2001;12:555–62.
10. Post FA, Holt SG. SG H. Recent developments in HIV and the kidney. Curr Opin Infect Dis. 2009;22:43–8.
11. Roling J, Schmid H, Fischereder M, Draenert R, Goebel FD. HIV-associated renal diseases and highly active antiretroviral therapy-induced nephropathy. Clin Infect Dis. 2006;42:1488–95.
12. WHO. Consolidated guidelines on the use of antiretroviral drugs for treating and preventing HIV infection. Geneva: World Health Organization; 2013. http://www.who.int/hiv/pub/guidelines/arv2013. Accessed 26 Jan 2016.
13. Ministry of Health U. Addendum to the National Antiretroviral Treatment Guidelines. 2013. http://preventcrypto.org/wp-content/uploads/2012/07/Uganda-National-ART-Guidelines_2014.pdf. Accessed 15 Jan 2015.
14. Ministry of Health, Republic of Kenya, (NASCOP). NAaSCP: guidelines on use of antiretroviral drugs for treating and preventing HIV infection: a rapid advice. 2014. http://guidelines.health.go.ke:8000/media/Rapid_Advice_Booklet_2014_July_V5.pdf. Accessed 17 Feb 2016.
15. Ministry of Health and Social Welfare, Tanzania TURo. NACProgramme: the United Republic of Tanzania. National Guidelines for the Management of HIV and AIDS. Fifth Edition-May, 2015. http://www.nacp.go.tz/site/publications/care-and-treatment/NationalGuidelineforManagementHIV.pdf. Accessed 15 Feb 2016.
16. Jülg BD, Bogner JR, Crispin A, Goebel FD. Progression of renal impairment under therapy with tenofovir. AIDS. 2005;19:1332–3.
17. Zimmermann AE, Pizzoferrato T, Bedford J, Morris A, Hoffman R, Braden G. Tenofovir-associated acute and chronic kidney disease: a case of multiple drug interactions. Clin Infect Dis. 2006;42:283–90.
18. Gallant JE, Winston JA, DeJesus E, Pozniak AL, Chen S-S, Cheng AK, et al. The 3-year renal safety of a tenofovir disoproxil fumarate vs. a thymidine analogue-containing regimen in antiretroviral-naive patients. AIDS. 2008;22:2155–63.

19. Ryom L, Mocroft A, Kirk O, Worm SW, Kamara DA, Reiss P, et al. Association between antiretroviral exposure and renal impairment among HIV-positive persons with normal baseline renal function: the D: A: D Study. J Infect Dis. 2013;207:1359–69.
20. Labarga P, Barreiro P, Martin-Carbonero L, Rodriguez-Novoa S, Solera C, Medrano J, et al. Kidney tubular abnormalities in the absence of impaired glomerular function in HIV patients treated with tenofovir. AIDS. 2009;23:689–96.
21. Laprise C, Baril J-G, Dufresne S, Trottier H. Association between tenofovir exposure and reduced kidney function in a cohort of HIV-positive patients: results from 10 years of follow-up. Clin Infect Dis. 2012;56:567–75.
22. Oboho I, Abraham A, Benning L, Anastos K, Sharma A, Young M, et al. Tenofovir use and urinary biomarkers among HIV-infected women in the Women's Interagency HIV Study (WIHS). J Acquir Immune Defic Syndr. 2013;62:388–95.
23. Gupta SK. Tenofovir-associated Fanconi syndrome: review of the FDA adverse event reporting system. AIDS Patient Care STDS. 2008;22:99–103.
24. Cm W. HIV and the kidney: a spotlight on racial disparities. J Infect Dis. 2008;197:1490–2.
25. Mugyenyi P, Walker AS, Hakim J, Munderi P, Gibb DM, Kityo C, et al. Routine versus clinically driven laboratory monitoring of HIV antiretroviral therapy in Africa (DART): a randomised non-inferiority trial. Lancet. 2010;375:123–31.
26. Morgan D, Malamba SS, Maude GH, Okongo MJ, Wagner HU, Mulder DW, et al. An HIV-1 natural history cohort and survival times in rural Uganda. AIDS. 1997;11:633–40.
27. Shafer LA, Nsubuga RN, White R, Mayanja BN, Chapman R, O'Brien K, et al. Antiretroviral therapy and sexual behavior in Uganda: a cohort study. AIDS. 2011;25:671–8.
28. Mayanja BN, Todd J, Hughes P, Van der Paal L, Mugisha JO, Atuhumuza E, et al. Septicaemia in a population-based HIV clinical cohort in rural Uganda, 1996–2007: incidence, aetiology, antimicrobial drug resistance and impact of antiretroviral therapy. Trop Med Int Health Trop Med Int Health. 2010;15:697–705.
29. Iwuji CC, Mayanja BN, Weiss HA, Atuhumuza E, Hughes P, Maher D, et al. Morbidity in HIV-1-infected individuals before and after the introduction of antiretroviral therapy: a longitudinal study of a population-based cohort in Uganda. HIV Med. 2011;12:553–61.
30. Mayanja BN, Baisley K, Nalweyiso N, Kibengo FM, Mugisha JO, Van der Paal L, et al. Using verbal autopsy to assess the prevalence of HIV infection among deaths in the ART period in rural Uganda: a prospective cohort study, 2006–2008. Popul Health Metr. 2011;9:36.
31. Asiki G, Murphy G, Nakiyingi-Miiro J, Seeley J, Nsubuga RN, Karabarinde A, et al. The general population cohort in rural south-western Uganda: a platform for communicable and non-communicable disease studies. Int J Epidemiol. 2013;42:129–41.
32. French N, Nakiyingi J, Carpenter L, Lugada E, Watera C, Moi K, et al. 23-valent pneumococcal polysaccharide vaccine in HIV-1-infected Ugandan adults: double-blind, randomised and placebo controlled trial. Lancet. 2000;355:2106–11.
33. Ministry of Health, Uganda. Integrated national guidelines on antiretroviral therapy, prevention of mother to child transmission of HIV and on infant & young child feeding. First Edition, June 2011. http://www.emtct-iatt.org/wp-content/uploads/2014/05/GL_Integrated-National-Guidelines-on-ART-PMTCT-and-IYCF-June-2011-MOH-Uganda_0.pdf. Accessed 27 Sept 2015.
34. Asiki G, Murphy GA, Baisley K, Nsubuga RN, Karabarinde A, Newton R, et al. Prevalence of dyslipidaemia and associated risk factors in a rural population in South-Western Uganda: a community based survey. PLoS ONE. 2015;10(5):e0126166.
35. WHO. Chronic diseases and health promotion, STEPwise approach to chronic disease risk factor surveillance. http://www.who.int/chp/steps/nauru/en/. Accessed 23 Sept 2015.
36. Bennett DE, Camacho RJ, Otelea D, Kuritzkes DR, Fleury H, Kiuchi M, et al. Drug resistance mutations for surveillance of transmitted HIV-1 drug-resistance: 2009 update. PLoS ONE. 2009;4:e4724.
37. Gifford RJ, Liu TF, Rhee SY, Kiuchi M, Hue S, Pillay D, et al. The calibrated population resistance tool: standardized genotypic estimation of transmitted HIV-1 drug resistance. Bioinformatics. 2009;25:1197–8.
38. Izzedine H, Isnard-Bagnis C, Hulot J-S, Vittecoq D, Cheng A, Jais CK, et al. Renal safety of tenofovir in HIV treatment-experienced patients. AIDS. 2004;18:1074–6.
39. Kyaw NTT, Harries AD, Chinnakali P, Antierens A, Soe KP, Woodman M, et al. Low incidence of renal dysfunction among HIV-infected patients on a Tenofovir-based first line antiretroviral treatment regimen in Myanmar. PLoS ONE. 2015;10:e0135188.
40. Nelson MR, Katlama C, Montaner JS, Cooper DA, Gazzard B, Clotet B, et al. The safety of tenofovir disoproxil fumarate for the treatment of HIV infection in adults: the first 4 years. AIDS. 2007;21:1273–81.
41. Madeddu G, Bonfanti P, Giuseppe V, Carradori S, Grosso C, Marconi P, et al. Tenofovir renal safety in HIV-infected patients: results from the SCOLTA project. Biomed Pharmacother. 2008;62:6–11.
42. O'Reilly JI, Ocama P, Opio CK, Alfred A, Paintsil E, Seremba E, et al. Risk factors and seroprevalence of hepatitis C among patients hospitalized at Mulago Hospital, Uganda. J Trop Med. 2011;2011:598341.
43. Walusansa V, Kagimu M. Screening for hepatitis C among HIV positive patients at Mulago hospital in Uganda. Afr Health Sci. 2009;9:143–6.

9

The role of the glycosyl moiety of myricetin derivatives in anti-HIV-1 activity in vitro

Joseph T. Ortega[1], Alirica I. Suárez[2], Maria L. Serrano[3], Jani Baptista[2], Flor H. Pujol[1] and Hector R. Rangel[1*]

Abstract

Background: Plant extracts are sources of valuable compounds with biological activity, especially for the anti-proliferative activity against pathogens or tumor cells. Myricetin is a flavonoid found in several plants that has been described as an inhibitor of Human immunodeficiency virus type 1 (HIV-1) through its action against the HIV reverse transcriptase, but myricetin derivatives have not been fully studied. The aim of this study was to evaluate the anti-HIV-1 activity of glycosylated metabolites obtained from *Marcetia taxifolia* and derived from myricetin: myricetin rhamnoside and myricetin 3-(6-rhamnosylgalactoside).

Methods: Compounds were obtained from organic extracts by maceration of aerial parts of *M. taxifolia*. All biological assays were performed in the MT4 cell line. Antiviral activity was measured as inhibition of p24 and reverse transcriptase with a fluorescent assay.

Results: Both flavonoids have antiviral activity in vitro, with an EC50 of 120 μM for myricetin 3-rhamnoside (MR) and 45 μM for myricetin 3-(6-rhamnosylgalactoside) (MRG), both significantly lower than the EC50 of myricetin (230 μM). Although both compounds inhibited the reverse transcriptase activity, with an IC50 of 10.6 μM for MR and 13.8 μM for MRG, myricetin was the most potent, with an IC50 of 7.6 μM, and an inhibition greater than 80%. Molecular docking approach showed correlation between the free energy of binding with the assays of enzyme inhibition.

Conclusions: The results suggest that glycosylated moiety might enhance the anti-HIV-1 activity of myricetin, probably by favoring the internalization of the flavonoid into the cell. The inhibition of the HIV-1 reverse transcriptase is likely responsible for the antiviral activity.

Keywords: HIV-1, Reverse transcriptase, Flavonoids, Myricetin, Glycosyl flavonoids, HIV RT docking

Background

The AIDS epidemic is the result of one of the most important viral infections affecting humans. As there is no vaccine currently available, the antiviral drugs constitute the only way to slow the progression of the disease [1, 2]. The appearance of drug resistance, serious side effects of existing drugs have promoted the search for new anti-HIV agents [3].

Plants are a rich source of new bioactive compounds [4]. Flavonoids, a large group of polyphenolic compound, are known for their bioactive properties and are widely distributed in the vegetal kingdom [5]. The range of their biological properties include anti-allergic, antibacterial, antidiabetic, anti-inflammatory and antiviral activities [6, 7].

The *Melastomataceae* are plants common in the tropical and mountainous areas. This family is abundantly distributed in South America, Southeast Asia and southern China [8]. *Marcetia* is a neotropical genus with 44 described species, distributed from Venezuela to Uruguay, with most of the species found in Southern Brazil and Uruguay [9]. The extract of *Marcetia taxifolia* has

*Correspondence: hrangel2006@gmail.com
[1] Laboratorio de Virología Molecular, Centro de Microbiología y Biología Celular, Instituto Venezolano de Investigaciones Científicas, Caracas, Venezuela

been shown to have antimicrobial activities, and the compounds responsible for this effect are flavonoids, particularly myricetin [10]. Pasetto et al. [11] and Ono et al. [12] determined that myricetin and quercetin inhibited HIV-1 proliferation and the HIV-1 reverse transcriptase (RT). The RT plays an essential role in the HIV life cycle and is one of the principal targets for several anti HIV-1 drugs in clinical use [13]. Some flavonoids have been characterized as nonnucleoside inhibitors (NNRTIs) that bind to a site in the p66 subunit of the HIV-1 RT p66/p51 heterodimer, situated approximately 10 Å from the RT active site [14, 15]. Ortega et al. [16], found that quercetin, a glycosylated derivative of myricetin, exhibited an improved antiviral activity and suggested that the enhanced activity was due to the glycosyl moiety.

The aim of this study was to evaluate the anti-HIV-1 activity in vitro of glycosylated metabolites of myricetin obtained from *Marcetia taxifolia* extracts: myricetin 3-rhamnoside (MR) and myricetin 3-(6-rhamnosylgalactoside) (MRG). These compounds contain one and two glycosides respectively, as substituents on the myricetin backbone (Fig. 1). In order to determine the possible role of the glycosyl moiety on antiviral activity we used a molecular docking approach to compare the binding of the glycosylated compounds and the aglycone myricetin to HIV-1 RT.

Methods

Plant material and extraction

The plant *Marcetia taxifolia* (A.St.-Hil.) DC., was collected in the Amazonas State of Venezuela, and its botanical identity was confirmed and authenticated by Dr. Stephen Tillett. A voucher of the collection was archived with the code MYF 28418 in the "Herbario Víctor Manuel Ovalles" of the School of Pharmacy, Universidad Central de Venezuela. Extraction and separation of compounds obtained from the aerial parts of *M. taxifolia* was performed as described previously [17]. Two glycosylated compounds derived from myricetin: myricetin 3-rhamnoside and myricetin 3-(6-rhamnosylgalactoside) were evaluated, along with the commercially available aglycone myricetin (Sigma-Aldrich, USA).

Cells and virus

HIV-1 (HTLV-IIIB/H9) and MT4 cells were obtained from the NIH AIDS Research and Reference Reagent Program. The cells were grown in RPMI-1640 medium supplemented with 10% FBS and penicillin/streptomycin and splitted every 3 days.

Cytotoxicity assay

MT4 cells were seeded in 96 wells/plate at a density of 30,000 cells/well, and different concentrations of the compounds were added. After 24 h the cultures were evaluated with MTT cell proliferation assay (Sigma-Aldrich, USA) to determine the percent of live cells under the different conditions evaluated.

Antiviral activity

Different concentrations of the compounds and HIV-1, at an MOI of 0.03, were added simultaneously to the wells of a 96 wells plate containing 30,000 cells/well. The virus production was evaluated at 72 h post infection by detecting the viral antigen p24 with an in-house ELISA [18]. The results were expressed relative to the control of untreated HIV-1 infected cells. Selectivity Index value (SI) was determined as the ratio of CC50 to EC50 for each compound.

RT inhibition assay

The inhibitory activity of compounds against HIV-1 RT was evaluated by using the EnzChek Reverse Transcriptase Assay kit (Molecular Probes, Inc., USA). Purified RT enzyme purchased from Worthington Biochemical Corporation and Nevirapine were used as controls for enzyme and antiviral drug respectively. Statistical analysis (ANOVA) of the results from at least three independent experiments was performed using

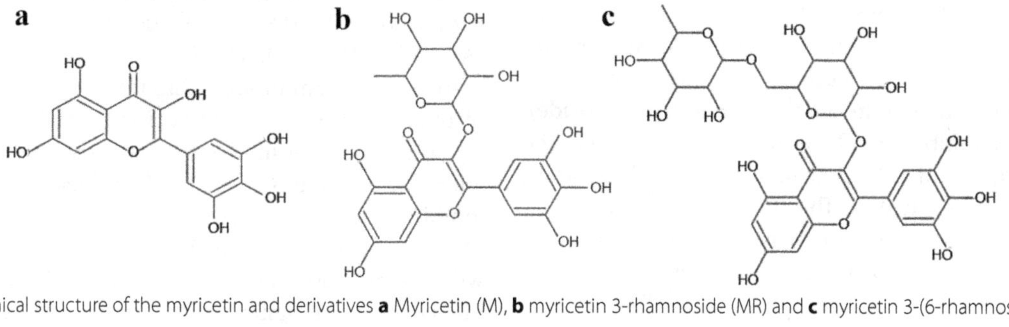

Fig. 1 Chemical structure of the myricetin and derivatives **a** Myricetin (M), **b** myricetin 3-rhamnoside (MR) and **c** myricetin 3-(6-rhamnosylgalactoside) (MRG)

Prism GraphPad 6 version 6.01 ($p \leq 0.05$ was used as the level of significance).

Molecular docking

The coordinates of wild-type HIV-1 reverse transcriptase (RT) bound with DNA and the NNRTI Nevirapine at 2.85 Å resolution was obtained from the protein data bank [19], PDB code 3V81 [20]. The inhibitor, the DNA molecule and all crystallographic water molecules were removed from the coordinate set: hydrogen atoms were added and partial charges were assigned to all atoms. The enzyme was then submitted to restrained molecular mechanics refinement with NAMD [21], using the CHARMM22 force field. The binding site was delimited according to previous studies reporting key residues of the enzyme and the 3D structure of each inhibitor was obtained from the PubChem database [22]. The molecular docking was performed with AutoDock 4/VegaZZ 3.1.0.21 and 30 runs were conducted for each compound. The results were prioritized according to the predicted free energy of binding in kcal/mol.

Results

Cytotoxicity and antiviral activity

The anti-HIV-1 activity in vitro was evaluated with a wide range of concentrations of the myricetin glycosylated compounds. The EC50 for myricetin 3-rhamnoside was 120 μM, for myricetin 3-(6-rhamnosylgalactoside) 45 and 230 μM for myricetin (Fig. 2a). Neither myricetin nor either of the myricetin derivatives used, exhibited significant cytotoxic activity at the concentrations tested (Fig. 2b). Because the CC50 for all the compounds assayed was out of the range of the evaluated concentrations, (maximum > 300 μM) an exact estimation of the selectivity index (SI) was impossible, and instead a crude estimation was performed by assigning the CC50 as > 300 μM and then calculating the EC50 for each compound. The estimated CC50 values thereby obtained were: $IS_M > 1.3$, $IS_{MR} > 2.6$ and $IS_{MRG} > 7$.

RT inhibition assay

The capacity of the compounds to inhibit HIV-1 RT was also evaluated. Figure 3 shows that at a concentration higher than 7.5 μM, myricetin 3-rhamnoside was more potent than myricetin 3-(6-rhamnosylgalactoside), reaching an inhibitory effect over 65%. However, the aglycone myricetin exhibited more RT inhibition at all concentrations evaluated. The IC50 obtained for myricetin was 7.6 μM, while for myricetin 3-rhamnoside it was 10.6 μM, and for myricetin 3-(6-rhamnosylgalactoside) 13.8 μM.

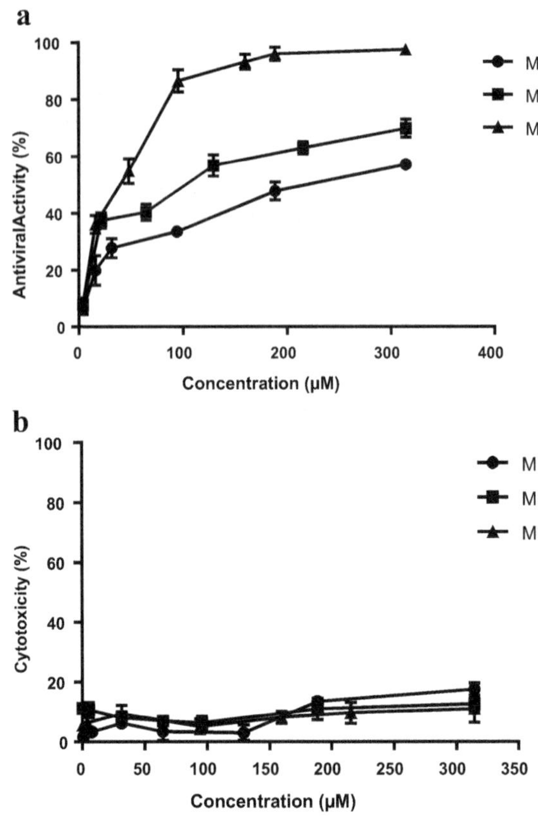

Fig. 2 Antiviral **a** and cytotoxic **b** activity of compounds evaluated. The percent of cytotoxicity of different concentrations of MR (Square), MRG (Triangle) and M (Circle) are shown as media ± SEM. Antiviral activity (solid lines) is expressed as the percent inhibition of p24 production relative to control. Results are media ± SEM (n = 3)

Molecular docking

The potential interactions of the active compounds with the RT enzyme were evaluated by molecular docking. Myricetin exhibited the lowest free energy of binding (− 6.95 kcal/mol), compared to glycosylated compounds (Table 1). In Fig. 4, which shows the interactions between myricetin and RT residues, there are five hydrogen bonds with residues Lys101 (A), Glu138 (B) and Ile180 (A) and electrostatic interactions Pi–Pi, Pi–Alkyl and Pi–sigma with residues Tyr188 (A), Leu100 (A), Val106 (A), Leu234 (A) and Val179 (A). Of the two myricetin glycosides, myricetin 3-rhamnoside exhibited the best free energy of binding to RT, (− 5.02 kcal/mol) and Fig. 4b shows the interactions of myricetin 3-rhamnoside with various amino acid residues in the binding pocket of RT NNRTI inhibitors. Four hydrogen bonds with residues Tyr318 (A), Lys101 (A) and Ile108 (A) were observed, along with electrostatic interactions such as Pi–Pi, Pi–Alkyl, Pi–sigma and Pi–anion with Tyr181 (A), Val 179 (A), Leu100 (A), Glu 138 (B), and Alkyl–Alkyl interactions

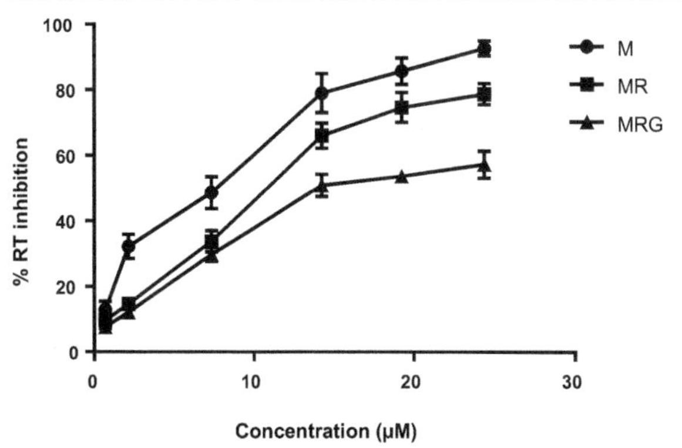

Fig. 3 Reverse transcriptase inhibition. The inhibitory effect of MR (Square) MRG (Triangle) and M (Circle) on recombinant Reverse Transcriptase enzyme (0.25 UI/ml), is expressed as the activity of the treated enzyme relative to control w/o treatment. All results were normalized to respective control (reaction buffer)

with the residues Lys103 (A), Val106 (A), Val179 (A) and Pro236 (A). Myricetin 3-(6-rhamnosylgalactoside) showed a higher free energy of binding to RT (2.38 kcal/mol) and fewer interactions than seen with myricetin 3-rhamnoside, two hydrogen bonds with residues Lys101 (A) and Glu138 (A) and several electrostatic interactions Pi–cation and, Pi–Alkyl that occurred with the residues Leu100, Pro321, and Lys101.

Discussion

Because of several reports describing the activity of other flavonoids against HIV-1 [23–25] we evaluated the activity of glycosylate flavonoids obtained from *M. taxifolia*. The results showed that the antiviral potency of myricetin derived compounds was related to the number of glycosyl residues on the molecule supporting the notion that the addition of glycosides to myricetin could modulate the anti-HIV-1 activity of these compounds.

Flavonoids are generally found in plants and fruits as glycosides and less commonly as aglycones [26]. The glycosilated flavonoids obtained from the diet are hydrolyzed in the intestine and then transported into the cells and systemic circulation. However, it has been described that glycosylated flavonoids may be a substrate of sodium-dependent glucose transporters (SGLT1) in the cell membrane of enterocytes [27, 28] and then, once inside the cell, the glycosides are cleaved by a cytosolic beta-glycosidase [29]. This process could contribute to their accumulation within the cell. Consistent with this possibility, it has been shown that two glycosyl derivatives of quercetin (guajaverin and avicularin) have higher antiviral activity than quercetin [16]. Similar results were obtained in this study, with a reduction of two to five-fold of the EC50 with the addition of glycosyl moieties to myricetin.

In contrast to the results observed with the inhibition of HIV-1 replication, RT inhibition was inversely proportional to the glycosylation grade of myricetin [myricetin (R = aglycone) > myricetin 3-rhamnoside (R = mono-glycosylated) > myricetin 3-(6-rhamnosylgalactoside) (R = Bi-glycosylated)]. These results are in concordance with the free energy of binding obtained in silico, where myricetin exhibited the lowest free energy and MRG the highest. The analysis of the resulting complexes clearly reveals that the binding interactions of these compounds occurred with the residues of the hydrophobic NNRTI-binding pocket, described by Sarafianos et al. [30] as containing residues Leu100, Lys101, Lys103, Val106, Tre107, Val108, Val179, Tyr181, Tyr188, Val189, Gly190, Phe227,

Table 1 Docking analysis of the evaluated compounds

Mol ID	EC_{50} (Elisa p24)	EB[a]	RT interactions	Residues (H-bonds) Number of H bonds
M	230	− 6.95	vdW: Lys102 (A), Lys103 (A), Tyr181 (A), Phe227 (A), His235 (A)	Lys101 (A), Ile180 (A) Glu138 (B), Leu100 (A), Pro236 (A)
			Pi interactions: Leu100 (A), VAL106 (A), Tyr188 (A), Val179 (A), Leu 234 (A)	*5*
MR	120	− 5.02	vdW: Pro95 (A), Lys102 (A), Thr139 (B), Lys172 (A), Tyr188 (A), Phe227 (A), Trp229 (A), Leu234 (A), His235 (A)	Lys101 (A), Ile108 (A), Tyr318 (A)
			Pi interactions: Leu100 (A), Tyr181 (A), GLU138 (B), VAL179 (A)	*4*
			Alkil interactions: Lys102 (A), Val106 (A), Pro236 (A)	
MRG	45	2.38	vdW: Glu 28 (B) Lys 102 (A), Lys 103 (A), Val 106 (A), Ile 135 (A), Val 179 (A), Tyr 181 (A), Tyr 188 (A), Gly 190 (A) Asp 192 (A), Asp 320 (A)	Lys101, Glu138
			Pi interactions: Leu 100 (A), Pro 321 (A)	*2*

M myricetin, *MR* myricetin rhamnoside, *MRG* myricetin 3-(6-rhamnosylgalactoside). EC50: Antiviral activity (μM) measured by Elisa p24, *EB* free energy of binding (kcal/mol), *vdW* van der Waals interactions

[a] Note that the more positive the free energy of binding, the less likely the probability interaction

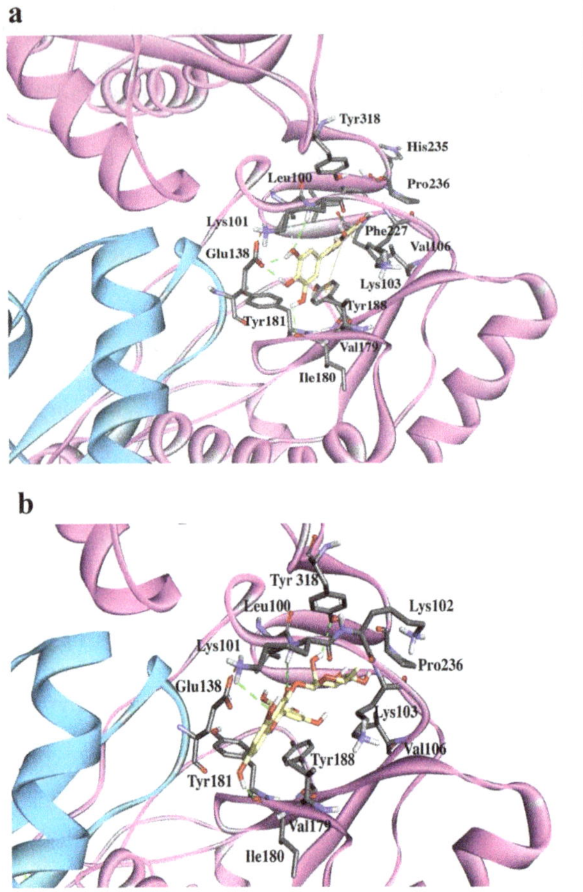

Fig. 4 Docking results. Best pose of M **a** and MR **b** into the no nucleoside binding pocket of HIV-1 RT. The ligand is shown in gold and residues involved in the interactions in gray. The hydrogen bonds are represented as a green dotted line

Trp229, Leu234, and Tyr318 of the p66 sub-unit and Glu138 of the p51 sub-unit. The analysis of the docked complexes emphasizes the relevant role of the H-bonds formed with residues Lys101, Ile 108, Ile 180, Tyr 318 and Glu 318. The results presented in this work are in agreement with those obtained by Syahdi in 2012 [31], which evaluated HIV RT docking of other flavonoids derived from plants and found that a hydrogen bond interaction with Lys101 is present on the docked pose with the lowest free energy of binding. From the docking analysis, myricetin might interact through five hydrogen bonds, while myricetin 3-rhamnoside through four hydrogen bonds and myricetin 3-(6-rhamnosylgalactoside) through only two. The number of hydrogen bonds formed is related to the free energy of binding found for each compound, and those molecules that can form a greater number of hydrogen bonds consequently create a more stable interaction.

Myricetin and the derivatives evaluates in this study have not been tested against HIV-1 resistant strains, nor mutant enzymes, in vitro to evaluate their capacity to inhibit viral replication of NNRTI resistant viruses. However, the docking study of myricetin on a RT enzyme with mutations conferring NNRTI resistance (L101I, K103N, and E138K) was performed with the protein models 1s1u, 1fkp and 2hny respectively. The analysis showed that the mutations did not result in significant changes in the free energy of binding levels, although with the L101I mutation, a small change in the orientation of myricetin in the binding pocket was observed. To better understand the possible effect of mutations, our laboratory is currently studying the interaction of myricetin in the NNRTI binding pocket through molecular dynamics simulations. We will also perform an in vitro analysis with NNRTI resistant strains of HIV-1 to determine the effect of the mutations on inhibitory action of these flavonoids derivatives.

Conclusions

The flavonoids are produced naturally as glycosides in plants and fruits but are found as aglycones in blood, as a consequence of the hydrolysis by glycosidases at the intestine lumen or inside the cell. The glycosylated flavonoids could be actively transported by SGLT1, with posterior hydrolysis within cytoplasm or they could be hydrolyzed at the cell surface and then enter the cell by diffusion. The existence of two different chemical forms of the flavonoid could generate a gradient constant favoring an increased concentration inside the cell.

The differences in the antiviral activity and the RT inhibition of the myricetin, MR and MRG together with the in silico analysis suggest that the glycosyl moiety could play a role in the entry of flavonoids into the cell and then, after enzymatic cleavage of the glycosyl moiety, the myricetin aglycone would ultimately be responsible for anti-HIV activity. This activity is presumed to be mediated primarily by the inhibition of RT, although interaction with other targets can't be discarded with the results described. Further studies are required to clarify the role of the glycosides in the activity/transport of myricetin and other related flavonoids.

Abbreviations

HIV: human immunodeficiency virus; RT: reverse transcriptase; MOI: multiplicity of infection; M: myricetin; MR: myricetin 3-rhamnoside; MRG: myricetin 3-(6-rhamnosylgalactoside); EC50: half effective concentration; CC50: half cytotoxic concentration; IC50: half inhibitory concentration.

Authors' contributions

This study was conceived and designed by JTO, HRR, MLS and FHP. JTO, HRR and MLS implemented the study and analyzed results. AIS and JB purified and characterized the compounds. JTO and HRR drafted the manuscript. All authors read and approved the final manuscript.

Author details
[1] Laboratorio de Virología Molecular, Centro de Microbiología y Biología Celular, Instituto Venezolano de Investigaciones Científicas, Caracas, Venezuela. [2] Laboratorio de Productos Naturales, Facultad de Farmacia, Universidad Central de Venezuela, Caracas, Venezuela. [3] Unidad de Química Medicinal, Facultad de Farmacia, Universidad Central de Venezuela, Caracas, Venezuela.

Acknowledgements
We thanks to Dr. José Domingo Medina for providing Myricetin. Also, we thanks to Dr. Stephen Tillett from Herbario Víctor Manuel Ovalles, Pharmacy School (Universidad Central de Venezuela) for the botanical identification and Dr Howard Takiff for the revision of English.

Competing interests
The authors declare that they have no competing interests.

Funding
This study was supported by Grant 495 to HRR, from the Instituto Venezolano de Investigaciones Científicas, Caracas, Venezuela.

References

1. UNAIDS. UNAIDS report on the global AIDS epidemic Geneva: Joint United Nations Programme on HIV/AIDS (UNAIDS). 2012. http://www.unaids.org/sites/default/files/media_asset/20121120_UNAIDS_Global_Report_2012_with_annexes_en_1.pdf. Accessed Jan 2017.
2. Collaboration Antiretroviral Therapy Cohort. Life expectancy of individuals on combination antiretroviral therapy in high-income countries: a collaborative analysis of 14 cohort studies. Lancet. 2008;372(9635):293–9.
3. Cihlar T, Fordyce M. Current status and prospects of HIV treatment. Curr Opin Virol. 2016;26(18):50–6.
4. Mukhtar M, Arshad M, Ahmad M, Pomerantz RJ, Wigdahl B, Parveen Z. Antiviral potentials of medicinal plants. Virus Res. 2008;131:111–20.
5. Naithani R, Huma LC, Holland LE, Shukla D, McCormick DL, Mehta RG, Moriarty RM. Antiviral activity of phytochemicals: a comprehensive review. Mini Rev Med Chem. 2008;8(11):1106–33.
6. Orhan DD, Ozçelik B, Ozgen S, Ergun F. Antibacterial, antifungal, and antiviral activities of some flavonoids. Microbiol Res. 2010;165(6):496–504.
7. Rathee P, Chaudhary H, Rathee S, Rathee D, Kumar V, Kohli K. Mechanism of action of flavonoids as anti-inflammatory agents: a review. Inflamm Allergy Drug Targets. 2009;8(3):229–35.
8. Hokche DO, Ramírez N. Sistemas reproductivos en especies de Melastomataceae en la Gran sabana (Estado Bolívar, Venezuela). Acta Botanica Venezuelica. 2008;31:387–408.
9. Berry PE, Luckana N. Melastomataceae. In: Berry PE, Yatskievych K, Holst BK, editors. Flora of the Venezuelan Guayana. Liliaceae-Myrsinaceae. 6th ed. Louis: Missouri Botanical Garden, St; 2001. p. 263–383.
10. Leite TC, de Sena AR, Dos Santos Silva TR, Dos Santos AK, Uetanabaro AP, Branco A. Antimicrobial activity of *Marcetia* DC species (Melastomataceae) and analysis of its flavonoids by reverse phase-high performance liquid chromatography coupled-diode array detector. Pharmacogn Mag. 2012;8(31):209–14.
11. Pasetto S, Pardi V, Murata RM. Anti-HIV-1 activity of flavonoid myricetin on HIV-1 infection in a dual-chamber in vitro model. PLoS ONE. 2014;29:e115323.
12. Ono K, Nakane H, Fukushima M, Chermann JC, Barré-Sinoussi F. Differential inhibitory effects of various flavonoids on the activities of reverse transcriptase and cellular DNA and RNA polymerases. Eur J Biochem. 1990;190(3):469–76.
13. De Clercq E. Antiretroviral drugs. Curr Opin Pharmacol. 2010;10(5):507–15.
14. Li S, Hattori T, Kodama EN. Epigallocatechin gallate inhibits the HIV reverse transcription step. Antivir Chem Chemother. 2011;21(6):239–43.
15. Sluis-Cremer N, Tachedjian G. Mechanisms of inhibition of HIV replication by nonnucleoside reverse transcriptase inhibitors. Virus Res. 2008;134(1–2):147–56.
16. Ortega JT, Estrada O, Serrano M, Contreras W, Orsini G, Pujol FH, Rangel HR. Glycosylated flavonoids from *Psidium guineense* as major inhibitors of HIV replication in vitro. Nat Prod Commun. 2017;12(7):1049–52.
17. Baptista J, Chavez K, Torrico F, Trejo E, García C, Urbina J, Carrasco J, Taddei A, Tillet S, Suarez AI. Constituyentes químicos y actividad antiinflamatoria de *Marcetia taxifolia*. CIENCIA. 2016;24(2):82–94.
18. Quintero A, Fabbro R, Maillo M, Barrios M, Milano MB, Fernández A, Williams B, Michelangeli F, Rangel HR, Pujol FH. Inhibition of hepatitis B virus and human immunodeficiency virus (HIV-1) replication by *Warscewiczia coccinea* (Vahl) Kl. (Rubiaceae) ethanol extract. Nat Prod Res. 2011;25(16):1565–9.
19. Berman H, Westbrook J, Feng G, Gilliland T, Bhat H, Weissig IN, Shindyalov PE. Bourne: the protein data bank. Nucleic Acids Res. 2000;28:235–42.
20. Das K, Martinez SE, Bauman JD, Arnold E. HIV-1 reverse transcriptase complex with DNA and nevirapine reveals non-nucleoside inhibition mechanism. Nat Struct Mol Biol. 2012;19(2):253–9.
21. Phillips J, Braun R, Wang W, Gumbart J, Tajkhorshid E, Villa E, Chipot C, Skeel R, Kale L, Schulten K. Scalable molecular dynamics with NAMD. J Comput Chem. 2005;26:1781–802.
22. Kim S, Thiessen PA, Bolton EE, Chen J, Fu G, Gindulyte A, Han L, He J, He S, Shoemaker BA, Wang J, Yu B, Zhang J, Bryant SH. PubChem substance and compound databases. Nucleic Acids Res. 2016;44(D1):D1202–13.
23. Jeong JJ, Kim DH. 5,7-Dihydroxy-6-methoxy-flavonoids eliminate HIV-1 D3-transfected cytoprotective macrophages by inhibiting the PI3K/Akt signaling pathway. Phytother Res. 2015. doi:10.1002/ptr.5388.
24. Namazi R, Zabihollahi R, Behbahani M, Rezaei A. Inhibitory activity of avicennia marina, a medicinal plant in persian folk medicine, against HIV and HSV. Iran J Pharm Res. 2013;12(2):435–43.
25. Sauter D, Schwarz S, Wang K, Zhang R, Sun B, Schwarz W. Genistein as antiviral drug against HIV ion channel. Planta Med. 2014;80(8–9):682–7.
26. Serra H, Mendes T, Bronze MR, Simplicio AL. Prediction of intestinal absorption and metabolism of pharmacologically active flavones and flavanones. Bioorg Med Chem. 2008;16:4009–18.
27. Walgren RA, Lin JT, Kinne RK, Walle T. Cellular uptake of dietary flavonoid quercetin 4′-beta-glucoside by sodium-dependent glucose transporter SGLT1. J Pharmacol Exp Ther. 2000;294(3):837–43.
28. Passamonti S, Terdoslavich M, Franca R, Vanzo A, Tramer F, Braidot E, Petrussa E, Vianello A. Bioavailability of flavonoids: a review of their membrane transport and the function of bilitranslocase in animal and plant organisms. Curr Drug Metab. 2009;10:369–94.
29. Tapiero H, Tew KD, Naguyen Ba G, Mathé G. Polyphenols: do the play a role in the prevention of human pathologies? Biomed Phamacother. 2002;56:200–2007.
30. Sarafianos SG, Marchand B, Das K, Himmel DM, Parniak MA, Hughes SH, Arnold E. Structure and function of HIV-1 reverse transcriptase: molecular mechanisms of polymerization and inhibition. J Mol Biol. 2009;385(3):693–713.
31. Syahdi RR, Mun'im A, Suhartanto H, Yanuar A. Virtual screening of Indonesian herbal database as HIV-1 reverse transcriptase inhibitor. Bioinformation. 2012;8(24):1206–10.

10

Molecular diagnosis of central nervous system opportunistic infections and mortality in HIV-infected adults

Rongrong Yang[1†], Hong Zhang[1†], Yong Xiong[1*], Xien Gui[1], Yongxi Zhang[1], Liping Deng[1], Shicheng Gao[1], Mingqi Luo[1], Wei Hou[2] and Deyin Guo[2]

Abstract

Background: CSF PCR is the standard diagnostic technique used in resource-rich settings to detect pathogens of the CNS infection. However, it is not currently used for routine CSF testing in China. Knowledge of CNS opportunistic infections among people living with HIV in China is limited.

Methods: Intensive cerebrospiral fluid (CSF) testing was performed to evaluate for bacterial, viral and fungal etiologies. Pathogen-specific primers were used to detect DNA from cytomegalovirus (CMV), herpes simplex virus (HSV), varicella-zoster virus (VZV), Epstein-Barr virus (EBV), human herpesvirus 6 (HHV-6) and John Cunningham virus (JCV) via real-time polymerase chain reaction (PCR).

Results: Cryptococcal meningitis accounted for 63.0% (34 of 54) of all causes of meningitis, 13.0% (7/54) for TB, 9.3% (5/54) for Toxoplasma gondii. Of 54 samples sent for viral PCR, 31.5% (17/54) were positive, 12 (22.2%) for CMV, 2 (3.7%) for VZV, 1 (1.9%) for EBV, 1 (1.9%) for HHV-6 and 1 (1.9%) for JCV. No patient was positive for HSV. Pathogen-based treatment and high GCS score tended to have a lower mortality rate, whereas patients with multiple pathogens infection, seizures or intracranial hypertension showed higher odds of death.

Conclusion: CNS OIs are frequent and multiple pathogens often coexist in CSF. Cryptococcal meningitis is the most prevalent CNS disorders among AIDS. The utility of molecular diagnostics for pathogen identification combined with the knowledge provided by the investigation may improve the diagnosis of AIDS related OIs in resource-limited developing countries, but the cost-efficacy remains to be further evaluated.

Keywords: AIDS, Central nervous system diseases, Cerebrospinal fluid

Background

Central nervous system (CNS) infectious is a major cause of morbidity and mortality among people living with human immunodeficiency virus (HIV) [1, 2]. Symptomatic neurological diseases happened in about 40–70% of HIV/AIDS patients during the course of their illness [1], and about 10–20% HIV/AIDS patients have neurologic symptoms as an initial manifestation [2, 3]. Studies indicated that opportunistic infections are the most common causes of neurologic diseases in HIV/AIDS patients in developing countries [4–8]. In China, lumbar puncture (LP) is a routine practice and cerebrospinal fluid (CSF) is commonly collected for patients with suspected diagnosis of CNS infection. However, the available and frequently-used means of diagnosis are generally limited to CSF routine and biochemical tests, Gram stain, India ink stain, cryptococcal antigen (CrAg) detection, and bacterial/fungal cultures. As a result, country-specific data in our hospital regarding prevalence of CNS disorders are sparse, and many patients remain misdiagnosed and inadequately treated.

In resource-rich settings, the standard diagnostic technique used to identify the presence of viral, parasitic, and

*Correspondence: yongxiong64@163.com
†Rongrong Yang and Hong Zhang contributed equally to this article
[1] Department of Infectious Diseases, Zhongnan Hospital of Wuhan University, 169 Donghu Road, Wuhan 430071, China

specific bacterial infection of the CNS disorders is CSF polymerase chain reaction (PCR); however, in China in HIV-infected patients, CSF PCR is not currently used for routine tests. The prevalence data regarding CNS infectious diagnosed via PCR in China was particularly absent at present. In this study, CSF samples were tested for CMV, HSV, VZV, EBV, HHV-6 and JCV via PCR. The prevalence of CNS OIs in HIV-infected Chinese adults and their impact on patient outcomes were determined.

Methods

Patients population

This hospital-based study was conducted at Zhongnan Hospital of Wuhan University, China, between 1 December 2012 and 30 September 2014. Patients were eligible for the study if they had: (1) confirmed with HIV infection; (2) three or more symptoms of meningitis and/or encephalitis (headache, seizure, nausea/vomiting, alteration in consciousness, photophobia, or a focal neurological deficit); and (3) agreed to do a lumbar puncture(LP), as determined by the attending physician. Exclusion criteria for enrollment included: (1) patients with delirium, such as sepsis due to a non-neurological infection or metabolic abnormality; (2) patients with peripheral neuropathy and psychosis rather than medical explanation for their symptoms; or (3) patients with a documented immunosuppressive except for HIV infection or neurosurgical illness. Meningitis was diagnosed if there was a combination of meningeal irritation symptoms and signs and the presence of more than five white blood cells in CSF obtained by lumbar puncture. Exclusion criteria included malignancies, various inflammatory conditions, sarcoidosis, and infectious secondary to procedures. Meningoencephalitis was defined as any brain parenchymal involvement (e.g. seizures), behavioral change, confusion, dysphasia and other cortical deficits, with signs of meningeal irritation. Encephalitis was defined as fever with altered sensorium with CSF pleocytosis and raised protein with or without focal neurological signs in whom malaria, bacterial or fungal meningitis were excluded. Trained radiologists and neurologists were also invited to help identifying patients with a suspected diagnosis of meningitis, encephalitis or meningoencephalitis. The study was approved by Zhongnan Hospital of Wuhan University Ethics Committee.

Demographic information, such as age, gender, marital status, risk factors, duration between HIV infection and hospital admission, clinical features and past medical history were collected on a standardized report form by the trained physician. In China, lumbar puncture (LP) is routine practice for patients with a suspected CNS infection prior to antibiotic treatment. Other important medical assessment were computed tomography (CT) or magnetic resonance imaging (MRI) for patients with a focal brain lesion or suspected brain hemorrhage. But whether the imaging examination ultimately used depends on the patients' or their family members' willingness and attitude.

CSF testing

All CSF samples were collected via lumbar puncture and stored at −20 °C for molecular diagnostics. DNA was isolated by using the easyMAG Instrument (bioMérieux). Primers amplifying a conserved sequence of viral DNA polymerase (BALF5) gene and a fluorogenic probe were used at a primer concentration of 0.9 μM and a probe concentration of 0.25 μM. Amplification was carried out in an ABI PRISM 7900 HT Sequence Detector (PE Applied Biosystems) and the standard curve was created with Sequence Detection System software by plotting the CT values against known CMV, EBV, JCV, VZV, HHV-6, HSV or TB-DNA concentrations. The assay has a detection limit of 500 genome equivalents/ml.

Statistical analysis

Continuous data are presented as mean ± standard deviation (for normally distributed variables) or median and interquartile range or IQR (for variable influenced by extreme values). Categorical data are presented as numbers with proportions. *P*-values were 2-sided and considered statistically significant if <0.05. Statistical analyses were performed using SPSS for Windows, version 19.0 (SPSS, Chicago, IL).

Results

Patient characteristics

In this study, 57 patients with CNS diseases out of 658 hospitalized AIDS (≥14 years old) were admitted to Zhongnan Hospital of Wuhan University with a complaint of new or recurrent neurological or psychiatric symptoms were included (Fig. 1). Of these 57 patients, complete clinical information was available in 54 (94.7%). Forty-one cases of meningitis, six cases of encephalitis and seven cases of meningoencephalitis were found in this series. Characteristics of the 54 patients are shown in Table 1. The mean age was 38 years and 64.8% of participants were male. The main occupational population was farmer (70.4%). And the main HIV acquisition route was sexual contact (79.6%). At the time of enrollment, a median duration of 45 days was observed. The median $CD4^{+}$ T cell count was 31 cells/μl.

Pathogen(s) detecting in CSF

Pathogens were detected in 47 (87.0%) CSF samples. The number of patients diagnosed with one or more pathogens is shown in Table 2. *Cryptococcus neoformans* was

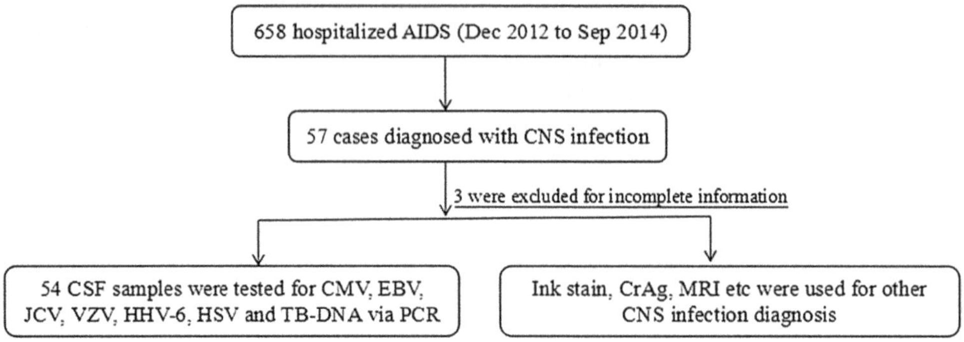

Fig. 1 Study profile

Table 1 Patient demographics (N = 54)

Feature	No (%)
Age (years), mean (SD)	38 (11.2)
Male	35 (64.8)
Occupation	
Farmers	38 (70.4)
Clerk	8 (14.8)
Businessman	4 (7.4)
Others	4 (7.4)
HIV transmission route	
Sex	43 (79.6)
Blood donation/transfusion	6 (11.1)
IDU	2 (3.7)
Unknown	3 (5.6)
Days since HIV diagnosis, median (IQR)	45 (1–732)
$CD4^+$ T cells/μl, median (IQR)	31 (21–83)

SD standard deviation

the most common pathogen found (63.0%) and the most common copathogen (22.2%). There were high rates of detection of CMV (22.2%) and tuberculosis (13.0%). We also detected VZV (3.7%), JCV (1.9%), EBV (1.9%) and HHV-6 (1.9%) in this patient population. No case of HSV were detected by PCR.

Results of PCR positive pathogen(s) detected by other methods

Of the 34 cases with cryptococcus, three were negative on India Ink (8.8%), and four were negative on CrAg (11.8%).

Of five PCR diagnosed toxoplasmosis in this series, all responded clinically and radiographically within four weeks of initiation of pyrimethamine and clindamycin combination therapy.

Among the 12 CMV-DNA positive patients, 8 (66.7%) serum samples were negative for CMV-DNA and the average level of CMV-DNA in CSF was 2.80 ± 1.15 Log_{10}copies/ml.

Among five patients diagnosed toxoplasmosis, brain CT or MRI was used for four patients. The representative ring enhancing lesions were found in all the four patients.

For the EBV-DNA positive patient, mass lesions were not found. For the JCV-DNA positive patient, typical

Table 2 Characteristics of patients with CSF pathogen(s)

Pathogens	Individual CSF prevalence	1 pathogen	No. of cases	2 pathogens	No. of cases	3 pathogens	No. of cases
Crypto[a]	34/54 (63.0%)	Crypto	22	Crypto/CMV	7	Crypto/TB/CMV	2
				Crypto/VZV	1	Crypto/TB/HHV-6	1
				Crypto/JCV	1		
CMV	12/54 (22.2%)	CMV	2	CMV/TB	1		
TB	7/54 (13.0%)	TB	3				
Toxop	5/54 (9.3%)	Toxop	5				
VZV	2/54 (3.7%)	VZV	1				
JCV	1/54 (1.9%)	JCV	0				
EBV	1/54 (1.9%)	EBV	1				
HHV-6	1/54 (1.9%)	HHV-6	0				
HSV	0/54 (0%)	HSV	0				
Total	63 pathogens	34/54 (63.0%)		10/54 (18.5%)		3/54 (5.6%)	

white matter changes were found, which was consistent with the PCR for JCV.

Among 12 CMV-DNA positive patients, brain CT or MRI was used for 6 patients and none was found with brain parenchymal lesion.

Risk factors associated with mortality

In our study population, the total mortality rate was 22.2% (12/54). Table 3 summarizes the potential risk factors of death in our study population. The odds of death together with 95% confidence intervals were reported for each covariate. In the multivariate analysis, pathogen-based treatment and high glasgow coma scale (GCS) score were associated with lower odds of death. Conversely, patients with multiple pathogens infection, seizures or intracranial hypertension showed higher odds of death.

Discussion

This hospital-based study provides information about the spectrum of pathogens causing CNS infections and mortality among people living with HIV in Zhongnan Hospital of Wuhan University in central China. The spectrum of HIV-associated central nervous system disorders may be influenced by differences in the epidemiology.

We identified a microbiologic diagnosis for clinical meningitis in a cohort of HIV-infected Chinese inpatients. Our data suggested that the most common pathogen causing meningitis is Cryptococcus neoformans. The most common viral pathogen causing meningitis is CMV and that the most common bacterial pathogen is TB. Our finding highlighted the utility of molecular diagnostics for improving pathogen identification for CNS infections.

The HIV epidemic has caused a marked increase in cases of cryptococcal meningitis such that it has become the leading cause of meningitis among patients living with HIV [9–11]. We found that cryptococcal meningitis caused the majority of meningitis among hospitalized AIDS patients, which accounted for 63.0% of all causes of meningitis in this study. In a review, the total cryptococcal meningitis prevalence was 52.0% in sub-Saharan Africa [12]. Our relatively high prevalence may be attributable to different methodologies and tests used for assessing prevalence; differences in host factors; or geographic variations in the epidemiology of cryptococcal meningitis.

The prevalence of toxoplasma gondii in this study are higher than previously reported from a study in Zambian [13]. In our study population, the median $CD4^+$ T-cell count was 31 cells/μl and all were newly diagnosed with HIV and without any prophylaxis treatment, whereas in Zambian [13] study, the enrollment $CD4^+$ T-cell count was 81 cells/μl in men and 99 cells/μl in women, and 118 (35.6%) patients were on cART for a median duration of 240 days. The patient population and the presence of anti-Toxoplasma treatment may account for the high present of *Toxoplasma gondii.*

Table 3 Variables associate with death in univariate and multivariate analysis

Variable	Univariate analysis		Multivariate analysis	
	Odds ratio (95% CI)	*P* value	Odds ratio (95% CI)	*P* value
Categorical				
Male	0.58 (0.30–1.32)	0.26		
cART status	0.48 (0.30–2.22)	0.56		
Multiple pathogens	0.33 (0.14–0.56)	<0.0001	0.46 (0.26–0.74)	0.002
Cryptococcal meningitis	1.32 (0.80–2.34)	0.22		
CMV	1.21 (0.58–2.33)	0.74		
Tuberculosis	0.63 (0.88–3.26)	0.30		
EBV	0.70 (0.44–1.33)	0.23		
Other pathogens	0.85 (0.44–1.63)	0.53		
Pathogen-based treatment	5.7 (2.0–17.6)	<0.0001	4.8 (2.4–16.5)	0.001
Seizures	0.87 (0.33–1.42)	0.08	0.52 (0.36–0.98)	0.04
Intracranial hypertension	0.27 (0.18–0.84)	0.04	0.33 (0.22–0.84)	0.03
Disturbance of consciousness	0.67 (0.43–1.04)	0.06	1.00 (0.46–2.18)	0.99
Continuous				
Age	0.36 (0.14–0.89)	0.08	0.56 (0.32–1.02)	0.25
GCS	0.22 (0.12–0.32)	<0.0001	0.42 (0.21–0.80)	0.001
CD4 count	0.66 (0.45–1.24)	0.68		

GCS Glasgow coma scale

Cytomegalovirus is a ubiquitous agent that can cause infection at any time during the course of life and commonly infects individuals from diverse geographical and socio-economic backgrounds [14, 15]. By serology, a study reports that 93.9% of the HIV infection patients were positive for anti-CMV IgG antibody [16]. But in most patients, the diseases caused by CMV is so mild that it is overlooked. AIDS patients are commonly positive for CMV when sick with other illnesses. Diagnosis of CMV infection from tissue biopsies is considered the gold standard with specificity for histopathological evaluation near 100% but with low sensitivity (23.2%) [17]. In this study through PCR for CMV-DNA, 12 out of 54 (22.2%) CSF samples were positive. Whether the CMV is truly pathogenic or simply an innocent bystander remains to be further identified. Among the 12 patients with CMV-DNA positive in CSF, 8 (66.7%) serum samples were negative for CMV-DNA and the average level of CMV-DNA in CSF was 2.80 ± 1.15 Log_{10} copies/ml. Among 12 CMV-DNA positive patients, brain CT or MRI was used for six patients. None patient was found with brain parenchymal lesion. These features supported a low CMV burden which is combination with the negative PCR in the blood favored the argument of CMV being a bystander.

Cerebral toxoplasmosis is a very relevant neurological disease in individuals with AIDS [18]. In this study, toxoplasma is the fourth most common pathogen in CNS disorders. Among five patients diagnosed toxoplasmosis, brain CT or MRI was used for four patients. The representative ring enhancing lesions were found in all the four patients. The limited data imply PCR for the diagnosis of toxoplasmosis was accurate and reliable. Of 5 PCR diagnosed toxoplasmosis in this series, all responded clinically and radiographically within four weeks of initiation of pyrimethamine and clindamycin combination therapy. Although DNA positive in serum or cerebrospinal fluid can be diagnosed as Toxoplasma infection, the policy of empiric treatment of suspected Toxoplasma encephalitis is still satisfactory and recommendable. For patients with AIDS and suspected Toxoplasma encephalitis, early diagnosis and initiation of empiric treatment and antiretroviral therapy are important for good prognosis.

EBV is consider to be associated with primary CNS lymphoma in HIV infected patient, though further diagnostics for evaluation are lacking in this study. Detection of EBV DNA from a CSF sample may represent replication of EBV within B lymphocytes, and it was also closely related to an increased risk of death [19]. Neuroimaging was not obtained as part of this study. However, in the EBV PCR-positive patients with neuroimaging, mass lesions were not found. Therefore, we speculated that EBV might be a non-pathogenic marker of immunodepression, being shed from activated B-cells trafficking into the CSF during meningitis. Further investigation on the significance of EBV in the CSF is needed. Quantitative and comparison values from the CSF and serum is necessary to distinguish those with CNS lymphoma from those with non-pathogenic presence of EBV.

HIV strain and host susceptibility factors were thought to be less tendentious to infection by JCV, the pathogen of progressive multifocal leukoencephalopathy (PML). Indeed, the JCV CSF-positive patient had neurological symptoms consistent with PML. The sole JCV-DNA positive patients received brain imaging examination, white matter changes were found, which was consistent with the PCR for JCV.

Seroprevalence of CNS HSV infection has previously been documented at 47.2% in an urban Zambian population [20]. However, HSV DNA was not detected in any CSF samples in our study population. This is likely because the sample in our series is small and because our study used a different detection method (HSV-DNA PCR in CSF) as the Zambian population [20] (HSV IgG ELISA in serum).

In our study population, the total mortality rate was 22.2% (12/54). This rate of mortality is lower than reported in Zambian at the beginning of the AIDS epidemic [13]. Our study was not designed for long-term follow-up. It is possible that death occurred in the post-hospitalization period due to loss of follow-up, poor compliance with treatment, and poor access to emergency health services. As expected, the actual mortality was higher than 22.2%.

Our study shows that numerous pathogens can be found in the CSF of HIV-infected patients presenting with neurological symptoms in China, and the mortality of this population is very high. There was a high prevalence of co-infection in the CSF, indicative of severe immunodepression in this population. This finding warrant a more in dept study in the future since in resource-limited settings, patients present with advance immunodepression and the high morbidity and mortality associated with this condition will continue to bring great challenges to clinicians. Multiple pathogens infection in CNS disorder patients will be an important topic to assess with further study in larger cohorts and with subsequent validation of results.

Diagnostic testing for a broad array of CSF pathogens may be helpful in resource-limited settings to avoid unnecessary treatments and achieve better prognosis. For TB diagnosis, the Xpert MTD/RIF assay is a fully automated nucleic acid amplification testing (NAAT) that can deliver a result for MTB and rifampin resistance in about 2 h. On the basis of studies in countries with high tuberculosis burden, Xpert has been endorsed by the World Health Organization and widely deployed [21–28]. In contrast to other NAATs, Xpert can be performed on-demand by personnel with minimal training [28, 29]. The present study supports analysed suggesting that Xpert implementation in the United States is efficient and cost-effective [30]. Therefore, in resource-limited countries, establishment of Xpert is one of the ways to attempt improving the clinical diagnosis level about TB infection in CNS among AIDS patients.

Our study had some limitations. First, the generalizability of our research finding is limited. Since our hospital is the sole comprehensive hospital well-known for AIDS treatment in Hubei province, we can make some general assumptions regarding CNS infection in a province in China. Second, the number of specific pathogens for PCR testing was limited and there are other possible etiologies of CNS infection, but were not assessed in our study. Last but not least, the detection samples associated with the study were limited to CSF, which may be incomplete for diagnosis since pathogens can present in the CSF transiently. For many types of CNS infections, serologic detection on the presence of virus-specific IgM antibodies in serum or a rise in antibody titer can be useful; this study did not include serologic assays.

In this series, in addition to the molecular testing, Cryptococcus can be diagnosed with India Ink and CrAg, TB can be diagnosed with Xpert, and Toxoplasmosis can frequently be managed using an empirical strategy. Meanwhile, some pathogens such as EBV and JCV have no specific, effective treatment, while others such as CMV and HHV-6 require specialized therapies that are frequently unavailable in a resource limited setting. Disease burden, economic pressure, health resource and severity of diseases are critical factors which can effect the cost-efficacy of running a molecular laboratory. In China, we believed that the molecular testing can only be recommended under conditioned circumstances, rather than prioritized under all circumstances.

In conclusion, this study provides baseline data regarding the etiology distribution of CNS infections among hospitalized patients living with HIV/AIDS in a comprehensive Chinese hospital. It reported that the most etiology was cryptococcal meningitis (63.0%). Even as high as 22.2% of CMV DNA positive rate was found in this study, more than half were proved to be an innocent bystander. During periods of severe immunosuppression, AIDS patients with unrecognized CNS opportunistic infections are at high risk of death; thus, efforts should be focused in improving rates of pathogen diagnosis in this vulnerable group. CSF PCR, which is the standard diagnostic technique used in resource-rich settings to detect etiology infections of the CNS, is not currently used for suspected CNS disorder patients in China. Due to limited resources, whether CSF PCR should be prioritized needs to consider the patients' economic ability.

Abbreviations

CNS: central nervous system; AIDS: acquired immunodeficiency syndrome; CMV: cytomegalovirus; EBV: Epstein-Barr virus; JCV: JC polyomavirus; VZV: varicella-zoster virus; HHV-6: human herpesvirus 6; HSV: herpes simplex viruses; CSF: cerebrospinal fluid.

Authors' contributions

RRY, HZ and YX devised the study, advised on data analysis and participated in interpreting the data and reviewing the manuscript. XE Gi,YXZ, LPD, SCG and MQL advised on data analysis and participated in interpreting the data and reviewing the manuscript. WH and DYG participated in its design and coordination and helped to draft the manuscript. All authors read and approved the final manuscript.

Author details

[1] Department of Infectious Diseases, Zhongnan Hospital of Wuhan University, 169 Donghu Road, Wuhan 430071, China. [2] Basic Medical College of Wuhan University, Wuhan, China.

Acknowledgements

We would like to acknowledge and thank all staff in the Department of Infectious Diseases, Zhongnan Hospital of Wuhan University.

Competing interests

The authors declare that they have no competing interests.

Funding

This study was supported by the National Science and Technology Major Project of China (2014ZX10001003).

References

1. Weisberg LA. Neurologic abnormalities in human immunodeficiency virus infection. South Med J. 2001;94(3):266–75.
2. Levy RM, Bredesen DE. Central nervous system dysfunction in acquired immunodeficiency syndrome. J Acquir Immune Defic Syndr. 1988;1(1):41–64.
3. Sacktor N, Lyles RH, Skolasky R, Kleeberger C, Selnes OA, Miller EN, et al. HIV associated neurologic disease incidence changes: multicenter AIDS Cohort Study, 1990–1998. Neurology. 2001;56(2):257–60.
4. Bhigjee AI, Naidoo K, Patel VB, Govender D. Intracranial mass lesions in HIV-positive Patients-the KwaZulu/Natal experience. Neuroscience AIDS Research Group. S Afr Med J. 1999;89(12):1284–8.
5. Fragoso YD, Mendes V, Adamo AP, Bosco LP, Tavares CA. Neurologic manifestations of AIDS: a review of fifty cases in Santos, Sao Paulo, Brazil. Sao Paulo Med J. 1998;116(3):1715–20.
6. Isezuo SA, Sani AZ, Ezunu E, Maiyaki S, Njoku CH, Obembe A. Clinical neuropathy in HIV/AIDS: an eight-year review of hospitalized patients in Sokoto, northwestern Nigeria. Trop Doct. 2009;39(3):133–5.

7. Modi M, Mochan A, Modi G. Management of HIV-associated focal brain lesions in developing countries. QJM. 2004;97(7):413–21.
8. World Health Organization. WHO case definitions of HIV for surveillance and revised clinical staging and immunological classification of HIV-related disease in adults and children. Geneva: World Health Organization; 2007. p. 10–38.
9. Bekondi C, Bernede C, Passone N, Minssart P, Kamalo C, Mbolidi D, et al. Primary and opportunistic pathogens associated with meningitis in adults in Bangui, Central African Republic, in relation to human immunodeficiency virus serostatus. Int J Infect Dis. 2006;10(5):387–95.
10. Cohen DB, Zijlstra EE, Mukaka M, Reiss M, Kamphambale S, Scholing M, et al. Diagnosis of crytococcal and tuberculous meningitis in a resource-limited African setting. Trop Med Int Health. 2010;15(8):910–7.
11. Bisson GP, Lukes J, Thakur R, Mtoni I, MacGregor RR. Cryptococcus and lymphocytic meningitis in Botswana. S Afr Med J. 2008;98(9):724–5.
12. Veltman JA, Bristow CC, Klausner JD. Meningitis in HIV-positive patients in sub-Saharan Africa: a review. J Int AIDS Soc. 2014;17:19184.
13. Siddiqi OK, Ghebremichael M, Dang X, Atadzhanov M, Kaonga P, Khoury MN, et al. Molecular diagnosis of central nervous system opportunistic infections in HIV-infected Zambian adults. Clin Infect Dis. 2014;58:1771–7.
14. Akinbami AA, Akanmu AS, Adeyemo TA, Wright KO, Dada MO, Dosunmu AO. Cytomegalovirus anti-bodies among healthy blood donors at Lagos University Teaching Hospital. S Afr Med J. 2009;99(7):528–30.
15. Spector SA, Wong R, Hsia K, et al. Plasma cytomegalovirus(CMV) DNA load predicts CMV disease and survival in AIDS patients. J Clin Invest. 1998;101:497–502.
16. Fowotade A, Okonko IO, Agbede OO, Suleiman ST. High seropositivity of IgG and IgM antibodies against cytomegalovirus (CMV) among HIV-1 seropositive patients in Ilorin. Nigeria. Afr Health Sci. 2015;15(1):1–9.
17. Kotler DP, Reka S, Borcich A, Cronin WJ. Detection, localization, and quantitation of HIV-associated antigens in intestinal biopsies from patients with HIV. Am J Pathol. 1991;139:823–30.
18. Manzardo C, Del Mar Ortega M, Sued O, Garcia F, Moreno A, Miro JM. Central nervous system opportunistic infections in developed countries in the highly active antiretroviral therapy era. J Neurovirol. 2005;11(suppl 3):72–82.
19. Kelly MJ, Benjamin LA, Cartwright K, et al. Epstein-Barr virus coinfection in cerebrospinal fluid is associated with increased mortality in Malawian adults with bacterial meningitis. J Infect Dis. 2012;205:106–10.
20. Weiss HA, Buve A, Robinson NJ, et al. The epidemiology of HSV-2 infection and its association with HIV infection in four urban African population. AIDS. 2001;15(suppl 4):s97–108.
21. Denkinger CM, Schumacher SG, Boehme CC, Dendukuri N, Pai M, Steingart KR. Xpert MTB/RIF assay for the diagnosis of extrapulmonary tuberculosis: a systematic review and meta-analysis. Eur Respir J. 2014;44(2):435–46.
22. Steingart KR, Schiller I, Horne DJ, Pai M, Boehme CC, Dendukuri N. Xpert MTB/RIF assay for pulmonary tuberculosis and rifampicin resistance in adults. Cochrane Database Syst Rev. 2014;4:CD009593.
23. World Health Organization. Tuberculosis diagnostics: Xpert MTB/RIF test. http://www.who.int/tb/publications/Xpert_factsheet.pdf. Accessed 21 Nov 2014.
24. Zwerling A, White RG, Vassall A, Cohen T, Dowdy DW, Houben RM. Modeling of novel diagnostic strategies for active tuberculosis-a systematic review: current practices and recommendations. PLoS ONE. 2014;9:e110558.
25. Langley I, Lin HH, Squire SB. Cost-effectiveness of Xpert MTB/RIF and investing in health care in African. Lancet Glob Health. 2015;3:e83–4.
26. Lawn SD, Mwaba P, Bates M, et al. Advances in tuberculosis diagnostics: the Xpert MTB/RIF assay and future prospects for a point-of-care test. Lancet Infect Dis. 2013;13:349–61.
27. Creswell J, Codlin AJ, Andre E, et al. Results from early programmatic implementation of Xpert MTB/RIF testing in nine countries. BMC Infect Dis. 2014;14:2.
28. Cowan JF, Michel C, Manhica I, et al. Implementing rapid testing for tuberculosis in Mozambique. Bull World Health Organ. 2015;93:125–30.
29. Boehme CC, Nabeta P, Hillemann D, et al. Rapid molecular detection of tuberculosis and rifampin resistance. N Engl J Med. 2010;363:1005–15.
30. Cowan JF, Chandler AS, Kracen E, Park DR, Wallis CK, Liu E, Song C, Persing DH, Fang FC. Clinical impact and cost-effectiveness of Xpert MTB/RIF testing in hospitalized patients with presumptive pulmonary tuberculosis in the United States. Clin Infect Dis. 2017;64(4):482–9.

11

Joint longitudinal data analysis in detecting determinants of CD4 cell count change and adherence to highly active antiretroviral therapy at Felege Hiwot Teaching and Specialized Hospital, North-west Ethiopia (Amhara Region)

Awoke Seyoum[1*], Principal Ndlovu[2] and Zewotir Temesgen[3]

Abstract

Background: Adherence and CD4 cell count change measure the progression of the disease in HIV patients after the commencement of HAART. Lack of information about associated factors on adherence to HAART and CD4 cell count reduction is a challenge for the improvement of cells in HIV positive adults. The main objective of adopting joint modeling was to compare separate and joint models of longitudinal repeated measures in identifying long-term predictors of the two longitudinal outcomes: CD4 cell count and adherence to HAART.

Methods: A longitudinal retrospective cohort study was conducted to examine the joint predictors of CD4 cell count change and adherence to HAART among HIV adult patients enrolled in the first 10 months of the year 2008 and followed-up to June 2012. Joint model was employed to determine joint predictors of two longitudinal response variables over time. Furthermore, the generalized linear mixed effect model had been used for specification of the marginal distribution, conditional to correlated random effect.

Results: A total of 792 adult HIV patients were studied to analyze the longitudinal joint model study. The result from this investigation revealed that age, weight, baseline CD4 cell count, ownership of cell phone, visiting times, marital status, residence area and level of disclosure of the disease to family members had significantly affected both outcomes. From the two-way interactions, time * owner of cell phone, time * sex, age * sex, age * level of education as well as time * level of education were significant for CD4 cell count change in the longitudinal data analysis. The multivariate joint model with linear predictor indicates that CD4 cell count change was positively correlated ($p \leq 0.0001$) with adherence to HAART. Hence, as adherence to HAART increased, CD4 cell count also increased; and those patients who had significant CD4 cell count change at each visiting time had been encouraged to be good adherents.

Conclusion: Joint model analysis was more parsimonious as compared to separate analysis, as it reduces type I error and subject-specific analysis improved its model fit. The joint model operates multivariate analysis simultaneously; and it has great power in parameter estimation. Developing joint model helps validate the observed correlation between the outcomes that have emerged from the association of intercepts. There should be a special attention and intervention for HIV positive adults, especially for those who had poor adherence and with low CD4 cell count

*Correspondence: bisrategebrail@yahoo.com
[1] Department of Statistics, Bahir Dar University, Bahir Dar, Ethiopia

change. The intervention may be important for pre-treatment counseling and awareness creation. The study also identified a group of patients who were with maximum risk of CD4 cell count change. It is suggested that this group of patients needs high intervention for counseling.

Keywords: HAART, Multivariate longitudinal data, Joint model, Adherence, CD4 cell count change

Background

Sub-Saharan Africa has the most serious HIV and AIDs epidemic in the world. In 2013, approximately 24.7 million people were living with HIV, accounting for 71% of the global total. In the same year, there were around 1.5 million new HIV infections and 1.1 million AIDs-related deaths. The 2013 report indicates that, in sub-Saharan African countries, the prevalence rate among both female and male sex workers was still high (13%) [1]. Ethiopia, as one of these countries has been affected by the epidemic with a prevalence of 1.5% [2]. Its burden has been high in the Amhara Region, including the catchment area of Felege Hiwot Teaching and Specialized Hospital [3]. Because of its large population size, the Amhara region has the largest Prevalence of human immunodeficiency virus [3]. Although the HIV prevalence shows a decreasing rate, still it bears a significant proportion of the epidemic burden as compared to the national and worldwide encumbrance [4]. HIV affects the CD4 cell count in the human body, so it can be employed to make appropriate decisions for the initiation of HAART and proper management of the progression of the infection [5, 6]. Patients' CD4 cell count should recover/rebound/at least to the lower limit of the CD4 cell count for the general healthy adult population (500 cells/mm^3), which, otherwise, can be an indication of immunologic failure [7].

In addition to HIV, there are also other factors affecting CD4 cell count changes. Some of these are demographic variables such as age (older ages are predictors of lower count response to HAART) [7, 8], sex (females experience better CD4 count response to HAART compared to males) [9, 10], and residence area (rural patients who start ART with a deteriorated CD4 cell count at the initiation of HAART poorly respond to HAART [11]. Previous studies also indicate that WHO's clinical stage is an independent predictor of CD4 cell count at enrolment [12]. Other investigators state that there is a positive association between baseline CD4 cell count and its size after initiation of treatment [13, 14]; however, this result was inconsistent with the result of other studies [8]. Identifying factors which influence the level of CD4 cell count other than HAART helps health professionals and patients to facilitate proper management and monitoring of health care interventions to be effective. Moreover, it helps check whether or not HIV patients who initiate HAART with baseline CD4 cell count $\leq$200 cells/mm^3 recover to the normal range of CD4 cell count after commencement of HAART [7].

On the other hand, the principal factors associated with non-adherence appear to be patient-related factors including substance and alcohol abuse [15]. However, other factors such as inconvenient dosing frequency, dietary restrictions, pill burden and side-effects, poor patient–care service provider relationships and poor care service provision may also contribute to the failure of adherence [16]. Another study disclosed that different factors such as sex, residence area, and ownership of cell phone contributed to patents' irregular use of medications [17]. Another investigation indicated that patients' current substance use concerning HAART, their beliefs about the necessity of HAART, and their trust in the HIV care provider are determinants for their non-adherence [18].

In HAART treatment, the number of CD4 cell count and adherence to HAART are measured repeatedly over time [15]. Patients' improvement of adherence to HAART provides progression of CD4 cell count in the blood of HIV patients; and this increment of CD4 cell count at every visiting time encourages the patient to be a good adherent to HAART [19]. Hence, the above findings indicated that there are discrepancies among the findings of different studies. This discrepancy of findings suggests that identifying and overcoming the factors that reduce adherence to antiretroviral agents is of utmost importance for prolonged CD4 cell count progression and viral load suppression [15].

A number of key issues are raised in the study of adherence to antiretroviral therapy and CD4 cell count change, determinants that affect jointly, and the development of interventions. Addressing these issues may provide valuable information about which patients are most at risk for non-adherence and about how adherence can be improved. It is well known that non-adherence in the treatment of HIV compromises the effectiveness of therapy or progression of CD4 cell count change [20].

In many practical situations, we observed two or more longitudinal outcomes that need joint modeling of the response variables to identify predictors that affected jointly. Joint models are used to describe the joint behavior of the two response variables simultaneously. These responses may have varied characteristics; that is, they might be binary, ordinal or continuous in nature.

Many previous studies had employed joint models of longitudinal outcomes and time to event [21–24]. Many of these methods were used for the joint modeling of longitudinal data and survival process outcomes, which have typically allowed a univariate outcome and a solitary event time. These studies did not consider two longitudinal values observed repeatedly from the same subject and lacked multivariate analysis of two repeatedly observed results. Joint modeling between two longitudinal outcome variables has advantages in reducing type I error rates in multiple tests with repeated observation on the same subject and improves efficiency in estimating parameters [25]. Thus, the current study was conducted with the objective of reviewing Generalized Linear Mixed Model (GLMM) approach that can be extended for multivariate longitudinal data by assuming separate random effect on each outcome variable, and then combining them by imposing a joint multivariate distribution on the random effect. This approach has an advantage of having additional correlation emerging from the longitudinal data structure that can be modeled with the same frame-work, and compare the separate and joint models with respect to parameter estimation in longitudinal data analysis. To the best of our knowledge, no other study has been conducted to assess factors affecting jointly these two longitudinal inter-related outcomes (CD4 cell count & adherence to HAART) around the study area.

Methods and data analysis

Study design

A retrospective cohort study was conducted to assess joint predictors of CD4 cell count change and adherence to HAART among adult HAART users enrolled in the first 10 months of 2008 and followed-up to June 2012. Joint modeling between count and ordinal responses was conducted.

Study area and population

The study was conducted at Felege-Hiwot Teaching and Specialized Hospital located in North-western Ethiopia, Amhara Region. The population of the study included HIV positive adults who initiated HAART treatment at Felege-Hiwot Teaching and Specialized Hospital.

Sample size and sampling procedure

From the total HIV positive adults who started HAART in the hospital from September 2008 to June 2012, 792 were selected using residence-based stratified random sampling technique. Patients with a minimum of 2 visits and a maximum of 23 visits were included in the study.

Data collection procedures

The study exclusively used secondary data. Therefore, a data extraction check-list was designed and used to adopt the routinely collected data. A baseline CD4 cell count data was identified and collected from the registration documents of HAART attendants. The first month adherence was also considered as covariate for longitudinal joint study. Similarly, other characteristics like socio-demographic variables, visiting times and clinical data were also collected from the registration documents of patients. The data were collected by health care service providers after they had been given adequate orientation about the variables included in the study.

Data structure, compilation and analysis strategy

Secondary data were entered and analyzed using SAS version 9.2 software. For the sample to be included in the study, CD4 cell count measurement just before the initiation of HAART was considered as a covariate so that there could be at least two visit responses after the initiation of HAART for analysis.

Quality of data

The quality of the data was controlled by data controllers from ART section of the hospital. The controllers were taken intensive training by the Ministry of Health for different services. The data extraction tools and the variables included in the study were tested for consistency of understanding and the completeness of the data items on 45 random samples. Necessary amendments were made on the final data collection sheet.

Variables included in the study

The longitudinal response variables for current study were CD4 cell count change and adherence to HAART. The two response variables are different in nature. CD4 cell count change is defined as the difference between CD4 cells/mm^3 in the current visiting time and CD4 cells/mm^3 in visiting times immediately prior to the current response. Hence, $Y_{ij} - Y_{ij-1}$, where y_{ij} is CD4 cell count result for the current visit and Y_{ij-1} is the CD4 cell count for the visit immediately prior to current visit which is discrete or count response. On the other hand, the adherence data obtained from the hospital is categorized as poor, fair and good adherence which is ordinal in nature, and measured with pills count. A patient is poor adherent if his/her performance is less than 85% of the prescribed medication; and he/she is a fair adherent if his/her performance is between 85 and 95% of the prescribed medication. If a patient's adherence performance is at least 95% of the prescribed medication, such patient is categorized as a good adherent. The trend of adherence to HAART was tested using Cochran–Armitage test.

On the other hand, the predictor variables for the two responses were age in years, sex (male, female), marital status (living with partner, living without partner), ownership of cell phone (yes, no), weight in kilogram, baseline CD4 cell count in cells/mm^3, disclosure of the disease to families (yes, no), residence area (rural, urban),WHO stages (stage I, stage II, stage III, stage IV), level of income (low, middle, high) visiting times (1, 2,..., 23) and first month adherence to HAART (poor, fair, good).

The impact of dropouts on the analysis

Patients who defaulted from HAART treatment will develop drug resistant virus and ultimately results in treatment failure and high risk of illness and death because of destruction of CD4 cell count by HIV. Non-adherence, therefore, reduces CD4 cell count; and this demands joint attention to maximally benefit from HAART. A logistic regression was conducted to assess whether or not missing values were affected by previous results; and this indicated that dropouts were independent of the previous outcomes ($\chi_1^2 = 0.2018$, $p = 0.654$). Dropout patients did not have reasons attributable to their progression rate of their previous visits; therefore dropout trend was Missed Completely at Random (MCAR). The trend of missing observation was assessed using a logistic regression model. Missing data were handled using multiple imputation technique.

A Chi square test of association and independent sampled t test were used for the comparison of baseline characteristics that will be included and excluded in the analysis for categorical and continuous variables, respectively. In model selection, we considered all predictors in the model, and fitted each product term obtained from predictor variables one at a time. This is important to assess the interaction effects of predictors on the variable of interest. A generalized linear mixed regression model (Quasi–Poisson) analysis was conducted to assess separate parametric estimation for the change of CD4 cell count [14]; and ordinal logistic regression was employed for separate data analysis of adherence to HAART [26]. The type of covariance structure and the magnitude of residual errors were also considered in model selection. In this regard, the model with the least within individual residual variability was selected.

Multivariate GLMM formulation of joint models

Since the specification of the joint distribution of the two responses is not straight forward, we can have two approaches for the formulation of joint multivariate models. The first approach is based on a conditioning argument that allows joint distribution to factor out in marginal and conditional component, where the conditioning can be done either on discrete or continuous outcome (avoiding direct specification of joint modeling) with introduction of probit approach. This approach does not directly lead to marginal inference, and the correlation between the two outcomes cannot be directly estimated. The second is direct formulation of joint modeling for both response variables with the introduction of Placket–Dale approach (Placket latent variable) assumption for modeling bivariate outcomes [27].

Instead of using a latent variable approach, one can directly specify the joint distribution for both outcomes through mixed model with specification of the marginal distribution, conditional on the correlated random effect. The generalized linear mixed model (GLMM) forms a very general class of subject-specific model which is used for univariate repeated measures. Joint model can be measured repeatedly over time or may be observed within a hierarchical trend. A GLMM can be easily adapted to situation where various outcomes are observed.

To obtain valid inferences, the joint model could account for the correction among the outcomes and effects of different factors. The joint generalized linear mixed model assumes that each outcome and the univariate models are combined through specification of joint multivariate distribution for all random effects. Furthermore, the mixed model can be applied with specification of marginal distribution, which is conditional on correlated random effect. To assess the association between CD4 cell count change and adherence to HAART for the data obtained at Felege-Hiwot Teaching and Specialized Hospital, the joint generalized linear mixed model was fitted. In this model, the correlation between the two responses is specified through the random effect structure assuming separate random intercept for each outcome and combining them by imposing joint multivariate distribution on the random intercept.

Results

The baseline characteristics of patients included in the analysis indicates that the median age of patients was 36 years old (IQR 28–48). Of all the patients studied 50.6% were females, 40.1% were living in rural area, 55.2% were living without partners, 52.7% did not disclose the disease to family members living together and only 68.2% had good adherence in the first month treatment. Over 50% of the patients had attended their secondary education and over 50% of them had no cell phone. The average baseline CD4 cell count for all patients was 134 (IQR 113–180) and the average CD4 cell count change for the first month was 15.9 cell/mm^3 (IQR 8–26). The average CD4 cell count change at all visits varies from 15.9 cells/mm^3 at the 1st visit to 28 cells/mm^3 at the 23rd visit. The corresponding standard deviations were 18 cells/mm^3 at the first visit and 27 cells/mm^3 at the last visit of the study period. Hence, the distribution at each visit shows that there were over-dispersion (variance > mean), and over-dispersed count response regression models should be considered for marginal analysis of CD4 cell count change data.

To fit the joint models of CD4 cell count change and adherence to HAART, first Quasi–Poisson for CD4 cell count change [14, 28] and ordinal logistic regression model for adherence to HAART data were considered separately [29]. Hence the parameter estimation for marginal models with log and cumulative logit link (Table 1) and conditional independence random-effect models (Table 2) were developed [30]. In addition, the parameter estimation for linear predictor or models which consist of the same variables already identified from GLMM models were developed (Table 3).

Table 1 indicates the separate or joint marginal models for CD4 cell count change and adherence to HAART using Quasi–Poisson regression and ordinal logistic regression. As indicated in the Table 1, age, weight, initial CD4 cell count and ownership of cell phone significantly affected both outcomes. From the two-way interaction, time * level of education, time * sex, age * sex as well as age * level of education were significant for both outcome variables. The separate models shown in Table 1 were univariate distributions. Table 2, on the other hand, shows the combination of the separate models by imposing joint multivariate distribution on the random effect. The analysis was done using generalized log likelihood function with Laplace approximation. The conditional independence of random-effect models considered in this analysis shows that the GLMM approach can be extended to multivariate longitudinal data by assuming separate random effect for each outcome and combining them by imposing a joint multivariate distribution on the random effects. The SAS procedure using general log-likelihood function allows one to impose the joint multivariate distribution on the random effects from the two separate models. The results obtained from fitting a joint model for the two response variables of uncorrelated random intercept using the GLIMMIX procedure were used as initial parameter estimates.

Table 2 shows the conditional independence random intercept model. As indicated in the Table 2, patients' age, weight, initial CD4 cell count, visiting time, ownership of cell phone and sex were jointly and significantly associated with both response variables. The same sign in parametric estimation indicates that the two outcomes are positively correlated to each other. Since the conditional independence assumption might be too restrictive, we, therefore, attempted to relax the conditional independence assumption by re-fitting the joint random intercepts model with possible correlated errors. However, the conditional independence approach, which we attempted, failed to converge the model. During this time, introducing conditional dependence of one response in terms of the other using linear predictor is important [31]. This approach is also helpful to validate the observed correlation between the two outcomes emerging from the association of the random intercepts. We fitted a generalized linear mixed model for CD4 cell count change as response variable including adherence to HAART in the linear predictor. The result is presented in Table 3 below. The result indicates that CD4 cell count change is positively correlated ($p \leq 0.0001$) with adherence to HAART.

As shown in Table 3, age, weight, baseline CD4 cell count, visiting times, marital status, sex, residence area, ownership of cell phone, disclosure of the disease to family members and first month adherence have significantly affected CD4 cell count change. Hence, as age of a patient increased by 1 year, the log of change of CD4 cell count decreased by 3.3% cell/mm^3 keeping the other variables constant [ARR = 0.0327, 95% CI (0.0098, 0.0899); p = 0.0264]. As the number of visiting times increased by one unit, the log of change of CD4 cell count increased by 2.4% [ARR = 1.0240, 95% CI (1.0206, 1.0276); p < 0.0001]. The analysis revealed that the rate of change of CD4 cell count for patients without ownership of cell phone was 2.9% less as compared to patients with ownership of cell phone [ARR = 0.0290, 95% CI (0.0172, 0.0870); p < 0.0001]. The log of change of CD4 cell count for patients with fair adherence at a given visiting time was 2.9% less than those patients who had good adherence [ARR = 0.0290133, 95% CI (0.00974, 0.043931); p < 0.0001] and the log of change of CD4 cell count for patients with poor adherence at visiting time, t was 5.7% less than those of good adherent patients [ARR = 0.0573, 95% CI (0.0214, 0.0706); p < 0.0001]. From the two way interaction effects; time * ownership of cell phone, time * sex, time * level of education, age * sex, age * level of education were significantly and jointly affected both responses through linear link (refer Table 3).

Interaction effects of ownership of cell phone and visiting times

For a unit increase of visiting time, the rate of change of CD4 cell count for patients without owner of cell phone was 5.2% less than patients with owner of cell phone [ARR = 0.0518, 95% CI (0.0443, 0.0996); p < 0.0001]. Figure 1 indicates that the log of change of CD4 cell count for patients with owner of cell phone was by far better than those patients without cell phone as visiting time increased.

Interaction effect between sex of patients and follow-up visits

As visiting times of adult patients increased by one unit, the log of change of CD4 cell count for female patients was 0.3% greater than male patients [ARR = 1.0027, 95% CI (1.0016, 1.0038); p < 0.0001]. From Fig. 2, we saw that as visiting time increased, the log of change of CD4 cell

Table 1 Parameter estimates and corresponding standard errors of joint marginal model/separate analysis for CD4 cell count change data and adherence to HAART with un-structured working covariance

Parameter	CD4 cell count change			Adherence to HAART		
	Estimate	St. error	p value	Estimate	St. error	p value
Intercept	4.0066	0.0329	<0.0001	0.8921	0.2428	0.0002
Age	−0.0002	0.0007	0.0264*	−0.0111	0.0029	0.0001*
Weight	−0.0006	0.0002	0.0020*	0.0158	0.0027	<0.0001*
Initial CD4 cell count	0.0048	0.0002	<0.0001*	0.0410	0.0013	<0.0001*
Time	0.0238	0.0017	<0.0001*	−0.0429	0.0012	<0.0001*
Marital status (ref. = without part)						
Living with part	0.0064	0.0034	0.0464*	−0.0241	0.0481	0.6156
Sex (ref. = male)						
Female	−0.0131	0.0039	0.0009*	−0.4548	0.1036	<0.0001*
Area (ref. = urban)						
Rural	0.0213	0.0105	0.0425*	0.1517	0.1029	0.1405
Education (ref. = tertiary)						
No education	−0.0410	0.0059	<0.0001*	−0.0970	0.1480	0.5123
Primary education	−0.0406	0.0065	<0.0001*	0.0970	0.1646	0.5555
Secondary educ.	−0.0577	0.0055	<0.0001*	0.1135	0.1423	0.4248
Level of income (ref. = high income)						
Middle income	−0.0099	0.0054	0.0679	−0.1055	0.0772	0.1715
Low income	−0.0106	0.0041	0.0095*	0.1661	0.0572	0.0037*
Owner of cell phone (ref. = with phone)						
Without cell phone	−0.0204	0.0038	<0.0001*	0.6957	0.0975	<0.0001*
Level of disclosed the disease (ref. = yes)						
No	−0.0062	0.0034	0.0715	0.2834	0.0484	<0.0001*
WHO stages (ref. = stage IV)						
Stage I	0.1191	0.0077	<0.0001*	−0.1978	0.1101	0.0725
Stage II	0.1239	0.0064	<0.0001*	0.2195	0.0904	0.0152*
Stage III	0.1006	0.0063	<0.0001*	0.1500	0.0886	0.0904
Time * ownership of cell phone (ref. = yes)						
Time * no	−0.0099	0.0013	<0.0001*	−0.0094	0.0077	0.2236
Time * area (ref. = urban)						
Time * rural	−0.0024	0.0020	0.2192	0.0033	0.0082	0.2236
Time * sex (ref. = male)						
Time * female	0.0027	0.0006	<0.0001*	0.0226	0.0067	0.0007*
Time * education (ref. = tertiary)						
Time * no educ.	0.0062	0.0007	<0.0001*	0.0300	0.0114	0.0085*
Time * primary educ.	0.0086	0.0008	<0.0001*	0.0315	0.0128	0.0138*
Time * secondary educ.	0.0067	0.0007	<0.0001*	0.0376	0.0111	0.0007*
Age * sex (ref. = male)						
Age * female	−0.0046	0.0004	<0.0001*	0.0078	0.0081	0.0345*
Age * education (ref. = tertiary)						
Age * no educ.	−0.0045	0.0006	<0.0001*	−0.0752	0.0098	<0.0001*
Age * primary educ.	−0.0022	0.0007	0.0015*	−0.1197	0.0115	<0.0001*
Age * secondary educ.	−0.0036	0.0006	<0.0001*	−0.0501	0.0102	<0.0001*
Age * area (ref. = urban)						
Age * rural area	−0.0025	0.0004	<0.0001*	0.0014	0.0065	0.8275
Mar. stat * level of exposedness (ref. = closed)						
Mar. stat * disclosed the disease	0.0067	0.0007	0.0652	0.2001	0.0989	0.0430*

* Significant p values

Table 2 Parameter estimates and corresponding standard errors for conditional independence random intercept model with CD4 cell count change data and adherence to HAART

Parameter	CD4 cell count change			Adherence to HAART		
	Estimate	St. error	p value	Estimate	St. error	p value
Intercept	4.0066	0.0329	<0.0001	0.8921	0.2428	0.0002*
Age	−0.0002	0.0007	0.0264*	−0.0111	0.0029	0.0001*
Weight	−0.0006	0.0002	0.0020*	0.0158	0.0027	<0.0001*
Initial CD4 cell count	0.0048	0.0002	<0.0001*	0.0410	0.0013	<0.0001*
Time	0.0238	0.0017	<0.0001*	0.0129	0.0312	<0.0001*
Marital status (ref. = without part)						
Living with part	0.0064	0.0034	0.0464*	−0.0241	0.0481	0.6156
Sex (ref. = male)						
Female	−0.0131	0.0039	0.0009*	−0.4548	0.1036	<0.0001*
Area (ref. = urban)						
Rural	0.0213	0.0105	0.0425*	0.1517	0.1029	0.1405
Education (ref. = tertiary)						
No education	−0.0410	0.0059	<0.0001*	−0.0970	0.1480	0.5123
Primary education	−0.0406	0.0065	<0.0001*	0.0970	0.1646	0.5555
Secondary educ.	−0.0577	0.0055	<0.0001*	0.1135	0.1423	0.4248
Level of income (ref. = high income)						
Middle income	−0.0099	0.0054	0.0679	−0.1055	0.0772	0.1715
Low income	−0.0106	0.0041	0.0095*	0.1661	0.0572	0.0037*
Owner of cell phone (ref. = with phone)						
Without cell phone	−0.0204	0.0038	<0.0001*	0.6957	0.0975	<0.0001*
Level of disclosure (ref. = disclosed)						
Closed the disease	−0.0062	0.0034	0.0715	0.2834	0.0484	<0.0001*
WHO stages (ref. = stage IV)						
Stage I	0.1191	0.0077	<0.0001*	−0.1978	0.1101	0.0725
Stage II	0.1239	0.0064	<0.0001*	0.2195	0.0904	0.0152*
Stage III	0.1006	0.0063	<0.0001*	0.1500	0.0886	0.0904
Time * ownership of cell phone (ref. = yes)						
Time * no	−0.0099	0.0013	<0.0001*	−0.0094	0.0077	0.0236*
Time * area (ref. = urban)						
Time * rural	−0.0024	0.0020	0.2192	0.0033	0.0082	0.0236*
Time * sex (ref. = male)						
Time * female	0.0027	0.0006	<0.0001*	0.0226	0.0067	0.0007*
Time * education (ref. = tertiary)						
Time * no educ.	0.0062	0.0007	<0.0001*	0.0300	0.0114	0.0085*
Time * primary educ.	0.0086	0.0008	<0.0001*	0.0315	0.0128	0.0138*
Time * secondary educ.	0.0067	0.0007	<0.0001*	0.0376	0.0111	0.0007*
Age * sex (ref. = male)						
Age * female	−0.0046	0.0004	<0.0001*	0.0078	0.0081	0.0345*
Age * education (ref. = tertiary)						
Age * no educ.	−0.0045	0.0006	<0.0001*	−0.0752	0.0098	<0.0001*
Age * primary educ.	−0.0022	0.0007	0.0015*	−0.1197	0.0115	<0.0001*
Age * secondary educ.	−0.0036	0.0006	<0.0001*	−0.0501	0.0102	<0.0001*
Age * area (ref. = urban)						
Age * rural area	−0.0025	0.0004	<0.0001*	0.0014	0.0065	0.8275
Mar. stat * level of exposedness (ref. = closed)						
Marital stat * disclosed the disease	0.0067	0.0007	0.0652	0.2001	0.0989	0.0430*

* Significant p values

Table 3 Parameter estimates for joint model of CD4 cell count change data using linear predictor

Parameter	Estimate	St. error	Adjusted rate ratio (ARR)	Wald 95% CI		p value
Intercept	4.0066	0.0029	54.9596	51.5318	58.6156	<0.0001
Age	−3.4201	0.0001	0.0327	0.0098	0.0899	0.0264*
Weight	0.0036	0.0001	1.0036	0.0021	1.0045	0.0820
Baseline CD4 cell count	0.0048	0.0002	1.0048	1.0035	1.0061	<0.0001*
Time	0.0238	0.0007	1.0240	1.0206	1.0277	<0.0001*
Marital status (ref. = without part)						
Patients living with partner	0.0064	0.0014	1.0064	0.9998	1.0132	0.0564
Sex (ref. = male)						
Female	0.0131	0.0005	1.0132	0.0124	1.0155	0.0659
Area (ref. = urban)						
Rural	−2.65	0.0005	0.0706	0.9558	1.0982	0.0525
Education (ref. = tertiary)						
No educ.	−4.02	0.0019	0.0183	0.9487	1.0298	0.0627
Primary educ.	−3.45	0.0005	0.0317	0.9480	1.9725	0.0801
Secondary educ.	−2.86	0.0015	0.0573	0.9337	1.0481	0.0568
Level of income (ref. = high income)						
Middle income	−4.12	0.0014	0.0162	0.9797	1.0007	0.0679
Low income	−3.63	0.0001	0.0265	0.9816	1.0974	0.0095
Owner of cell phone (ref. = yes)						
No	−3.54	0.0018	0.0290	0.0172	0.0870	<0.0001*
First month adherence level (ref. = good adherence)						
Fair adherence	−3.54	0.0002	0.0290	0.0097	0.0439	<0.0001*
Poor adherence	−2.86	0.0091	0.0573	0.0214	0.0706	<0.0001*
Level of disclosed the disease (ref. = yes)						
No	−2.6	0.0014	0.0743	0.9871	1.0995	0.0715
WHO stages (ref. = stage IV)						
Stage I	0.1191	0.0007	1.1265	0.1097	1.1436	0.0651
Stage II	0.1239	0.0014	1.1319	0.1173	1.0461	0.0612
Stage III	0.1006	0.0023	1.1058	0.0923	1.0196	0.0851
Time * owner of cell phone (ref. = yes)						
Time * no	−2.96	0.0003	0.0518	0.0443	0.0996	<0.0001*
Time * area (ref. = urban)						
Time * rural	−2.4	0.0010	0.0907	0.9937	1.0004	0.0792
Time * sex (ref. = male)						
Time * female	0.0027	0.0002	1.0027	1.0016	1.0038	<0.0001*
Time * education (ref. = tertiary)						
Time * no educ.	−4.00	0.0007	0.0183	0.0082	0.0452	<0.0001*
Time * primary educ.	−3.83	0.0002	0.0124	0.0044	0.0360	<0.0001*
Time * secondary educ.	−3.43	0.0001	0.0086	0.0053	0.0147	<0.0001*
Age * sex (ref. = male)						
Age * female	−3.421	0.0002	0.0326	0.0144	0.0662	<0.0001*
Age * education (ref. = tertiary)						
Age * no educ.	0.042	0.0002	1.0433	1.0126	1.0799	<0.0001*
Age * primary educ.	0.032	0.0001	1.0325	1.0112	1.0601	0.0015*
Age * secondary educ.	0.023	0.0004	1.0232	1.0093	1.0594	<0.0001*
Age * area (ref. = urban)						
Age * rural area	0.0025	0.0002	1.0025	0.0017	1.0034	0.08621

* Significant at 5% level of confidence for joint model

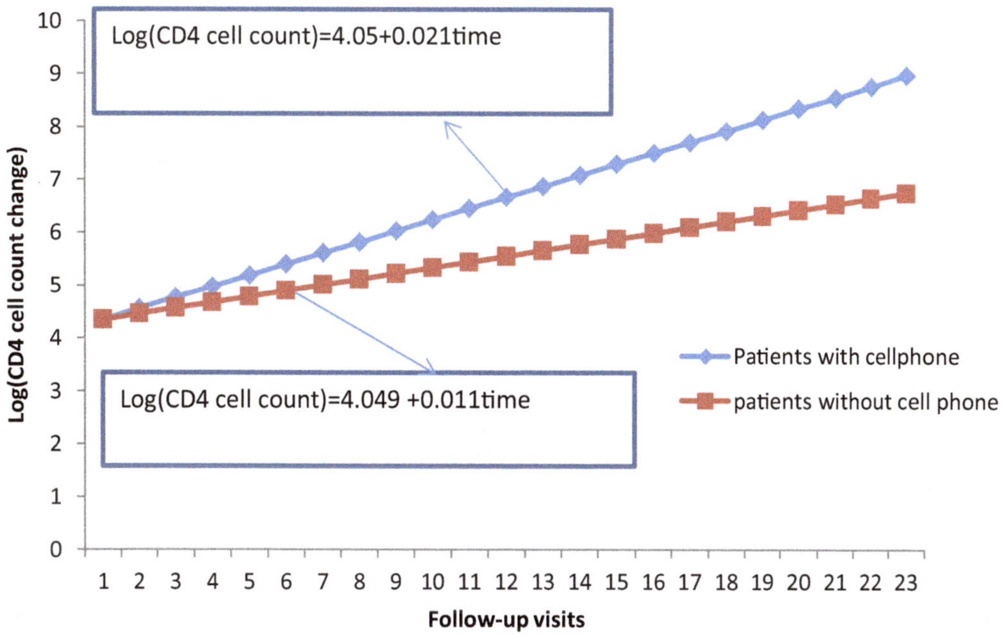

Fig. 1 Interaction plot between ownership of cell phone and follow-up visits

count for female patients is greater than that of male patients.

Interaction effect between age and sex of patients

From Table 3, it is indicated that as age of patients increased by 1 year, the decreasing rate of change of CD4 cell count for female patients was 3.3% less than male patients [ARR = 0.0326, 95% CI (0.0144, 0.0662); $p < 0.0001$]. Hence, as age of patients increased, the decreasing rate for female patients was less probable as compared to male patients (refer to Fig. 3).

Interaction effect between level of education and visiting times

As visiting time of patients increased by one unit, the rate of change of CD4 cell count for non-educated patients

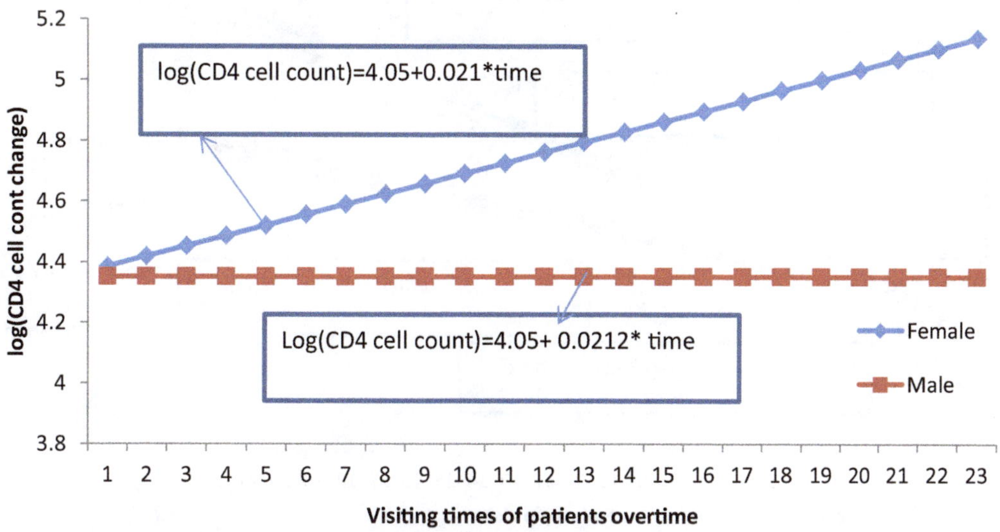

Fig. 2 Interaction plot between sex of patients and their follow-ups

was 1.8% less than those of tertiary educated patients [ARR = 0.0183, 95% CI (0.0082, 0.0452); $p < 0.0001$]. Similarly comparing primary educated patients with tertiary level, the log of change of CD4 cell count for primary educated patients was 1.2% less than tertiary levels [ARR = 0.0124, 95% CI (0.0044, 0.03662); $p < 0.0001$] and the log of change of CD4 cell count for secondary educated patients was 0.8% less than tertiary educated patients [ARR = 0.0086, 95% CI (0.0053, 0.0147); $p < 0.0001$] (refer to Table 3). Figure 4 indicates that as visiting time of patients increased, patients with tertiary education perform high log of CD4 cell count change as compared to the other group.

Interaction effect between level of education and age of patients

It is known from the literature that as age of patients increase, the log of change of CD4 cell count decrease.

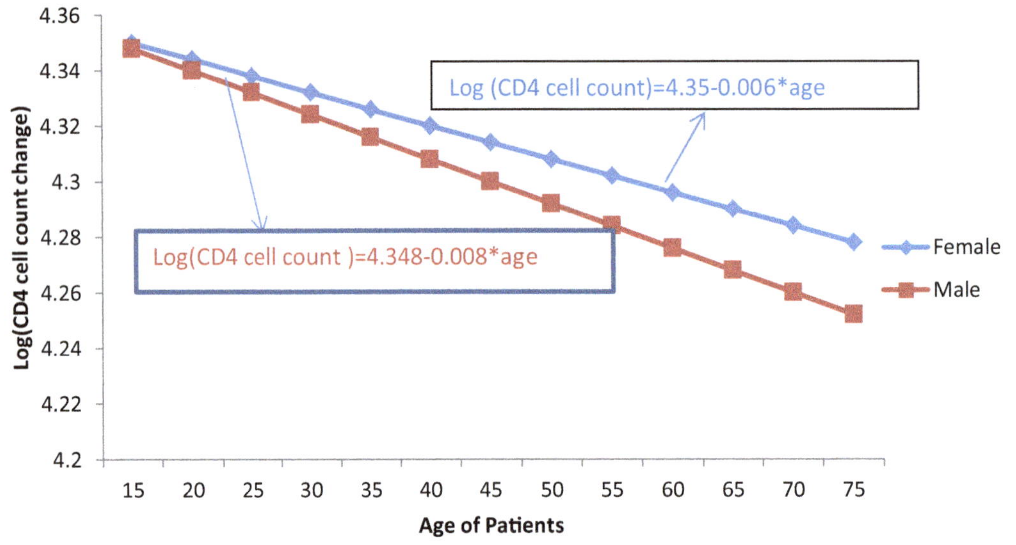

Fig. 3 Interaction plot between sex and age of patients

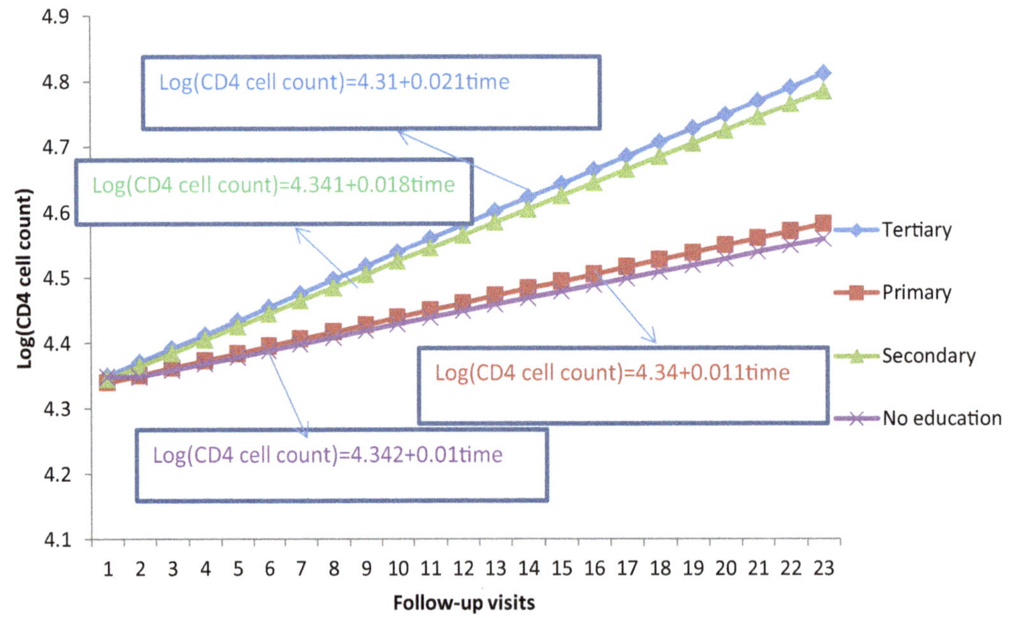

Fig. 4 Interaction plot between level of education and follow-up visits

However, the decreasing rate for different level of education was different from the current analysis. Hence as age of a patient increased by 1 year, the decreasing rate of CD4 cell count for non-educated patient was 4.3% greater as compared to tertiary educated patients [ARR = 1.0433, 95% CI (1.0126, 1.0799); p < 0.0001]; the log of change CD4 cell count for primary educated patients was 3.2% greater than tertiary educated patients [ARR = 1.0325, 95% CI (1.0112, 1.0601); p = 0.0015]; and decreasing rate of CD4 cell count for secondary educated patients was 2.3% greater than tertiary educated patients [ARR = 1.0232, 95% CI (1.0093, 0.0594); p < 0.0001]. Figure 5 indicates that as age of patients increase, the decreasing rate of tertiary educated patients was lower than other groups.

Discussion

We have presented a general approach to the joint analysis of two longitudinal response variables assuming their separate analysis. The results in this study indicated that the separate models which did not include patients' specific effects were not significantly different from joint models developed with the assumption of separate analysis. As indicated above the joint models were formed by imposing the joint multivariate distribution of random effect, Hence, the results of both separate and joint analysis were consistent. However, the joint models were simpler as compared to the separate models as their effective member of parameters was smaller. In other words, the reduction of the number of effective parameters ensures that joint models were more parsimonious/less complex in parameter estimation of longitudinal data analysis. This result complies with previous researches [30, 32, 33]. Furthermore, joint models were advantageous for answering multivariate questions at the same time. They also helped assess the correlation between the two response variables and gave ample opportunity to see predictors of the two response variables jointly.

The result in this study indicated that CD4 cell count change and adherence to HAART had been influenced jointly by some of the covariates like age, weight, baseline CD4 cell count, visiting times, sex, ownership of cell phone, first month adherence and level of disclosing the disease to family members and by their interaction effects (refer to Table 3). Recent findings from longitudinal study [34] also proved that CD4 cell count change was affected by many of these covariates. This finding suggests that the hospital should advise adult HIV patients to adhere the prescribed medication on time to achieve high CD4 cell count change. Patients, who had cell phone, had more probability to adhere the prescribed medication than patients who had not. This result is supported by another study [17]. Hence alarm of cell phone/memory aids/can be used to remember patients the time for taking pills and visiting health institutions.

As ages of patients increase, CD4 cell count and adherence to HAART decrease. But, the decreasing rate of these response variables for patients with tertiary education is

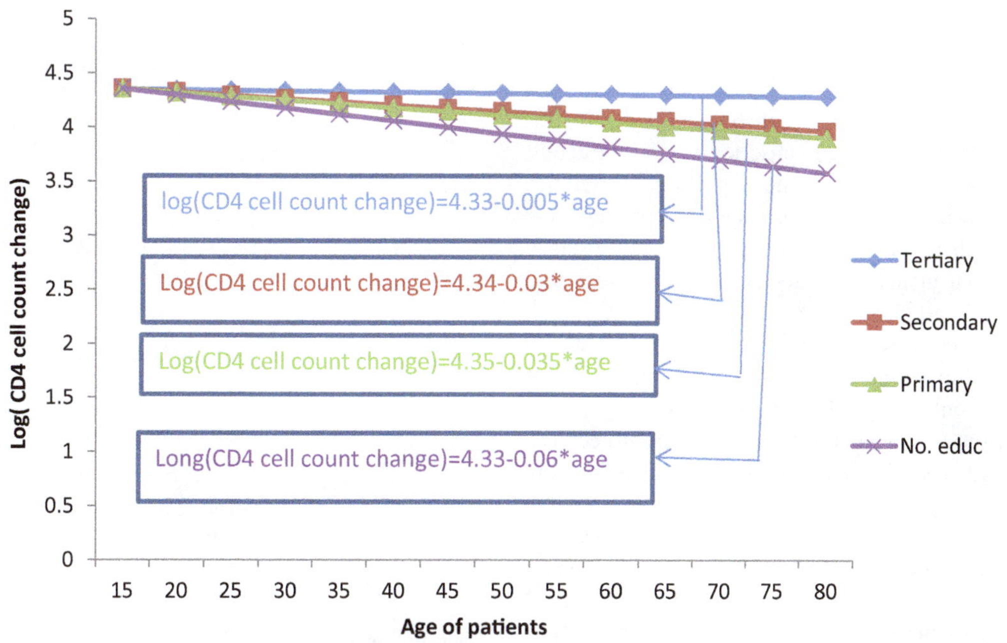

Fig. 5 Interaction plot between level of education and age of patients

less likely as compared to that of the others. This might occur because as patients become more educated, they may have better care of their health. This result has been supported by previous study [16]. Patients with high initial CD4 cell count adhere the prescribed medication more; and these results in high rate of change of CD4 cell count through time. This result suggests that patients should start their HAART without keeping the cut-off points (200 cell/mm^3). This result is supported by previous study [35] on the impact of adherence on CD4 cell count change.

The two responses were higher for urban adult patients than rural areas through time. The reason for this might be the long distance of the rural areas from health institutions, and patients in these areas may come after high destruction of CD4 cells by HIV. There are discordant other findings concerning this. For instance, the result of this study agrees with a previous study [36]. However, another study indicates that rural patients' adherence to HAART is better through time, and this implies that they have better CD4 cell count [37]. Therefore, this issue needs further investigation for reliable information.

Patients who lived with a partner had more probability to adhere the prescribed medication and had high CD4 cell count change as compared to patients who lived without partners. This can be associated with lack of social support for patients living without partner. This result had been supported by former research [17]. The result of this study also indicates that female patients had more probability to adhere the prescribed medication than males, and through time they had achieved high rate of change of CD4 cell count. This result, however, is inconsistent with previous studies [38].

Limitations

The interactions between variables, which were not expected during the data collection process, were identified during data analysis. The cause for these interaction occurrences was not detected and explained. Adherence to HAART, which was one of the response variables, was measured in pill count technique. This technique had a disadvantage that include patients' switching of medicines between bottles and discarding pills before visits [27]. Despite its limitations, pill count technique has strong linear relationship with viral load [39]. The result in this analysis is true only for adult patients; that is, it may have different outcomes when patients with all ages are considered. This could be a potential area for further investigation.

Conclusions

Longitudinal joint models fitted for the joint data analysis under this investigation. Generalized linear mixed model was extended to multivariate cases in the data analysis process. This had been done using marginal/separate analysis as well as conditional independent random effect models and a random intercept model with correlated residual error structure. Developing joint models has helped validate the observed correlation between the outcomes emerging from the association of intercepts. The result under this investigation indicated that some covariates were significantly associated with the change of CD4 cell count; and the development of joint model for the two responses gave powerful estimation as compared to the separate or marginal model. The result of this study identified a certain group of patients who were with maximum risk of CD4 cell count change, but who had poor adherence performance. This group of patients needs high intervention in counseling and awareness creation.

Abbreviations

AIC: Akaike Information Criteria; BIC: Bayesian Information Criteria; CI: confidence interval; CD4: classification determinant four; HAART: highly active antiretroviral therapy; HIV: human immune deficiency virus; WHO: World Health Organization; MLE: maximum likelihood estimator; GLM: generalized linear model; GLMMs: generalized linear mixed modes; MCAR: missed completely at random; ARR: adjusted rate ratio; IQR: inter quartile range.

Authors' contributions

The principal author wrote the proposal, developed data collection format, supervised the data collection process and analyzed the data in consultation with the second and the third authors. The second and the third authors edited the document and gave critical comments. All authors read and approved the final manuscript.

Authors' information

Awoke Seyoum is an Assistant Professor of the department of statistics at Bahir Dar University, Ethiopia, He had previous three publications, currently a Ph.D. student with close supervision of the two professors.

Principal Ndlovu is an Associate Professor of the department of statistics at UNISA, South Africa. He is a senior staff in the department and has more than 8 publications.

Zewotir Temesgen is a senior Professor at School of Mathematics, Statistics and Computer Science, University of KwaZulu Natal, South Africa. He has more than 65 publications in peer reviewed journals.

Author details

[1] Department of Statistics, Bahir Dar University, Bahir Dar, Ethiopia. [2] Department of Statistics, UNISA, Pretoria, South Africa. [3] School of Mathematics, Statistics and Computer Science, University of KwaZulu Natal, Durban, South Africa.

Acknowledgements

Amhara Region Health Research & Laboratory Center at Felege-Hiwot Referral Hospital, Ethiopia, is gratefully acknowledged for the data they supplied for our health research. Prof. Abiy Yigzaw is also highly acknowledged for final edition of the manuscript related to language usage, spelling and grammar.

Competing interests

The authors declare that they have no competing interests.

agreed with its submission to AIDS Research and Therapy. We agreed about authorship and order of authors for this manuscript.

References

1. East S, Africa S-S. Towards universal access: scaling up priority HIV/AIDS interventions in the health sector. Europe. 2010;85:000.
2. Hladik W, et al. HIV/AIDS in Ethiopia: where is the epidemic heading? Sex Transm Infect. 2006;82(suppl 1):i32–5.
3. Gezie LD. Predictors of CD4 count over time among HIV patients initiated ART in Felege Hiwot Referral Hospital, northwest Ethiopia: multilevel analysis. BMC Res Notes. 2016;9(1):377.
4. REPoRTInG H. Global update. 2014.
5. Mellors JW, et al. Plasma viral load and CD4+ lymphocytes as prognostic markers of HIV-1 infection. Ann Intern Med. 1997;126(12):946–54.
6. van Leth F, et al. Comparison of first-line antiretroviral therapy with regimens including nevirapine, efavirenz, or both drugs, plus stavudine and lamivudine: a randomised open-label trial, the 2NN Study. Lancet. 2004;363(9417):1253–63.
7. Kaufmann GR, et al. CD4 T-lymphocyte recovery in individuals with advanced HIV-1 infection receiving potent antiretroviral therapy for 4 years: the Swiss HIV Cohort Study. Arch Intern Med. 2003;163(18):2187–95.
8. Florence E, et al. Factors associated with a reduced CD4 lymphocyte count response to HAART despite full viral suppression in the EuroSIDA study. HIV Med. 2003;4(3):255–62.
9. Asfaw A, et al. CD4 cell count trends after commencement of antiretroviral therapy among HIV-infected patients in Tigray, Northern Ethiopia: a retrospective cross-sectional study. PLoS ONE. 2015;10(3):e0122583.
10. Smith CJ, et al. Factors influencing increases in CD4 cell counts of HIV-positive persons receiving long-term highly active antiretroviral therapy. J Infect Dis. 2004;190(10):1860–8.
11. Gea-Banacloche JC, Clifford LH. Immune reconstitution in HIV infection. AIDS. 1998;13:25–38.
12. Ebonyi AO, et al. Factors associated with a low CD4 count among HIV-1 infected patients at enrolment into HAART in Jos, Nigeria. Br J Med Med Res. 2014;4(13):2536.
13. Gandhi RT, et al. Effect of baseline-and treatment-related factors on immunologic recovery after initiation of antiretroviral therapy in HIV-1-positive subjects: results from ACTG 384. J Acquir Immune Defic Syndr. 2006;42(4):426–34.
14. Seyoum A, Zewotir T. Quasi–Poisson versus negative binomial regression models in identifying factors affecting initial CD4 cell count change due to antiretroviral therapy administered to HIV-positive adults in North-west Ethiopia (Amhara region). AIDS Res Ther. 2016;13(1):36.
15. Chesney MA. Factors affecting adherence to antiretroviral therapy. Clin Infect Dis. 2000;30(Supplement 2):S171–6.
16. Langebeek N, et al. Predictors and correlates of adherence to combination antiretroviral therapy (ART) for chronic HIV infection: a meta-analysis. BMC Med. 2014;12(1):142.
17. Maqutu D, et al. Determinants of optimal adherence over time to antiretroviral therapy amongst HIV positive adults in South Africa: a longitudinal study. AIDS Behav. 2011;15(7):1465–74.
18. Mitiku H, Abdosh T, Teklemariam Z. Factors affecting adherence to antiretroviral treatment in harari national regional state, Eastern Ethiopia. ISRN AIDS. 2013;2013:960954.
19. AIDSinfo A. Guidelines for the use of antiretroviral agents in HIV-1-infected adults and adolescents. 2013.
20. Low-Beer S, et al. Adherence to triple therapy and viral load response. J Acquir Immune Defic Syndr. 2000;23(4):360–1.
21. Tsiatis AA, Davidian M. Joint modeling of longitudinal and time-to-event data: an overview. Stat Sin. 2004;14(3):809–34.
22. Chakraborty A, Das K. Inferences for joint modelling of repeated ordinal scores and time to event data. Comput Math Methods Med. 2010;11(3):281–95.
23. Li N, et al. Joint modeling of longitudinal ordinal data and competing risks survival times and analysis of the NINDS rt-PA stroke trial. Stat Med. 2010;29(5):546–57.
24. Hickey GL, et al. Joint modelling of time-to-event and multivariate longitudinal outcomes: recent developments and issues. BMC Med Res Methodol. 2016;16(1):117.
25. Ayele D, Zewotir T, Mwambi H. Modelling the joint determinants of a positive malaria Rapid Diagnosis Test result, use of mosquito nets and indoor residual spraying with insecticide. Occup Health South Africa. 2014;20(4):20–7.
26. Liu X. Ordinal regression analysis: fitting the proportional odds model using Stata, SAS and SPSS. J Modern Appl Stat Methods. 2009;8(2):30.
27. Maqutu D, Zewotir T. Optimal HAART adherence over time and time interval between successive visits: their association and determinants. AIDS Care. 2011;23(11):1417–24.
28. Ver Hoef JM, Boveng PL. Quasi–Poisson vs. negative binomial regression: how should we model overdispersed count data? Ecology. 2007;88(11):2766–72.
29. Das S, Rahman RM. Application of ordinal logistic regression analysis in determining risk factors of child malnutrition in Bangladesh. Nutr J. 2011;10(1):1.
30. Seid A, et al. Joint modeling of longitudinal CD4 cell counts and time-to-default from HAART treatment: a comparison of separate and joint models. Electron J Appl Stat Anal. 2014;7(2):292–314.
31. Gueorguieva RV, Agresti A. A correlated probit model for joint modeling of clustered binary and continuous responses. J Am Stat Assoc. 2001;96(455):1102–12.
32. Tsay RS, Tiao GC. Consistent estimates of autoregressive parameters and extended sample autocorrelation function for stationary and nonstationary ARMA models. J Am Stat Assoc. 1984;79(385):84–96.
33. Verbeke G, Davidian M. Joint models for longitudinal data: introduction and overview. 2009.
34. Guo X, Carlin BP. Separate and joint modeling of longitudinal and event time data using standard computer packages. Am Stat. 2004;58(1):16–24.
35. MODEL GEE. Longitudinal study of change in CD4+ cell counts on HIV-positive patients initiated on antiretroviral therapy at The Comprehensive Care Centre in Kenyatta National Hospital. Nairobi: University of Nairobi; 2014.
36. Maqutu D, Zewotir T, North D. Determinants of adherence to antiretroviral therapy amongst HIV positive adults in South Africa: a longitudinal study.
37. Birbeck GL, et al. Antiretroviral adherence in rural Zambia: the first year of treatment availability. Am J Trop Med Hyg. 2009;80(4):669–74.
38. Escobar I, et al. Factors affecting patient adherence to highly active antiretroviral therapy. Ann Pharmacother. 2003;37(6):775–81.
39. Bangsberg DR, et al. Adherence to protease inhibitors, HIV-1 viral load, and development of drug resistance in an indigent population. Aids. 2000;14(4):357–66.

12

HIV treatment simplification to elvitegravir/cobicistat/emtricitabine/tenofovir disproxil fumarate (E/C/F/TDF) plus darunavir: a pharmacokinetic study

Marianne Harris[1,2,3,4*], Bruce Ganase[2], Birgit Watson[1], P. Richard Harrigan[1,4], Julio S. G. Montaner[1,4] and Mark W. Hull[1,4]

Abstract

Background: As a simplification strategy for treatment-experienced HIV-infected patients who have achieved virologic suppression on a multi-drug, multi-class antiretroviral regimen, the aim of this study was to evaluate the safety, efficacy, and pharmacokinetics of once-daily elvitegravir/cobicistat/emtricitabine/tenofovir disproxil fumarate (E/C/F/TDF) with darunavir.

Methods: A single arm, open-label 48-week study was conducted of regimen simplification to E/C/F/TDF plus darunavir 800 mg daily from stable therapy including two nucleoside/nucleotide reverse transcriptase inhibitors, a ritonavir-boosted protease inhibitor, and an integrase inhibitor. Participants had plasma HIV viral load consistently < 200 copies/mL for ≥ 6 months, estimated glomerular filtration rate (eGFR) ≥ 60 mL/min, and no genotypic resistance to major components of the study regimen. Plasma viral load was measured at weeks 2 and 4, then every 4 weeks throughout the study. Safety laboratory assessments were conducted at baseline and at weeks 12, 24, 36, and 48. Antiretroviral drug concentrations were measured at baseline and once ≥ 2 weeks after the regimen change.

Results: Ten HIV-infected adults (8 male and 2 female; median age 50.5 years) were enrolled. All maintained virologic suppression on the new regimen for 48 weeks. One subject experienced a decrease in eGFR from 62 mL/min at baseline to 52 mL/min at week 12; study medications were continued and his eGFR remained stable (50–59 mL/min) thereafter. No subjects discontinued study medications for renal function changes or other adverse events. Darunavir trough concentration were lower on the new regimen than on darunavir/ritonavir 800/100 mg ($n = 5$; $p < 0.05$).

Conclusions: Despite low darunavir trough concentrations, treatment simplification to a two-pill, once-daily regimen of E/C/F/TDF plus darunavir was safe and effective for 48 weeks among 10 selected treatment-experienced HIV-infected patients.

Keywords: HIV, Antiretrovirals, Elvitegravir, Cobicistat, Darunavir

Background

Despite the success of current highly active antiretroviral therapy regimens, some HIV-infected patients require regimens encompassing multiple drug classes because of transmitted or acquired drug-resistant virus [1, 2]. Such regimens usually include a ritonavir-boosted protease inhibitor and generally comprise several pills in two or more daily doses, making adherence a challenge for many patients [3]. For example, the TRIO regimen (raltegravir 400 mg twice daily, etravirine 200 mg twice daily, and

*Correspondence: mharris@cfenet.ubc.ca
[1] British Columbia Centre for Excellence in HIV/AIDS, Vancouver, BC, Canada

darunavir/ritonavir 600 mg/100 mg twice daily), which is effective and often used in patients harboring multi-drug resistant HIV, comprises six pills twice daily, and more if nucleoside reverse transciptase inhibitors (NRTIs) are taken as well (as was the case in the majority of subjects in the ANRS 139 TRIO study) [4]. Over the longer term, high pill burden is a major factor contributing to treatment fatigue among HIV-infected patients prescribed antiretroviral therapy, with important consequences including medication nonadherence and treatment failure [5].

In recent years, first-line regimens have included the use of a fixed-dose once-daily combination tablet consisting of the integrase inhibitor elvitegravir 150 mg (E) with a pharmacologic boosting agent (cobicistat 150 mg [C]) and two reverse transcriptase inhibitors (a nucleoside: emtricitabine or FTC 200 mg [F] and a nucleotide: tenofovir disoproxil fumarate 300 mg [TDF]) [6]. Cobicistat has been shown to also adequately boost plasma levels of protease inhibitors including darunavir [7]. In addition, there is evidence that once-daily boosted darunavir 800 mg is as effective as the twice-daily boosted darunavir 600 mg in treatment-experienced patients in the absence of darunavir resistance-associated mutations [8]. Pharmacokinetic studies support the use of once daily darunavir 800 mg in this population: 24-h post-dose minimum plasma concentrations of darunavir (when given with ritonavir 100 mg) remain above 55 ng/mL, the half maximal effective concentration (EC_{50}) for wild-type (non-protease inhibitor-resistant) virus [9]. The elvitegravir/cobicistat/emtricitabine/tenofovir DF (E/C/F/TDF) fixed-dose formulation may allow construction of a two-pill once-daily salvage regimen containing an integrase inhibitor, two nucleoside/nucleotides, and a boosted protease inhibitor: E/C/F/TDF and darunavir 800 mg. Since both E/C/F/TDF and darunavir are recommended to be taken once a day with food [6, 10], this constitutes a truly compact once-daily multi-class regimen.

Some early pharmacokinetic (PK) studies suggested that steady-state trough concentrations ($C_{trough,ss}$) of both darunavir and elvitegravir may be lower when E/C/F/TDF and darunavir are given together, compared to levels obtained when elvitegravir/cobicistat and darunavir (boosted either with cobicistat or ritonavir) are given separately [11, 12]. However, the clinical implications of a potential decrease in $C_{trough,ss}$ are unclear, particularly given the potency of boosted protease-inhibitor-based regimens. Given the potential benefits of treatment simplification in patients receiving complex salvage regimens, we undertook to evaluate the use of once-daily E/C/F/TDF with darunavir as a simplification strategy for treatment-experienced patients who had already achieved virologic suppression on a multi-drug, multi-class antiretroviral regimen, with one-time PK testing and longitudinal viral load monitoring. In view of the known potential for TDF to cause nephrotoxicity [13–15], we also monitored renal function and other safety parameters.

Methods

Study design

We conducted a single arm, open-label study of regimen simplification to E/C/F/TDF plus darunavir 800 mg daily from stable therapy including two nucleoside/nucleotide reverse transcriptase inhibitors, a ritonavir-boosted protease inhibitor (atazanavir or darunavir), and raltegravir or dolutegravir.

Study population

The study enrolled HIV positive adults ($\geq$ 19 years of age) with plasma viral load consistently < 200 copies/mL for $\geq$ 6 months. Subjects were excluded if they had prior documented virologic rebound > 1000 copies/mL on an integrase inhibitor-containing regimen; had evidence on any previous genotypic testing of resistance mutations which would compromise activity of elvitegravir, darunavir, or tenofovir; were currently receiving any nonnucleoside reverse transcriptase inhibitor (NNRTI); were pregnant or breast-feeding; or had any contraindications to tenofovir DF, emtricitabine, elvitegravir, or cobicistat (e.g. previous significant toxicity, intolerance, or were receiving medications with significant drug interactions with the study drugs). The eligibility criteria included having estimated glomerular filtration rate (eGFR) $\geq$ 70 mL/min, as recommended by the manufacturer of E/C/F/TDF [6]; however, waivers were allowed for participants with a stable eGFR $\geq$ 60 mL/min, based on available evidence indicating the safety of E/C/F/TDF in HIV-infected patients with this degree of mild renal impairment [16].

Determination of plasma concentration of study drugs

A plasma sample for measurement of darunavir $C_{trough,ss}$ (pre-dose) was collected at baseline before the switch in subjects receiving once-daily darunavir in their pre-switch regimen.

All subjects took study medication (E/C/F/TDF and darunavir) with food under observation in the clinic on Day 14 or later after starting the new regimen. Plasma samples for drug level testing were drawn immediately pre-dose ($C_{trough,ss}$) and at 1, 2, 3, 4, 5, 6, and 8 h post-dose, then once on the following day for a 24-h post-dose $C_{trough,ss}$. Plasma samples were frozen and stored at – 80 °C until analysis.

Darunavir in stored plasma samples was measured in the BC Centre for Excellence in HIV/AIDS Laboratory using a fully validated method [17]. Addition of elvitegravir and cobicistat to the method was partly validated, including selectivity, linearity, accuracy and recovery, inter- and intra-run repeatability, and stability. External controls were included for darunavir and elvitegravir, but were not available for cobicistat. Lower limits of quantification were 70 ng/mL for darunavir, 80 ng/mL for elvitegravir, and 50 ng/mL for cobicistat. Plasma tenofovir and emtricitabine levels were not measured.

Safety and efficacy assessments

Medical history and physical exam were conducted at baseline, and clinical adverse event assessment and medication update performed at weeks 2, 12, 24, 36, and 48. HIV plasma viral load (COBAS Ampliprep Taqman HIV-1 assay, Roche Diagnostics Systems, Laval, Quebec, Canada) was measured at baseline, at weeks 2 and 4, then every 4 weeks throughout the study. The following laboratory assessments were conducted at baseline and at weeks 12, 24, 36, and 48: CD4 cell counts (absolute and fraction), CD4/CD8 ratio, renal function (serum creatinine, eGFR, serum phosphorus, urinalysis, urine albumin to creatinine ratio [UACR]), AST, ALT, total bilirubin, fasting blood sugar, fasting lipid parameters (total cholesterol, LDL, HDL, total cholesterol/HDL, triglycerides, and apolipoprotein B [apoB]), high-sensitivity C-reactive protein (hsCRP), and pregnancy test for women of child-bearing potential .

Study endpoints and statistical analyses

The primary endpoint was the proportion of subjects with plasma viral load < 200 copies/mL at week 12 following the regimen switch, with secondary endpoints at weeks 24 and 48. The threshold of 200 copies/mL was chosen based on data showing that low level viremia between 50–199 copies/mL is not associated with virological failure or clinical outcomes [18], and is consistent with the definition of virologic failure in international antiretroviral treatment guidelines [19, 20]. Changes in CD4 cell count (absolute and fraction), CD4/CD8 ratios, creatinine, eGFR, serum phosphorus, ALT, AST, total bilirubin, fasting glucose and lipid parameters, and hsCRP between baseline and week 48 were determined using a Wilcoxon signed rank sum test with significance level 0.05. For subjects receiving once daily darunavir prior to switching to the study regimen, darunavir $C_{trough,ss}$ at baseline and day 14 were compared using Wilcoxon signed rank sum test. Elvitegravir and cobicistat concentrations were compared to historical controls.

No sample size calculation was performed for this study. A convenience sample of ten patients was enrolled.

Results

Baseline characteristics

Ten HIV-infected subjects, 8 men and 2 women, were enrolled and started study medications between October 2014 and February 2016 (Table 1). Median age was 50.5 years (range 33–71), weight was 87.5 kg (range 56–101.5), and CD4 cell count was 505 cells/mm^3 (range 50–1020). All had viral load < 40 copies/mL except one whose viral load was 134 copies/mL, considered to be within the limits of error of the assay [21]. Median eGFR at baseline was 81 mL/min (range 60–102). The two subjects who entered the study with eGFR < 70 mL/min had stable renal function, with mildly decreased eGFR between 60 and 70 mL/min for at least 6 months prior to the study baseline visit. All study subjects were receiving tenofovir DF and emtricitabine; 9 were receiving raltegravir and one dolutegravir; 7 were receiving ritonavir-boosted darunavir (6 once daily and one twice daily) and 3 were receiving ritonavir-boosted atazanavir. No subjects were receiving any concomitant medications that would be expected to affect the plasma levels of the antiretrovirals.

Archived antiretroviral drug resistance mutations

Nine subjects had evidence of archived drug-resistant virus on previous genotypic testing, all of whom had M184V/I (conferring resistance to lamivudine and emtricitabine) (Table 2). Five subjects had had thymidine analogue mutations including 41L and 215Y or F, associated with reduced susceptibility to tenofovir DF: enrolment in the study was judged to be safe for these subjects because the other study drugs (darunavir and elvitegravir) were fully active. Six subjects had resistance to NNRTIs, and four had protease-inhibitor-associated mutations, but retained susceptibility to darunavir.

Efficacy results

All 10 subjects had plasma viral load < 200 copies/mL at baseline and at every time point during the study. Nine subjects had viral load < 40 copies/mL at baseline, and viral load remained < 40 copies/mL in 9 at week 12, in 8 at week 24, and in 8 at week 48 (Fig. 1); the subject whose viral load was detectable at week 48 had a viral load of 41 copies/mL. Subject 10's viral load remained detectable at < 200 copies/mL at each time point during the study, and was 174 copies/mL at week 48 (Fig. 2). Among all 10 subjects, no significant changes were observed between baseline and week 48 in absolute CD4 cell count (median 505 and 440 cells/mm^3, respectively) (Fig. 3), CD4 fraction (median 25 and 26%, respectively), or CD4/CD8 ratio (median 0.61 and 0.63, respectively) ($p > 0.05$ for all).

Table 1 Baseline characteristics of study participants (n = 10)

Subject no.	Gender	Age, years	Weight, kg	eGFR, mL/min	Viral load, copies/mL	CD4, cells/mm³	Antiretroviral regimen (with tenofovir DF and emtricitabine)
1	Male	59	92.5	78	< 40	180	RAL 400 mg twice daily DRV 800 mg daily Ritonavir 100 mg daily
2	Male	47	89.5	60	< 40	510	RAL 400 mg twice daily DRV 800 mg daily Ritonavir 100 mg daily
3	Male	71	63	62	< 40	400	RAL 400 mg twice daily ATV 300 mg daily Ritonavir 100 mg daily
4	Male	55	101.5	85	< 40	900	RAL 400 mg twice daily DRV 800 mg daily Ritonavir 100 mg daily
5	Female	42	56	84	< 40	900	RAL 400 mg twice daily DRV 600 mg twice daily Ritonavir 100 mg twice daily
6	Male	33	85.5	102	< 40	410	RAL 400 mg twice daily ATV 300 mg daily Ritonavir 100 mg daily
7	Male	53	72	95	< 40	500	RAL 400 mg twice daily DRV 800 mg daily Ritonavir 100 mg daily
8	Male	56	95.5	74	< 40	700	DTG 50 mg daily DRV 800 mg daily Ritonavir 100 mg daily
9	Female	48	84	100	< 40	50	RAL 400 mg twice daily DRV 800 mg daily Ritonavir 100 mg daily
10	Male	47	98.5	75	134	1020	RAL 400 mg twice daily ATV 300 mg daily Ritonavir 100 mg daily

eGFR estimated glomerular filtration rate, *RAL* raltegravir, *DTG* dolutegravir, *DRV* darunavir, *ATV* atazanavir

Table 2 Archived antiretroviral drug resistance mutations among study participants

Subject no.	Major NRTI resistance mutations		Major NNRTI resistance mutations	Major PI resistance mutations
	Non-TAMs	TAMs		
1	184V	67N, 70R, 219Q	103N	ND
2	184V, 74V	67N, 70R, 219Q	181C, 190A	ND
3	184V	41L, 210W, 215Y	ND	ND
4	184V	70R	ND	ND
5	184V, 74I	41L, 67N, 70R, 215F, 219Q	103N	84V, 90M
6	184V	41L, 67N, 70R, 215Y, 219Q	103N, 181C, 190S	30N, 88D
7	184V	41L, 215Y	103N	54V, 82A
8	184V	41L, 215Y	98G[a]	46L
9	184I, 70E	ND	ND	ND
10	ND	ND	ND	ND

Reference: Stanford HIV Drug Resistance Database. Major HIV-1 Drug Resistance Mutations, Updated summary March 9, 2015. http://hivdb.stanford.edu

NRTI nucleoside analogue reverse transcriptase inhibitor, *TAMs* thymidine analogue mutations, *NNRTI* nonnucleoside analogue reverse transcriptase inhibitor, *PI* protease inhibitor, *ND* none detected

[a] Although not listed as major NNRTI mutation, 98G confers resistance to nevirapine

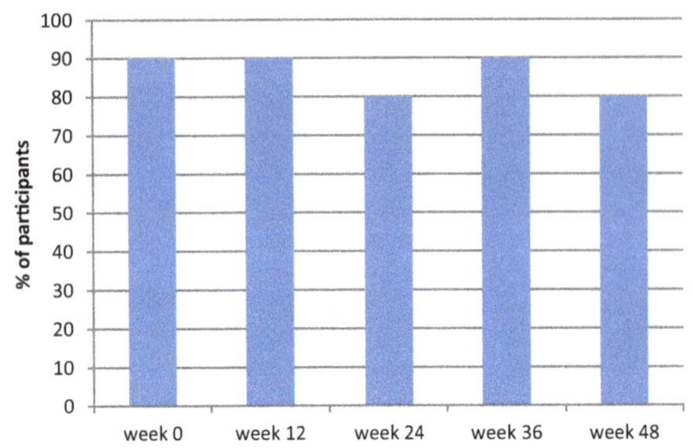

Fig. 1 Proportion of participants (n = 10) with plasma viral load < 40 copies/mL

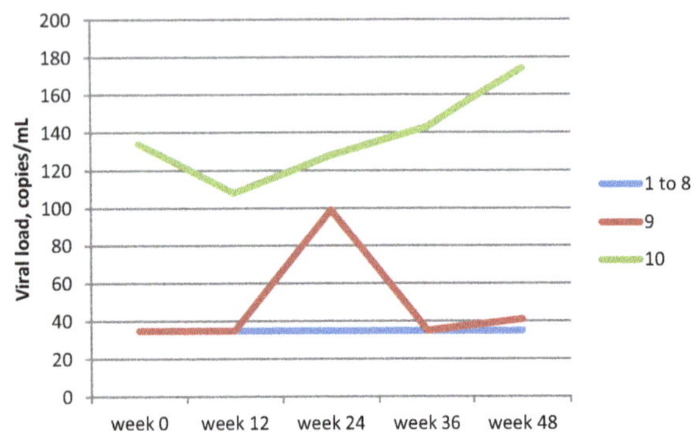

Fig. 2 Viral load of each study participant

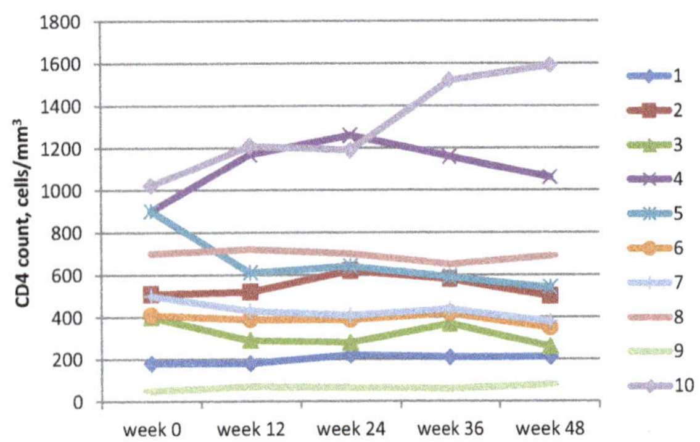

Fig. 3 CD4 cell count of each study participant

Safety results

In the group as a whole, no significant changes were observed between baseline and week 48 in creatinine, eGFR, serum phosphorus, ALT, AST, total bilirubin, glucose, lipid parameters, or hsCRP ($p > 0.05$ for all). No subjects discontinued study medications during the 48-week study for renal function changes or other adverse events. Subject three experienced a decrease in eGFR from 62 mL/min at baseline to 52 mL/min at week 12; study medications were continued and his eGFR remained stable (50–59 mL/min) thereafter. At study entry, this patient had been receiving a tenofovir DF-containing regimen for 29 months and had hypophosphatemia (serum phosphorus 0.66 mmol/L, lower limit of normal 0.80 mmol/L) and proteinuria (UACR 19.2 mg/mmol, upper limit of normal 2.0 mg/mmol), which persisted over the course of the study; at week 48, his serum phosphorus was 0.72 mmol/L and UACR was 33.9 mg/mmol. After week 48, study medications were discontinued and replaced with abacavir, lamivudine, raltegravir, and darunavir/ritonavir; 3 months later, his eGFR was 63 mL/min, serum phosphorus was 0.92 mmol/L, and UACR was 2.3 mg/mmol. No significant clinical or laboratory adverse events were observed in any other study subjects.

Pharmacokinetics of darunavir, elvitegravir, and cobicistat

Darunavir levels

Six subjects were receiving darunavir/ ritonavir once daily prior to study entry, of whom 5 had 24-h post-dose darunavir $C_{trough,ss}$ measured at both baseline and 2 weeks after the switch to E/C/F/TDF and darunavir (the other subject [number 7 in Tables 1 and 2] had taken his medications before the study baseline visit so a pre-dose sample could not be drawn). The median darunavir $C_{trough,ss}$ for these 5 subjects decreased from 981 ng/mL (range 667–1150) at baseline to 431 ng/mL (range 96–784) at week 2 ($p \leq 0.05$). Among all nine subjects who had plasma drug levels measured after the switch to E/C/F/TDF and darunavir (median 14 days, range 14–28 days after the switch; Subject 6 was not available for week 2 sampling), the median darunavir $C_{trough,ss}$ was 482 ng/mL (range 96–848).

Mean and median darunavir $C_{trough,ss}$ are shown in Table 3 for the purpose of comparison with data from the literature. The darunavir $C_{trough,ss}$ we observed with ritonavir prior to the switch to E/C/F/TDF tended to be lower than $C_{trough,ss}$ published in the literature for darunavir/ritonavir 800 mg/100 mg once daily [22, 23]. After the switch to E/C/F/TDF, the darunavir $C_{trough,ss}$ we observed were higher than the extrapolated $C_{trough,ss}$ reported in the presence of E/C/F/TDF by Ricard et al [12], but lower than the measured 24-h darunavir $C_{trough,ss}$ with the same regimen reported by Gutierrez-Valencia et al [24].

The maximum observed darunavir level at 2 weeks was 5840 ng/mL (median), range 3590–7840 ng/mL (n = 9), and was reached at a median of 2.5 h (range 1–5 h) after dosing. This is generally similar to published data for 60 subjects receiving darunavir 800 mg/cobicistat 150 mg with two nucleoside/nucleotide reverse transcriptase

Table 3 Plasma concentrations of darunavir and elvitegravir at 24 h post-dose

Study intervention	N	Darunavir $C_{trough,ss}$, ng/mL		Elvitegravir $C_{trough,ss}$, ng/mL		Refs.
		Median/mean	Range	Median/mean	Range	
DRV/rtv, pre-switch	5	981 (median) 932 (mean)	667–1150	– –	–	
E/C/F/TDF + DRV	9	482 (median) 490 (mean)	96–848	184 (median) 200 (mean)	< 80–435	
DRV/rtv 800/100 mg	335[a]	2041 (median)	368–7242	–	–	[22]
	119	1820 (mean)	IQR 1470–2460	–	–	[23]
DRV/cobi 800/150 mg	298[a]	2150 (mean)	SD 1320	–	–	[25]
	59	1311 (mean)	SD 969	–	–	[25]
	32	1319 (mean)	288–3641	–	–	[24]
E/C/F/TDF (no DRV)	419[a]	–	–	451 (mean)	58–2341	[26]
	32	–	–	250 (mean)	30–762	[24]
E/C/F/TDF + DRV	24	1294 (mean)	163–3641	234 (mean)	92–432	[24]
	8	273 (median)[b]	164–501 (IQR)[b]	–	–	[12]
E/C/F/TAF + DRV	15	1250 (mean)	NA	464 (mean)	NA	[36]

$C_{trough,ss}$ trough plasma concentration at steady-state, *DRV* darunavir, *rtv* ritonavir, *cobi* cobicistat, *E/C/F/TDF* elvitegravir/cobicistat/emtricitabine/tenofovir disproxil fumarate, *E/C/F/TAF* elvitegravir/cobicistat/ emtricitabine/ tenofovir alafenamide, *IQR* interquartile range, *SD* standard deviation, *NA* not available

[a] Population pharmacokinetic estimate; [b] estimated

inhibitors: mean darunavir C_{max} 7663 ng/mL (standard deviation 1920), median t_{max} 3.5 h (interquartile range [IQR] 2.5–4.3 h) [25].

Elvitegravir and cobicistat levels

Among the 9 subjects who had drug levels measured 2 weeks after switching to E/C/F/TDF and darunavir, the median elvitegravir $C_{trough,ss}$ was 184 ng/mL (range < 80–296).

Mean and median elvitegravir $C_{trough,ss}$ are shown in Table 3 for the purpose of comparison with data from the literature. Our observed elvitegravir $C_{trough,ss}$ were somewhat lower than the manufacturer's population pharmacokinetic estimates for E/C/F/TDF without darunavir [26], but generally similar to 24-h $C_{trough,ss}$ measured by Gutierrez-Valencia et al. among patients taking E/C/F/TDF either with or without darunavir [24].

The maximum observed elvitegravir level was 1230 ng/mL (median), range 651–2400 ng/mL (n = 9), and was reached at a median of 3 h (range 1–8 h) after dosing. In comparison, population PK data for E/C/F/TDF (n = 419) provide a mean C_{max} of 1731 ng/mL (standard deviation 23) with a t_{max} of 4.0 h [6, 26].

Cobicistat levels at 24 h post-dosing were < 50 ng/mL in all 9 of our study subjects with available drug levels. The maximum observed cobicistat level was 769 ng/mL (median), range 493–1090 ng/mL (n = 9), and was reached at a median of 2 h (range 2–4 h) after dosing. In published data for 60 subjects receiving darunavir 800 mg/cobicistat 150 mg with two nucleoside/nucleotide reverse transcriptase inhibitors, mean cobicistat C_{0h} was 76 ng/mL (standard deviation 186), mean C_{max} was 991 ng/mL (standard deviation 331), and median t_{max} was 3.5 h (IQR 2.0–4.5) [25].

Discussion

Among 10 treatment-experienced HIV-infected patients who had viral load consistently < 200 copies/mL on a multiple-class antiretroviral regimen, a switch to a two-pill once-daily regimen of E/C/F/TDF and darunavir was safe and effective in maintaining virologic suppression for 48 weeks. One patient had pre-existing TDF-related renal tubular toxicity which persisted but did not worsen on the study regimen, and improved when he was changed to a non-TDF-containing regimen after completion of the study.

Among the 5 patients receiving once-daily darunavir/ritonavir at baseline, darunavir $C_{trough,ss}$ levels were significantly lower after the switch to E/C/F/TDF plus darunavir (the median decreased from 981 to 431 ng/mL), and darunavir $C_{trough,ss}$ levels were low for all 9 subjects with drug levels available on E/C/F/TDF plus darunavir (median 482 ng/mL). Previous studies have shown darunavir $C_{trough,ss}$ to be lower when boosted with cobicistat than with ritonavir, both in healthy volunteers (21–24% lower with cobicistat) [27] and HIV-infected patients (30% lower with cobicistat) [24]. However, the magnitude of the effect we observed (> 50% reduction in darunavir $C_{trough,ss}$) was greater than that observed in the previous studies. This is particularly striking since our subjects' darunavir $C_{trough,ss}$ levels on darunavir /ritonavir (median 981 ng/mL) were already more than 50% lower than those reported in the literature for HIV-infected patients receiving darunavir /ritonavir [22, 23]. The reason for this is unclear, as drug–drug interactions are not expected between darunavir and either raltegravir or dolutegravir (taken concomitantly by 4 subjects and 1 subject, respectively) [28–30]. Possibly as a result of these low baseline levels, our patients' darunavir $C_{trough,ss}$ levels on E/C/F/TDF plus darunavir were less than 40% of those expected with darunavir /cobicistat without elvitegravir (darunavir $C_{trough,ss}$ approximately 1300 ng/mL) [24, 25]. The low darunavir $C_{trough,ss}$ seen in our patients on E/C/F/TDF plus darunavir support an earlier retrospective study that used extrapolated levels and suggested a significant drug–drug interaction between darunavir and E/C/F/TDF [12]; however, a subsequent larger study showed darunavir $C_{trough,ss}$ were similar in 24 patients receiving E/C/F/TDF plus darunavir as in 32 patients receiving darunavir /cobicistat without elvitegravir [24]. Although our study is small, we were able to prospectively measure darunavir $C_{trough,ss}$ in the same patients before and after the switch from darunavir/ritonavir to E/C/F/TDF plus darunavir, and to demonstrate a statistically significant decrease in darunavir $C_{trough,ss}$ after the switch. On the other hand, while the observed darunavir concentrations were low, they remained 2- to 15-fold higher than the protein-adjusted 50% inhibitory concentration (IC_{50}) for darunavir against wild-type virus (55 ng/mL) [31], and the study regimen maintained antiviral efficacy throughout the 48 week study in all 10 patients. As an alternative boosted protease inhibitor-elvitegravir combination regimen, atazanavir would not be an ideal option; coadministration with elvitegravir/cobicistat has been shown to result in significant lowering of atazanavir trough levels [32].

The elvitegravir $C_{trough,ss}$ in our patients receiving E/C/F/TDF plus darunavir (median elvitegravir $C_{trough,ss}$ 184 ng/mL, mean 200 ng/mL) were about 40% of those reported by the manufacturer for E/C/F/TDF without darunavir based on population PK analysis (mean 451 ng/mL) [26]. This is despite the fact that our patients were instructed to take their medications with food, and were observed to do so on the day prior to the 24-h post-dose draw, as recommended to optimize elvitegravir exposure from the coformulation [6, 33]. However, the elvitegravir concentrations we observed were similar those observed by Gutierrez-Valencia et al. in patients receiving E/C/F/TDF, either with darunavir (mean elvitegravir $C_{trough,ss}$ 234 ng/mL) or without darunavir (mean elvitegravir $C_{trough,ss}$ 250 ng/mL) [24]. Since we do not have elvitegravir levels in our patients in the absence of darunavir, we cannot comment on whether there is a significant drug–drug interaction which lowers elvitegravir $C_{trough,ss}$, but the study by Gutierrez-Valencia et al. suggests that this may not be the case [24]. In 7 of 9 subjects in our study, the observed elvitegravir $C_{trough,ss}$ were more than 2-fold above the protein-adjusted 95% inhibitory concentration (IC_{95}) for elvitegravir against wild type virus (45 ng/mL) [34]; the other two patients had elvitegravir $C_{trough,ss}$ of 82 and < 80 ng/mL. Nevertheless, virologic efficacy was maintained in all 10 patients.

Cobicistat $C_{trough,ss}$ were below the lower limit of the assay (< 50 ng/mL) in all cases, and consistent with previous studies utilizing cobicistat as a booster for either elvitegravir or darunavir or both. Tashima et al. reported mean 24-h cobicistat levels of 33 ng/mL (standard deviation 95) among 59 HIV-infected patients taking darunavir/cobicistat with emtricitabine and tenofovir DF [25]. Gutierrez-Valencia et al. reported mean 24-h cobicistat concentrations of 20.2 ng/mL (IQR 11.2–33.1) in patients taking E/C/F/TDF with darunavir, and similar concentrations among those taking E/C/F/TDF without darunavir [24]. While we were unable to quantify cobicistat levels below 50 ng/mL, it appears there was enough cobicistat present to adequately boost elvitegravir, so low cobicistat concentrations are unlikely to explain the low darunavir concentrations seen in our patients taking E/C/F/TDF plus darunavir. In any case, cobicistat $C_{trough,ss}$ is probably less important than area under the plasma concentration-time curve (AUC) in terms of its pharmacological boosting properties [35].

Limitations of our study include the small sample size, non-randomized design, and the lack of full validation for the elvitegravir and cobicistat assays, although the darunavir assay was fully validated. Also our study was conducted with the older E/C/F/TDF formulation. Further investigation of this approach may be warranted, including the new tenofovir alafenamide (TAF) formulation. PK data are available for 15 treatment-experienced HIV patients participating in a switch study to E/C/F/TAF plus darunavir; their mean darunavir $C_{trough,ss}$ was 1250 ng/mL and elvitegravir $C_{trough,ss}$ was 464 ng/mL (no range or IQR available) [36]. There is no reason to expect a substantial difference in the interactions between elvitegravir, cobicistat, and darunavir when coadministered with TAF vs. TDF. The main difference to be expected would be lower plasma tenofovir levels in the presence of darunavir with E/C/F/TAF than with E/C/F/TDF, due to P-glycoprotein induction by darunavir and the resultant decrease in intestinal absorption of TAF (a P-glycoprotein substrate) [10, 37]. Indeed, in the PK substudy of the E/C/F/TAF plus darunavir switch study, plasma concentrations of TAF were at the lower end of the efficacious range, and plasma tenofovir exposure was "markedly lower" than that observed with E/C/F/TDF in previous studies [36]. Nevertheless, simplification to E/C/F/TAF plus darunavir was shown to be safe and efficacious, maintaining virologic suppression (viral load < 50 copies/mL) in 94% of 89 participants in the study [36]. Since we did not measure plasma tenofovir levels in the present study, we are unable to say whether the same effect occurred in our cohort.

Conclusions

In conclusion, E/C/F/TDF plus darunavir was safe and effective as a treatment simplification option for 10 selected treatment-experienced HIV-infected patients. Although darunavir $C_{trough,ss}$ with E/C/F/TDF plus darunavir were lower than with ritonavir-boosted darunavir in this small study, virologic suppression was maintained in all subjects for 48 weeks.

Abbreviations

apoB: apolipoprotein B; AUC: area under the plasma concentration-time curve; C_{0h}: plasma concentration at 0 h; C_{max}: maximum plasma concentration; $C_{trough,ss}$: trough plasma concentration at steady state; EC_{50}: half maximal effective concentration; E/C/F/TDF: elvitegravir/cobicistat/emtricitabine/tenofovir disproxil fumarate; eGFR: estimated glomerular filtration rate; FTC: emtricitabine; hsCRP: high-sensitivity C-reactive protein; IC_{50}: 50% inhibitory concentration; IC_{95}: 95% inhibitory concentration; IQR: interquartile range; NNRTI: nonnucleoside reverse transcriptase inhibitor; NRTI: nucleoside reverse transcriptase inhibitor; PK: pharmacokinetics; TAF: tenofovir alafenamide; TDF: tenofovir disoproxil fumarate; t_{max}: time to maximum plasma concentration; UACR: urine albumin to creatinine ratio.

Authors' contributions

MH contributed to the design of the study and to data analysis and interpretation, and wrote the manuscript. BG enrolled and followed participants and collected data. BW performed the drug level assays and interpreted the data. PRH performed the drug level and genotypic assays and interpreted the data. JSGM contributed to the design of the study, data analysis and interpretation. MWH designed the study, recruited and followed study participants, and contributed to data analysis and interpretation. All authors read and approved the final manuscript

Author details

[1] British Columbia Centre for Excellence in HIV/AIDS, Vancouver, BC, Canada. [2] AIDS Research Program, St. Paul's Hospital, Vancouver, BC, Canada. [3] Department of Family Practice, Faculty of Medicine, University of British Columbia, Vancouver, BC, Canada. [4] Division of AIDS, Faculty of Medicine, University of British Columbia, Vancouver, BC, Canada.

Acknowledgements

The authors would like to thank the study participants, and Jill Jackson for obtaining regulatory and ethical approvals.

Competing interests

MH has received grants, paid to the institution, from the Canadian Institutes for Health Research (CIHR) and honoraria for consultancy and/or speaking engagements from Gilead Sciences Canada Inc., Merck Canada Inc., and ViiV Healthcare. BG and BW declare that they have no competing interests. PRH has received grants from Genome BC, Genome Canada, and CIHR, and limited unrestricted funding, paid to his institution, from AbbVie, Bristol-Myers Squibb, Gilead Sciences, Janssen, Merck, and ViiV. JSGM has received support, paid to the institution, from CIHR, the Public Health Agency of Canada, the British Columbia Ministry of Health, US National Institutes of Health (NIDA R01DA036307 and CTN 248), Johnson & Johnson, and Merck. MWH has received grants, paid to the institution, from the US National Institutes of Health (NIDA Grant 1-RO1DA031043-01), and has received consultancy and speaker's honoraria from Bristol-Myers Squibb, Merck, Gilead, Ortho-Janssen, and ViiV.

Funding

This study was supported by a grant from Gilead Sciences Canada, Inc. (IN-CA-236-1313). The funder was not involved in the design of the study; in the collection, analysis, or interpretation of data; or in writing the manuscript. The funder reviewed the manuscript and provided suggestions for revision prior to submission.

References

1. Harris M, Harrigan PR, Montaner JSG. Chapter 46: Antiretroviral Therapy of Drug-resistant HIV. In: Volberding PA, Sande MA, Lange J, Greene WC, Gallant JE, editors. Global HIV/AIDS medicine. Saunders: Elsevier; 2008. p. 537–45.
2. Wainberg MA, Zaharatos GJ, Brenner BG. Development of antiretroviral drug resistance. N Engl J Med. 2011;365:637–46.
3. Chesney MA. Factors affecting adherence to antiretroviral therapy. Clin Infect Dis. 2000;30(Suppl 2):S171–6.
4. Yazdanpanah Y, Fagard C, Descamps D, et al. High rate of virologic suppression with raltegravir plus etravirine and darunavir/ritonavir among treatment-experienced patients infected with multi-drug resistant HIV: results of the ANRS 139 TRIO trial. Clin Infect Dis. 2009;49:1441–9.
5. Claborn KR, Meier E, Miller MB, Leffingwell TR. A systematic review of treatment fatigue among HIV-infected patients prescribed antiretroviral therapy. Psychol Health Med. 2015;20:255–65.
6. Gilead Sciences Canada Inc. Stribild Product Monograph. Mississauga, Ontario, Canada; March 7, 2017.
7. Shah BM, Schafer JJ, Priano J, Squires KE. Cobicistat: a new boost for the treatment of human immunodeficiency virus infection. Pharmacotherapy. 2013;33:1107–16.
8. Cahn P, Fourie J, Grinzstejn B, et al. Week 48 analysis of once-daily vs. twice-daily drunavir/ritonavir in treatment-experienced HIV-1-infected patients. AIDS. 2011;25:929–39.
9. Boffito M, Miralles D, Hill A. Pharmacokinetics, efficacy, and safety of darunavir/ritonavir 800/100 mg once-daily in treatment-naïve and -experienced patients. HIV Clin Trials. 2008;9:418–27.
10. Janssen Inc. Prezista Product monograph. Toronto, Ontario, Canada; April 7, 2017.
11. Ramanathan S, Wang H, Szwarcberg J, Kearney BP. Safety/tolerability, pharmacokinetics and boosting of twice-daily cobicistat administered alone or in combination with darunavir or tipranavir. In: 13th International Workshop on Clinical Pharmacology of HIV Therapy. Barcelona, Spain. April 16-18, 2012. (poster P08).
12. Ricard F, Wong A, Lebouche B, et al. Low darunavir concentrations in patients receiving Stribild (elvitegravir/cobicistat/emtricitabine/tenofovir disproxil fumarate) and darunavir once daily. In: 16th International Workshop on Clinical Pharmacology of HIV and Hepatitis Therapy. May 26–28, 2015. Washington, DC, USA. (poster 50).
13. Ryom L, Mocroft A, Kirk O, et al. Association between antiretroviral exposure and renal impairment among HIV-positive persons with normal baseline renal function: the D: a: D study. J Infect Dis. 2013;207:1359–69.
14. Islam FM, Wu J, Jansson J, Wilson DP. Relative risk of renal disease among people living with HIV: a systematic review and meta-analysis. BMC Public Health. 2012;12:234.
15. Scherzer R, Estrella M, Li Y, Deeks SG, Grunfeld C, Shlipak MG. Association of tenofovir exposure with kidney disease risk in HIV infection. AIDS. 2012;26:867–75.
16. Post FA, Winston J, Andrade-Villanueva JF, et al. Elvitegravir/cobicistat/emtricitabine/ tenofovir DF in HIV-infected patients with mild-to-moderate renal impairment. J Acquir Immune Defic Syndr. 2015;68:310–3.
17. Gonzalez-Serna A, Swenson LC, Watson B, Auyeung K, Montaner J, Harrigan R. A single untimed plasma drug concentration measurement during low-level HIV viremia predicts virologic failure. Clin Microbiol Infection. 2016;22:1004.e9–16.
18. The Antiretroviral Therapy Cohort Collaboration. (ART-CC). Impact of low-level viremia on clinical and virological outcomes in treated HIV-1-infected patients. AIDS. 2015;29:373–83.
19. Panel on antiretroviral guidelines for adults and adolescents. Guideleins for the use of antiretroviral agents in HIV-1-infected adults and adolescents. Department of Health and Human Services. http://www.aidsinfo.nih.gov/ContentFiles/AdultandAdolescentGL.pdf. Accessed 13 Oct 2017.

20. Günthard HF, Saag MS, Benson CA, et al. Antiretroviral drugs for treatment and prevention of HIV infection in adults: 2016 recommendations of the international antiviral society-USA Panel. JAMA. J Am Med Assoc. 2016;316(2):191–210.
21. Lima V, Harrigan R, Montaner JS. Increased reporting of detectable plasma HIV-1 RNA levels at the critical threshold of 50 copies per milliliter with the Taqman assay in comparison to the Amplicor assay. J Acquir Immune Defic Syndr. 2009;51:3–6.
22. Sekar V, Vanden Abeele C, Van Baelen B, et al. Pharmacokinetic/pharmacodynamic analyses of once-daily darunavir in the ARTEMIS study. 15th Conference on Retroviruses and Opportunistic Infections. February 3–6, 2008. Boston, USA. (poster 769).
23. Gutierrez-Valencia A, Torres-Cornejo A, BenMarzouk-Hidalgo OJ, et al. Darunavir minimum plasma concentration and ritonavir-boosted darunavir monotherapy outcome in HIV-infected patients. Antivir Ther. 2014;19:443–7.
24. Gutierrez-Valencia A, Benmarzouk-Hidalgo OJ, Llaves S, et al. Pharmacokinetic interactions between cobicistat-boosted elvitegravir and darunavir in HIV-infected patients. J Antimicrob Chemother. 2017;72:816–9.
25. Tashima K, Crofoot G, Tomaka FL, et al. Cobicistat-boosted darunavir in HIV-1-infected adults: week 48 results of a Phase IIIb, open-label single-arm trial. AIDS Res Ther. 2014;11:39.
26. Ramanathan S, Wei X, Szwarcberg J, Chang S, Cheng AK, Kearney BP. Exposure-response analysis of once-daily elvitegravir administered as EVG/COBI/FTC/TDF single tablet regimen (Quad STR) in HIV-1 infected patients. In: 19th Conference on Retroviruses and Opportunistic Infections. March 5–8, 2012. Seattle, USA. (poster 622).
27. Kakuda TN, Opsomer M, Timmers M, et al. Pharmacokinetics of darunavir in fixed-dose combination with cobicistat compared with coadministration of darunavir and ritonavir as single agents in healthy volunteers. J Clin Pharm. 2014;54:949–57.
28. Jackson A, Watson V, Back D, et al. Plasma and Intracellular Pharmacokinetics of darunavir/ritonavir once daily and raltegravir once and twice daily in HIV-1 infected individuals. J Acquir Immune Defic Syndr. 2011;58(5):450–7.
29. Garvey L, Latc N, Erlwein OW, et al. The effects of a nucleoside-sparing antiretroviral regimen on the pharmacokinetics of ritonavir-boosted darunavir in HIV type-1-infected patients. Antivir Ther. 2010;15(2):213–8.
30. Song I, Min SS, Borland J, et al. The effect of lopinavir/ritonavir and darunavir/ritonavir on the HIV integrase inhibitor S/GSK1349572 in healthy participants. J Clin Pharmacol. 2011;51(2):237–42.
31. De Meyer S, Azijn H, Surleraux D, et al. TMC114, a novel human immunodeficiency virus type 1 protease inhibitor active against protease inhibitor-resistant viruses, including a broad range of clinical isolates. Antimicrob Agents Chemother. 2005;49:2314–21.
32. S Ramanathan, H Wang, T Stondell, A Cheng, and BP Kearney. Pharmacokinetics and Drug Interaction Profile of Cobicistat boosted-Elvitegravir with Atazanavir, Rosuvastatin or Rifabutin. In: 13th International Workshop on Clinical Pharmacology of HIV Therapy, Barcelona, Spain. April 16–18, 2012.
33. Cattaneo D, Baldelli S, Minisci D, et al. When food can make the difference: the case of elvitegravir-based co-formulation. Int J Pharm. 2016;512:301–4.
34. Ramanathan S, Mathias AA, German P, Kearney BP. Clinical pharmacokinetic and pharmacodynamic profile of the HIV integrase inhibitor elvitegravir. Clin Pharmacokinet. 2011;50(4):229–44.
35. Barcelo C, Gaspar F, Aouri M, et al. Population pharmacokinetic analysis of elvitegravir and cobicistat in HIV-1-infected individuals. J Antimicrob Chemother. 2016;71:1933–42.
36. Huhn GD, Tebas P, Gallant J, et al. A randomized, open-label trial to evaluate switching to elvitegravir/cobicistat/emtricitabine/tenofovir alafenamide plus darunavir in treatment-experienced HIV-1-infected adults. J Acquir Immune Defic Syndr. 2017;74:193–200.
37. Gilead Sciences Canada Inc. Genvoya Product Monograph. Mississauga, Ontario, Canada; May 24, 2017.

13

Hospital days attributable to immune reconstitution inflammatory syndrome in persons living with HIV before and after the 2012 DHHS HIV guidelines

Peter Liu[1*], Rebecca Dillingham[2] and Kathleen A. McManus[2]

Abstract

Background: Immune reconstitution inflammatory syndrome (IRIS) can manifest with initiation or reintroduction of antiretroviral therapy (ART) in persons living with HIV (PLWH). In 2012, updated United States treatment guidelines recommended initiation of ART for all PLWH regardless of CD4 count. The objectives of this study were to quantify hospital usage attributable to IRIS and assess the reasons for hospitalization in PLWH before and after the guideline update.

Methods: Subjects were PLWH between 18–89 years of age who were hospitalized between November 1, 2009 and July 31, 2014. Equivalent time periods before and after updated treatment guidelines were considered, and designated as Time Period 1 and Time Period 2, respectively. IRIS-attributable hospitalizations were identified by ICD9 codes and electronic medical record searches with subsequent review and confirmation. For hospitalizations that were not confirmed as being IRIS-attributable, primary discharge diagnoses were reviewed.

Results: A total of 278 PLWH were hospitalized 521 times throughout the study period. Time Period 1 had 9 PLWH with 12 IRIS-attributable hospitalizations while Time Period 2 had 6 PLWH with 9 IRIS-attributable hospitalizations. A larger proportion of IRIS-attributable hospital days was observed in Time Period 1 compared to Time Period 2 (7.5 vs 4.2%; $p < 0.001$). Median length of stay for IRIS-attributable hospitalizations was longer than for other diagnoses, particularly during Time Period 1 (12.0 vs 4.0; $p = 0.05$). The most common causes for hospitalizations in PLWH were non AIDS-defining infection, AIDS-defining malignancy, and gastrointestinal. PLWH who had HIV viral suppression (<200 copies/mL) accounted for 34 and 24% of hospitalizations in Time Periods 1 and 2 respectively.

Conclusions: Hospitalizations for PLWH continue at high rates and IRIS is a significant contributing factor. In our single-center study, there was a lower number of IRIS-attributable hospitalizations and IRIS-attributable hospital days in Time Period 2 compared with Time Period 1. The hospital burden of IRIS may decrease over time as more PLWH are started on ART earlier in the course of infection. This study highlights the continued importance of early diagnosis and linkage to care of those infected with HIV, so that morbidity and costs associated with IRIS continue to decline.

Keywords: Human immunodeficiency virus, HIV, Immune reconstitution inflammatory syndrome, IRIS, Hospitalization, Practice guidelines, United States Dept. of Health and Human Services, Acquired immunodeficiency syndrome, AIDS

*Correspondence: Peterliu53@gmail.com

[1] Department of Internal Medicine, University of Virginia, PO Box 801379, Charlottesville, VA 22908, USA

Background

Anti-retroviral therapy (ART) utilizes combination drug therapy to suppress replication of human immunodeficiency virus (HIV) and facilitates restoration of host immune function by increasing CD4 positive T-lymphocytes. The advent and wide usage of ART marked a paradigm shift in the management of persons living with HIV (PLWH) [1]. Multi-disciplinary efforts have yielded many novel agents that are both highly potent and generally well-tolerated making the use of ART more ubiquitous. As a result, the life expectancy for persons living with HIV (PLWH) has increased, and within this group, conditions experienced by the general population have become more prevalent [2–6].

While numerous clinical benefits are derived from ART, immune reconstitution inflammatory syndrome (IRIS) is a morbid complication that can manifest with initiation or reintroduction of ART. IRIS is broadly categorized into two pathophysiologic processes of 'unmasking' an untreated sub-clinical opportunistic infection (OI) or a 'paradoxical worsening' of a previously treated infection upon commencement of ART. Well described micro-organisms associated with IRIS include Mycobacterium tuberculosis, Cryptococcus, Cytomegalovirus (CMV), and Herpes virus, among others [7–16].

While the immuno-pathology of IRIS has yet to be completely defined, existing studies suggest that it is multifactorial and complex and includes elements of immune system dysregulation and restructuring of immune cell quantity and function [1, 7]. Several biomarkers have been identified as being disproportionately elevated in the setting of IRIS including TNF-α, IF-γ, and numerous interleukins [17–24]. Regulatory T- cells appear to demonstrate an impaired functional ability to abrogate over-exuberant immunological responses to antigenic stimuli despite an absolute quantitative expansion [25]. More recent studies also highlight the importance of innate immune system dysfunction with high pathogen burden in the development of IRIS [26, 27].

Clinicians are often confronted with the difficult task of discerning between IRIS and a more typical presentation of undertreated primary disease. The clinical manifestations and pathogenesis of IRIS are highly variable and related to the affected organ systems and causative pathogen [17–19, 22]. Further compounding the problem is the absence of clear diagnostic criteria for IRIS with the exception of pathogen-specific definitions that have been proposed for Mycobacterium tuberculosis and Cryptococcus IRIS [26]. Risk factors for IRIS must also be recognized. Numerous studies suggest that severe immunodeficiency and the presence of an OI at the time of ART initiation, particularly if accompanied by a high pathogen burden or disseminated disease, are important considerations [1, 7, 8, 11, 14, 15, 26]. The diagnostic complexity of IRIS in the face of the variable prevalence of underlying OIs have led to estimates of IRIS incidence ranging from 6–47% in PLWH [7, 28, 29].

In 2012, the United States Department of Health and Human Services (DHHS) published updated guidelines recommending the initiation of ART in all HIV infected individuals regardless of their CD4 count at the time of diagnosis [30]. While clinicians must still consider other factors including patient willingness and barriers to adherence, the anticipated population effect is that ART is being initiated earlier and often before severe immunodeficiency develops. To the best of our knowledge, the comparison of the burden of IRIS on the healthcare system as measured by hospital days related to IRIS before and after the 2012 HIV management guideline updates has not been investigated. In this study, we compare hospital days related to IRIS at our 604 bed tertiary-care hospital both before and after updated ART guidelines were published and describe the reasons for hospitalization in PLWH.

Methods

The Clinical Data Repository (CDR), an electronic real-time database of protected health information was used to identify subjects at the University of Virginia Medical Center (UVaMC), a 604 bed tertiary care referral hospital. Cases included persons between 18–89 years of age who were coded by the International Classification of Diseases, Ninth Revision (ICD9) as having a diagnosis of HIV/AIDS or who had a reactive HIV screening assay and were hospitalized at UVaMC between November 1, 2009 and July 31, 2014. Cases with hospitalizations possibly attributable to IRIS were identified by (1) ICD9 code 995.90 and (2) by use of a comprehensive electronic medical record search for the terms "Immune Reconstitution Inflammatory Syndrome" or "IRIS" in hospital notes. By these mechanisms, hospitalizations identified as possibly being attributable to IRIS were then manually reviewed and confirmed independently by two Infectious Diseases physicians who have considerable experience in caring for PLWH. Cases that were not consistent with IRIS despite being coded by ICD9 were excluded.

Equivalent time periods of 28.5 months before (November 1, 2009–March 15, 2012, designated as Time Period 1) and after (March 16, 2012–July 31, 2014, designated as Time Period 2) publication of updated treatment guidelines were considered. Electronic medical records were reviewed for clinical and demographic characteristics, reason for hospitalization, and length of stay.

Clinical characteristics including CD4 cell count and HIV–RNA Viral Load were defined as the values obtained during the examined hospitalization or the values that were taken before the hospitalization. Hepatitis B (HBV) co-infection was defined as a positive HBV surface antigen, HBV IgM core antibody, or detectable HBV Viral Load anytime during or prior to the examined hospitalization. Hepatitis C (HCV) co-infection was defined as a positive HCV antibody or detectable HCV Viral Load anytime during or prior to the examined hospitalization. Chronic HBV or HCV infection was defined as persistent detection of HBV surface antigen, HBV Viral Load, or HCV Viral Load on at least two occasions with one instance occurring during hospitalization or at the time of the laboratory result chronologically closest to the start of hospitalization.

The primary outcome considered was hospital usage related to IRIS measured by IRIS-attributable hospital days and the percentage of total hospital days for PLWH that were attributable to IRIS. Comparisons were made between Time Period 1 and Time Period 2. Reasons for non IRIS-attributable hospitalizations were ascertained from documentation of the primary discharge diagnoses from discharge summaries. Primary discharge diagnoses were then systematically grouped by organ system and diagnosis category for analysis. Categorizing documented diagnoses of AIDS-defining infection or AIDS-defining malignancy was based on the comprehensive list issued by the Centers for Disease Control and Prevention [31].

Clinical information about IRIS-attributable hospitalizations including type of IRIS and causative pathogen was obtained. Paradoxical IRIS cases were defined as cases in which worsening of a previously recognized OI was observed in temporal relation to recent ART implementation. Unmasking IRIS cases were defined as cases in which new onset of symptoms compatible with a previously unrecognized OI were seen in temporal relation to recent ART implementation [7–16]. Due to low numbers and unavailable data, statistical analyses were not performed.

Chi square analyses were performed on categorical data to determine statistically significant differences between groups. Fisher's Exact Test was utilized when a Chi square test had an expected value in any cell of less than five. Continuous data was analyzed by a t test to determine statistically significant differences between groups. When comparing medians, the Mann-Whitney U test was utilized. The significance threshold for all tests was set at .05.

Results

A total of 278 subjects were hospitalized 521 times throughout Time Periods 1 and 2. The entire study population included 69% male, 53% black, and 44% white subjects with a mean age of 47.5 years. Across the time periods, at the time of hospitalization, more than 40% of subjects had CD4 cell counts less than 200, while 31% had CD4 cell counts between 200 and 500, and 25% had CD4 cell counts greater than 500. Approximately 55% of subjects had HIV viral loads less than 200 copies/mL with 46% under 20 copies/mL, while 37% had poor HIV viral suppression with viral loads greater than 1000 copies/mL. Overall in the hospitalized PLWH, the rates of Hepatitis B and Hepatitis C Co-infection were 12 and 18%.

During Time Period 1, there were 151 subjects with 259 non IRIS-attributable hospitalizations, and 9 subjects with 12 IRIS-attributable hospitalizations (Table 1). The majority of patients hospitalized during Time Period 1, for either IRIS-attributable or non IRIS-attributable causes, were male and identified as Black or Hispanic. There were no significant differences in age, race/ethnicity, and rates of Hepatitis B or Hepatitis C co-infection in subjects admitted with IRIS compared to those admitted for alternate causes (Table 1). A greater proportion of subjects with IRIS-attributable hospitalizations (56%) compared to non IRIS-attributable hospitalizations (32%) had poor virologic control with HIV viral loads greater than 1000 copies/mL), but this difference was not statistically significant ($p = 0.54$). Subjects with IRIS-attributable hospitalizations were more likely to have CD4 cell counts less than 200 compared to subjects with non IRIS-attributable hospitalizations, 89 vs 39% ($p = 0.04$).

Time Period 2 had 112 subjects with 241 non IRIS-attributable hospitalizations and 6 subjects with 9 IRIS-attributable hospitalizations. The majority of subjects hospitalized during Time Period 2 were male. Subjects who had IRIS-attributable hospitalizations were more likely to identify as Black compared to those with non IRIS-attributable hospitalizations, 83 vs 47% ($p = 0.008$). The age, race/ethnicity, and rates of Hepatitis B or Hepatitis C co-infections were similar for those with IRIS and non IRIS-attributable admissions. A greater proportion of subjects admitted with IRIS had poor virologic control with HIV viral loads greater than 1000 copies/mL (66 vs 40%, $p = 0.04$). During Time Period 2, patients with IRIS-attributable hospitalizations had more advanced immunodeficiency with 83% having CD4 cell counts less than 200 compared to 36% in those admitted for reasons unrelated to IRIS, although this difference was not statistically significant (Table 1).

There were more hospital days attributable to IRIS in Time Period 1 compared to Time Period 2, 134 and 73 days respectively, while the number of hospital days for non IRIS-attributable hospitalizations was stable (Fig. 1). There was a decrease in the number of all-cause hospitalizations from Time Period 1 to Time Period 2, but a larger proportion of hospital days were IRIS-attributable

Table 1 Hospitalized patient clinical and demographic characteristics by IRIS and study period

	Total study duration n (%)	Subjects with Time Period 1 non IRIS-attributable hospitalization n (%)	Subjects with Time Period 1 IRIS-attributable hospitalization n (%)	p value	Subjects with Time Period 2 non IRIS-attributable hospitalization n (%)	Subjects with Time Period 2 IRIS-attributable hospitalization n (%)	p value
Total subjects	278	151	9		112	6	
Mean age	47.5	47.7	42.8	0.17	47.7	47.3	0.94
Sex[a]				0.73			0.66
Male	192 (69)	105 (70)	7 (78)		75 (67)	5 (83)	
Female	86 (31)	46 (30)	2 (22)		37 (33)	1 (17)	
Race/ethnicity				0.08			0.008
White	121 (44)	61 (40)	2 (22)		58 (52)	0 (0)	
Black	147 (53)	84 (56)	5 (56)		53 (47)	5 (83)	
Hispanic	5 (2)	4 (3)	1 (11)		0 (0)	0 (0)	
Other/unknown	5 (2)	2 (1)	1(11)		1 (1)	1 (17)	
CD4 count[b]				0.004			0.18
<200	112 (40)	59 (39)	8 (89)		40 (36)	5 (83)	
200–500	86 (31)	47 (31)	1 (11)		37 (33)	1 (17)	
>500	69 (25)	39 (26)	0 (0)		30 (27)	0 (0)	
HIV viral load[c]				0.54			0.04
<200	154 (55)	89 (59)	4 (44)		60 (54)	1 (17)	
200–1000	10 (4)	7 (5)	0 (0)		2 (2)	1 (17)	
>1000	103 (37)	49 (32)	5 (56)		45 (40)	4 (66)	
Hepatitis B co-infection[d]				0.47			0.21
Chronic infection	59 (21)	15 (10)	2 (22)		15 (13)	1 (17)	
Exposure and clearance	33 (12)	35 (23)	1 (11)		20 (18)	3 (50)	
No exposure or infection	162 (58)	88 (58)	5 (56)		67 (60)	2 (33)	
Hepatitis C co-infection[e]				0.58			1.00
Chronic infection	16 (6)	31 (21)	1 (11)		18 (16)	1 (17)	
Exposure and clearance	51 (18)	10 (7)	1 (11)		5 (4)	0 (0)	
No exposure or infection	189 (68)	99 (66)	6 (67)		79 (71)	5 (83)	

[a] In our health system, subjects self-identify as male or female. This information is recorded in the electronic health record

[b] Time Period 1: 154 had a CD4 cell count measured, Time Period 2: 113 had a CD4 cell count measured

[c] Time Period 1: 154 had a HIV Viral Load measured, Time Period 2: 113 had a HIV Viral Load measured

[d] Time Period 1: 146 had HBV serologies measured, Time Period 2: 108 had HBV serologies measured

[e] Time Period 1: 148 had HCV serologies measured, Time Period 2: 108 had HCV serologies measured

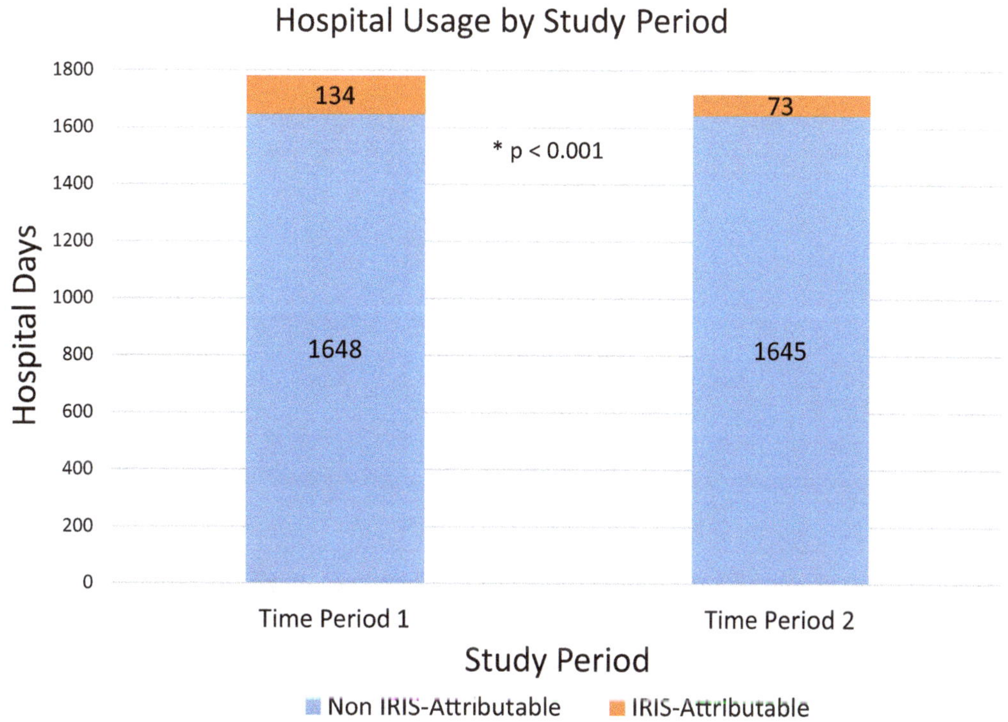

Fig. 1 A comparison of hospital days for IRIS-attributable and non IRIS-attributable hospitalizations stratified by Study Time Period

in Time Period 1 compared to the proportion in Time Period 2 (7.5 vs 4.2%, $p < 0.001$). The median length of stay for IRIS-attributable hospitalizations was longer than for other diagnoses in both Time Period 1 (12.0, interquartile range (IQR) 10 vs 4.0, IQR 5, $p = 0.05$) and Time Period 2 (5.5, IQR 8.25 vs 5.0, IQR 5.0, $p = 0.58$). The average length of stay for IRIS-attributable hospitalizations (11.1) was longer than for non IRIS-attributable hospitalizations (6.4) during Time Period 1. During Time Period 2, the average length of stay was 8.1 days for IRIS-attributable hospitalizations compared to 6.8 days for non IRIS-attributable hospitalizations.

Cases of paradoxical IRIS accounted for the majority of IRIS-attributable hospitalizations in both Time Period 1 (67%) and Time Period 2 (67%). Unmasking IRIS was observed in 33 and 22% of IRIS-attributable hospitalizations in Time Period 1 and Time Period 2 respectively. The most common causative pathogen of IRIS in Time Period 1 was Cryptococcus (42%), followed by Mycobacterium avium complex (17%), and JC Polyomavirus (17%). The most common causative pathogen of IRIS in Time Period 2 was Cryptococcus (22%), followed by Mycobacterium avium complex (22%) and Mycobacterium tuberculosis (11%). There was 1 case (8%) in Time Period 1 and 4 cases (44%) in Time Period 2 in which the causative pathogen was unknown. All cases of Cryptococcal IRIS (7, 100%) in our study manifest as paradoxical IRIS and 2 (50%) cases of MAC IRIS manifest as unmasking IRIS. During Time Period 1, 7 (58%) IRIS-attributable hospitalizations were for subjects on first-line ART, while 1 (8%) and 4 (33%) hospitalizations were for subjects on second-line and salvage ART respectively. During Time Period 2, 6 (67%) IRIS-attributable hospitalizations were for subjects on first-line ART, while 1 (11%) and 2 (22%) hospitalizations were for subjects on second-line and salvage ART respectively. Data regarding the exact duration of ART preceding IRIS-attributable hospitalizations and quantitative viral load trends were often unavailable due to prior care occurring at other institutions.

PLWH were hospitalized 271 times during Time Period 1 and 250 times during Time Period 2. IRIS-attributable hospitalizations accounted for 4.4% of hospitalizations in Time Period 1 and 3.6% of hospitalizations in Time Period 2. The most common cause for hospitalization in Time Period 1 was non-AIDS-defining infection accounting for 19.6% of hospitalizations. This was followed by gastrointestinal, AIDS-defining malignancy, and AIDS-defining infection. The most common cause for hospitalization in Time Period 2 was non-AIDS-defining infection accounting for 19.2% of hospitalizations. This was followed by AIDS-defining malignancy, gastrointestinal, and pulmonary (Tables 2, 3). During Time Period 1, 93 hospitalizations (34%) were for PLWH who had HIV Viral Loads less than 200 copies/mL, while 61 hospitalizations

Table 2 Reason for hospitalization by organ system and diagnosis category

Diagnosis category	Number of admissions for PLWH in Time Period 1 (Nov. 1, 2009–Mar. 15, 2012) n (%)
Total admissions	271 (100)
1. Non-AIDS-defining infection	53 (19.6)
2. Gastrointestinal	30 (11.1)
3. AIDS-defining malignancy[a]	21 (7.7)
4. AIDS-defining infection[b]	17 (6.3)
5. Orthopedic	17 (6.3)
6. Pulmonary	16 (5.9)
7. Renal	13 (4.8)
8. Hematologic	13 (4.8)
9. Cardiovascular	12 (4.4)
10. IRIS	12 (4.4)
11. Psychological	12 (4.4)
12. Non-AIDS-defining malignancy	11 (4.1)
13. Neurological	8 (3.0)
14. Substance abuse	8 (3.0)
15. Symptom based	8 (3.0)
16. Other	8 (3.0)
17. Obstetric	7 (2.6)
18. Endocrine	5 (1.8)
19. Trauma	0 (0)

[a] AIDS Defining Malignancy category includes Invasive Cervical CA, Kaposi Sarcoma, Burkitt Lymphoma, Immunoblastic Lymphoma, Primary CNS Lymphoma

[b] AIDS Defining Infection category includes Candidiasis of the esophagus, bronchi, trachea, or lungs, invasive cervical cancer, disseminated or extrapulmonary Coccidioidomycosis, extrapulmonary Cryptococcosis, chronic Cryptosporidiosis, Cytomegalovirus disease (other than liver, spleen, or nodes), Cytomegalovirus retinitis, HIV related encephalopathy, chronic ulcers, bronchitis, pneumonitis, or esophagitis due to Herpes simplex, disseminated or extrapulmonary Histoplasmosis, chronic Isosporiasis, Kaposi's Sarcoma, Burkitt's Lymphoma, Immunoblastic Lymphoma, Primary CNS Lymphoma, disseminated or extrapulmonary disease due to non-tuberculous Mycobacterium, Mycobacterium tuberculosis of any site, Pneumocystis jirovecii pneumonia, recurrent pneumonia, Progressive Multifocal Leukoencephalopathy, recurrent Salmonella septicemia, Toxoplasmosis, HIV wasting syndrome [30]

Table 3 Reason for hospitalization by organ system and diagnosis category

Diagnosis category	Number of admissions for PLWH in Time Period 2 (Mar. 16, 2012–July 31, 2014) n (%)
Total admissions	250 (100)
1. Non-AIDS-defining infection	48 (19.2)
2. AIDS-defining malignancy[a]	35 (14.0)
3. Gastrointestinal	24 (9.6)
4. Pulmonary	24 (9.6)
5. AIDS-defining infection[b]	20 (8.0)
6. Cardiovascular	15 (6.0)
7. Neurological	13 (5.2)
8. Renal	12 (4.8)
9. Substance abuse	12 (4.8)
10. IRIS	9 (3.6)
11. Symptom based	8 (3.2)
12. Orthopedic	7 (2.8)
13. Non-AIDS-defining malignancy	7 (2.8)
14. Psychological	4 (1.6)
15. Obstetric	4 (1.6)
16. Hematologic	3 (1.2)
17. Other	3 (1.2)
18. Trauma	2 (0.8)
19. Endocrine	0 (0)

[a] AIDS Defining Malignancy category includes Invasive Cervical CA, Kaposi Sarcoma, Burkitt Lymphoma, Immunoblastic Lymphoma, Primary CNS Lymphoma

[b] AIDS Defining Infection category includes Candidiasis of the esophagus, bronchi, trachea, or lungs, invasive cervical cancer, disseminated or extrapulmonary Coccidioidomycosis, extrapulmonary Cryptococcosis, chronic Cryptosporidiosis, Cytomegalovirus disease (other than liver, spleen, or nodes), Cytomegalovirus retinitis, HIV related encephalopathy, chronic ulcers, bronchitis, pneumonitis, or esophagitis due to Herpes simplex, disseminated or extrapulmonary Histoplasmosis, chronic Isosporiasis, Kaposi's Sarcoma, Burkitt's Lymphoma, Immunoblastic Lymphoma, Primary CNS Lymphoma, disseminated or extrapulmonary disease due to non-tuberculous Mycobacterium, Mycobacterium tuberculosis of any site, Pneumocystis jirovecii pneumonia, recurrent pneumonia, Progressive Multifocal Leukoencephalopathy, recurrent Salmonella septicemia, Toxoplasmosis, HIV wasting syndrome [31]

(24%) during Time Period 2 were for PLWH with similar viral suppression.

Discussion

In this retrospective study, there was a statistically significant decrease in hospital usage related to IRIS following the release of updated HIV treatment guidelines by the DHHS in 2012 with the proportion of hospital days attributable to IRIS in Time Period 2 being 4.2% compared to Time Period 1 of 7.5% (Chi square $p < 0.001$). The United States treatment guidelines issued by the DHHS prior to 2012 recommended ART for all patients with CD4 counts <350, however, the panel was divided on the strength of recommendation for patients with CD4 counts between 350 and 500, and half viewed ART as optional for patients with CD4 counts >500 [32]. With the 2012 guideline updates recommending the initiation of ART for PLWH regardless of the CD4 cell count at the time of diagnosis, it is plausible that a greater proportion of PLWH are being initiated on ART earlier in the course of HIV infection before progressive immunodeficiency develops and the likelihood of acquiring opportunistic infections rises.

The majority of subjects with an IRIS-attributable hospitalization in our cohort had CD4 cell counts less than 200 (mean 112) and detectable HIV Viral Loads in excess of 1000 copies/mL. This finding is similar to that of numerous prior studies which report on the association of severe immunodeficiency and the development of IRIS in PLWH [1, 7, 8, 26]. In a retrospective multicenter study evaluating the incidence and risk factors associated with Cryptococcal IRIS, Lortholary et al found that lower CD4 cell counts (<7 × 10^6 cell/L, lower quartile) was an independent risk factor for the occurrence of IRIS [31]. In a separate study on M. *tuberculosis* IRIS in PLWH, Breton et al found that PLWH who developed IRIS had lower baseline CD4 cell counts (median 75), and that IRIS was associated with more pronounced reductions in HIV-1 RNA levels and increases in CD4 cell count percentages after 1 month of ART [34].

During both Time Period 1 and Time Period 2, subjects who identified as either Black or Hispanic were more likely to have IRIS compared to subjects who identified as White. Although findings have been heterogeneous, racial disparities, as it pertains to the care of PLWH and complications of HIV infection have been well described [35, 36]. In a multi-center analysis involving more than 10,000 subjects by Gebo et al, being of African American ethnicity was associated with a lower likelihood of receiving ART compared to Whites [37]. Similarly, in an analysis by Novak and colleagues, being of nonwhite race/ethnicity was significantly associated with the development of IRIS compared to non-Hispanic Whites (Adjusted OR: 1.50, $p = 0.009$) [28]. Reasons for these disparities are likely multi-factorial and include differences in access to care or insurance, variations in healthcare literacy, potential language barriers, stigma, and differences in rates of co-existing substance abuse [37–42].

The precise measurable impact of IRIS on PLWH and the healthcare system remain uncertain. Estimates on the incidence of IRIS range from 6–47% related to variable definitions of IRIS and the diversity of settings in which studies take place with different resources and prevalence of OIs [7, 28, 29, 32–34]. Yet while the majority of IRIS events are self-limiting, fatalities, particularly when pathogen specific IRIS involves the central nervous system are well documented [7, 22, 28, 33, 43]. Moreover, the morbidity and use of healthcare resources associated with IRIS are significant.

The median length of stay for subjects with IRIS-attributable hospitalizations was 8 days longer than for non IRIS-attributable hospitalizations during Time Period 1. The reasons for this are likely multiple. First, IRIS is a diagnostically complex entity without clear pathognomonic features, and exclusion of progression or inadequate treatment of an underlying primary OI is required. Second, the management of IRIS events are not standardized. Finally, PLWH who experience IRIS events often comprise a population with higher acuity of illness owing to associations with poorer baseline immunologic parameters and virologic control.

During both Time Period 1 and Time Period 2, Cryptococcus species and Mycobacterium avium complex (MAC) were the most frequent causes of IRIS-attributable hospitalizations. Cryptococcal IRIS was associated with paradoxical IRIS, and MAC with unmasking IRIS, although the latter was not exclusively observed. The relatively high rate of paradoxical Cryptococcal IRIS may be due to several factors. The incidence of paradoxical Cryptococcal IRIS is relatively high and has been reported at frequencies of 10–42% in ART naïve PLWH [23, 44, 45]. Compared to other etiologies of IRIS which can be self-limiting, Cryptococcal meningitis IRIS carries a high rate of morbidity and mortality which may necessitate hospital admission [45]. Moreover, prolonged or recrudescence of symptoms, which is not unusual for Cryptococcal IRIS, led to recurrent admissions in our study. One patient with paradoxical Cryptococcal IRIS accounted for 3 IRIS-attributable hospitalizations in Time Period 1, while a different patient accounted for 2 IRIS-attributable hospitalizations in Time Period 2.

With widely expanding usage of ART and the ease of several once daily regimens now available as first-line treatments, PLWH are living longer, but hospitalizations for PLWH continue at rates higher than the general population [46]. Over the course of our 57 month study period, PLWH were hospitalized 521 times with IRIS accounting for 4.4% of hospitalizations in the pre-guideline period and 3.6% of hospitalizations in the post-guideline period (Tables 2, 3). Importantly, 34% of hospitalizations in Time Period 1 and 24% of hospitalizations in Time Period 2 were for PLWH who demonstrated HIV viral suppression with HIV Viral Loads quantitated as undetectable or less than 200 copies/mL. This parallels findings from other studies that show higher rates of hospitalization in PLWH compared to the general population, even amongst those with viral suppression [46, 47].

The leading reason for hospitalization in both study periods was non-AIDS-defining infection accounting for greater than 19% of hospitalizations throughout. This is similar to findings in several other studies reporting on the causes for hospitalization in PLWH [46, 47]. Following non-AIDS-defining infection, gastrointestinal reasons represented the second most common cause of hospitalization in Time Period 1 (11.1%), and the third most common cause in Time Period 2 (9.6%). Gastrointestinal causes, particularly pancreatitis and liver disease have also been found to be common causes for admission in other studies examining hospitalization trends among PLWH [46, 47]. Co-existing substance abuse and hepatitis co-infection, which remains prevalent among PLWH, may be at least in part responsible for this trend.

AIDS-defining malignancy comprised a significant proportion of hospitalizations for PLWH in both the pre-guideline and post-guideline period accounting for 7.7 and 14.0% of admissions respectively. This is in contrast to lower rates that are reported in other studies including a large 8 year analysis of a United States military cohort in which hospitalizations for AIDS-defining malignancy was observed at a rate of only 2.3 per 1000 person-years [46]. While the high proportion of admissions related to AIDS-defining malignancy we observed is surprising, the majority of these hospitalizations were for a minority of the study population. In Time Period 1, 5 subjects accounted for the 21 hospitalizations for AIDS-defining malignancy, and in Time Period 2, 9 subjects accounted for 35 such hospitalizations. Moreover, the majority of these hospitalizations were for pre-scheduled chemotherapeutic admissions.

Limitations of this study include the retrospective study design and reliance on the accuracy of medical record documentation. Without universally accepted definitions for IRIS, we, like others, have relied on expert opinion for diagnostic purposes. IRIS events requiring inpatient care are an uncommon occurrence, and as such, the number of cases in our study was relatively low. Nevertheless, we did observe a reduction in the burden of IRIS on the healthcare system in the Time Period 2 compared to Time Period 1, and our study adds to the literature as the first to examine such a trend. While guideline updates were undoubtedly significant, other factors that were not evaluated in our study may have influenced our findings, such as rates of retention in care, rates of ART compliance, and growth of expertise with recognition of IRIS. Finally, PLWH who experienced IRIS events that were managed in the outpatient setting and who may have required significant healthcare resource allocation, were not captured in our study.

Future multi-center studies could elucidate whether fewer IRIS events requiring hospitalization is occurring on a broader scale. Further evaluation of the demographic characteristics, immunologic recovery and viral suppression trends, and ART regimens that are associated with an IRIS event would be informative. Continued efforts to clarify the complex pathogenesis of IRIS will be instructive as more standardized definitions of IRIS are developed.

Conclusions

Hospitalizations continue at high rates for PLWH compared to the general population, and IRIS is an important contributing factor [46–50]. In our single center study, we observed a decrease in the burden of IRIS on the healthcare system as measured by a reduction in the percentage of IRIS-attributable hospital days in Time Period 2 compared with Time Period 1. As a greater proportion of PLWH are started on ART earlier in the course of HIV infection, immunologic control and suppression of viral replication may more readily occur prior to acquisition of OIs thereby reducing the risk of IRIS. Efforts to recognize and diminish healthcare disparities in HIV care must continue, so that individual and population-level benefits derived from early ART can be achieved across all groups.

Abbreviations

IRIS: immune reconstitution inflammatory syndrome; ART: antiretroviral therapy; PLWH: persons living with HIV; HIV: human immunodeficiency virus; OI: opportunistic infection; CMV: cytomegalovirus; DHHS: United States Department of Health and Human Services; CDR: Clinical Data Repository; UVaMC: University of Virginia Medical Center; ICD9: International Classification of Diseases, Ninth Revision; HBV: Hepatitis B; HCV: Hepatitis C; IQR: interquartile range; MAC: mycobacterium avium complex.

Authors' contributions

PL, KM, and RD participated in the design of the study, drafting of the manuscript, and table/figure design. PL and KM performed analysis of data. RD further contributed with statistical analysis. All authors read and approved the final manuscript.

Author details

[1] Department of Internal Medicine, University of Virginia, PO Box 801379, Charlottesville, VA 22908, USA. [2] Division of Infectious Diseases and International Health, University of Virginia, PO Box 801379, Charlottesville, VA 22908, USA.

Acknowledgements

Not applicable.

Competing interests

The authors declare that they have no competing interests.

Funding

This work was supported by the Agency for Healthcare Research and Quality (Grant F32HS024196). The content of this article is solely the responsibility of the authors and does not necessarily represent the official views of the Agency for Healthcare Research and Quality.

References

1. Shelburne S, Hamill R, Rodriguez-Barradas M. Immune reconstitution inflammatory syndrome: emergence of a unique syndrome during highly active antiretroviral therapy. Medicine. 2002;81(3):213–27.
2. May M, Gompels M, Delpech V. Impact on life expectancy of HIV-1 positive individuals of CD4+ cell count and viral load response to antiretroviral therapy. AIDS. 2014;28:1193–202.
3. Wandeler G, Johnson LF, Egger M. Trends in life expectancy of HIV-positive adults on antiretroviral therapy across the globe: comparisons with general population. Curr Opin HIV AIDS. 2016;11(5):492–500 **[Epub ahead of print]**.
4. Teeraananchai S, Kerr S, Ruxrungtham K. Life expectancy of HIV-positive people after starting combination antiretroviral therapy: a meta-analysis. HIV Med **[Epub ahead of print]**.
5. Deeks S, Phillips A. HIV infection, antiretroviral treatment, ageing, and non-AIDS related morbidity. BMJ. 2009;338:a3172. doi:10.1136/bmj.a3172.
6. Serrano-Villar S, Perez-Elias M, Dronda F. Increased Risk of Serious Non-AIDS-Related Events in HIV-Infected Subjects on Antiretroviral Therapy Associated with a Low CD4/CD8 Ratio. PLoS One. 2013;9(1):e85798. doi:10.1371/journal.pone.0085798.
7. Muller M, Wandel S, Colebunders R. Incidence and lethality of immune reconstitution disease in HIV-infected patients starting antiretroviral therapy: systematic review and meta-analysis. Lancet Infect Dis. 2010;10(4):251–61.
8. French M, Price P, Stone S. Immune restoration disease after antiretroviral therapy. AIDS. 2004;18(12):1615–27.

9. DeSimone J, Pomerantz R, Babinchak T. Inflammatory reactions in HIV-1-infected persons after initiation of highly active antiretroviral therapy. Ann Intern Med. 2000;133(6):447–54.
10. French M, Lenzo N, John M. Immune restoration disease after the treatment of immunodeficient HIV-infected patients with highly active antiretroviral therapy. HIV Med. 2001;1(2):107–15.
11. Jevtovic D, Salemovic D, Ranin J. The prevalence and risk of immune restoration disease in HIV-infected patients treated with highly active antiretroviral therapy. HIV Med. 2005;6(2):140–3.
12. Ratnam I, Chiu C, Kandala N. Incidence and risk factors for immune reconstitution inflammatory syndrome in an ethnically diverse HIV type 1–Infected cohort. Clin Infect Dis. 2006;42(3):418–27.
13. Park WB, Choe PG, Jo JH. Tuberculosis manifested by immune reconstitution inflammatory syndrome during HAART. AIDS. 2007;21(7):875–7.
14. Jenny-Avital E, Abadi M. Immune reconstitution cryptococcosis after initiation of successful highly active antiretroviral therapy. Clin Infect Dis. 2002;35(12):128–33.
15. Davies M, Meintjes G. Assessing the contribution of the immune reconstitution inflammatory syndrome to mortality in developing country antiretroviral therapy programs. Clin Infect Dis. 2009;49(6):973–5.
16. Seydi M, Manga N, Dieng A. Immune reconstitution syndrome during antiretroviral therapy in senegal. Infect Dis Med. 2009;39(5):350–1.
17. Mayer K, French M. Immune reconstitution inflammatory syndrome: a reappraisal. Clin Infect Dis. 2009;48(1):101–7.
18. Mahnke Y, Greenwald J, DerSimonian R. Selective expansion of polyfunctional pathogen-specific CD4+ T cells in HIV-1-infected patients with immune reconstitution inflammatory syndrome. Blood. 2012;119(13):3105–12.
19. Kestens L, Seddiki N, Bohjanen P. Immunopathogenesis of immune reconstitution disease in HIV patients responding to antiretroviral therapy. Curr Opin HIV AIDS. 2008;3(4):419–24.
20. Tadokera R, Meintjes G, Skolimowska K. Hypercytokinaemia accompanies HIV-tuberculosis immune reconstitution inflammatory syndrome. Eur Respir J. 2011;37(5):1248–59.
21. Boulware D, Meya D, Bergemann T. Clinical features and serum biomarkers in HIV immune reconstitution inflammatory syndrome after cryptococcal meningitis: a prospective cohort study. PLOS Med. 2010;7(12):e1000384.
22. Shelburne S, Darcourt J, White C. The role of immune reconstitution inflammatory syndrome in AIDS-related *cryptococcus neoformans* disease in the era of highly active antiretroviral therapy. Clin Infect Dis. 2005;40(7):1049–52.
23. Sharma S, Soneja M. HIV & immune reconstitution inflammatory syndrome (IRIS). Indian J Med. 2011;134:866–77.
24. Piliero P, Fish D, Preston S. Guillain-barré syndrome associated with immune reconstitution. Clin Infect Dis. 2003;36(9):111–1114.
25. Seddiki N, Sasson S, Santner-Nanan B. Proliferation of weakly suppressive regulatory CD4+ T cells is associated with over-active CD4+ T-cell responses in HIV-positive patients with mycobacterial immune restoration disease. Eur J Immunol. 2009;39(2):391–403.
26. Walker N, Scriven J, Meintjes G. Immune reconstitution inflammatory syndrome in HIV-infected patients. HIV AIDS Res Palliat Care. 2015;7:49–64.
27. Barber D, Andrade B, Sereti I. Immune reconstitution inflammatory syndrome: the trouble with immunity when you had none. Nat Rev Microbiol. 2012;10(2):150–6.
28. Novak R, Richardson J, Buchacz K. Immune reconstitution inflammatory syndrome: incidence and implications for mortality. AIDS. 2012;26(6):721–30.
29. Marais S, Meintjes G, Pepper D. Frequency, severity, and prediction of tuberculous meningitis immune reconstitution inflammatory syndrome. Clin Infect Dis. 2013;56(3):450–60.
30. Guidelines for the use of antiretroviral agents in HIV-1 infected adults and adolescents. Department of Health and Human Services. http://aidsinfo.nih.gov/contentfiles/adultandadolescentgl003093.pdf. Accessed 27 Mar 2017
31. Center for Disease Control and Prevention (CDC). AIDS-defining Conditions. Morbidity and Mortality Weekly Report. Retrieved from https://www.cdc.gov/mmwr/preview/mmwrhtml/rr5710a2.htm. Accessed 5 Dec 2008
32. Panel on antiretroviral guidelines for adults and adolescents. Guidelines for the use of antiretroviral agents in HIV-1-infected adults and adolescents. Department of Health and Human Services. 1 Dec 2009;1–161. Available at http://www.aidsinfo.nih.gov/ContentFiles/AdultandAdolescentGL.pdf.
33. Lortholary O, Arnuad F, Mamain N. Incidence and risk factors of immune reconstitution inflammatory syndrome complicating HIV-associated cryptococcosis in France. AIDS. 2005;19(10):1043–9.
34. Breton G, Duval X, Estellat C. Determinants of immune reconstitution inflammatory syndrome in HIV Type 1-infected patients with tuberculosis after initiation of antiretroviral therapy. Clin Infect Dis. 2004;39(11):1709–12.
35. Johnson E, Roediger M, Landrum M. Race/ethnicity and HAART initiation in a military HIV infected cohort. AIDS Res Ther. 2014;11:10.
36. Turner B, Cunningham W, Duan N. Delayed medical care after diagnosis in a US national probability sample of persons infected with human immunodeficiency virus. Arch Intern Med. 2000;160:2614–22.
37. Gebo K, Fleishman J, Conviser R. Racial and Gender Disparities in Receipt of Highly Active Antiretroviral Therapy Persist in a Multistate Sample of HIV Patients in 2001. J Acquir Immune Defic Syndr. 2005;38(1):96–103.
38. Earnshaw V, Bogart L, Dovidio J. Stigma and racial/ethnic HIV disparities: moving toward resilience. Am Psychol. 2013;68(4):225–36.
39. Pellowski J, Kalichman S, Matthews K. A pandemic of the poor: social disadvantage and the U.S. HIV epidemic. Am Psychol. 2013;68(4):197–209.
40. Losina E, Schackman B, Sadownik S. Racial and gender disparities in life expectancy losses among HIV-infected persons in the United States: impact of risk behavior, late initiation, and early discontinuation of antiretroviral therapy. Clin Infect Dis. 2009;49(10):1570–8.
41. Haines C, Fleishman J, Yehia B. Closing the gap in antiretroviral initiation and viral suppression: time trends and racial disparities. J Acquir Immune Defic Syndr. 2016;73(3):340–7.
42. McManus K, Rhodes A, Bailey S. Affordable care act qualified health plan coverage: association with improved HIV viral suppression for AIDS drug assistance program clients in a medicaid nonexpansion state. CID. 2016;63(3):396–403.
43. Hoyo-Ulloa I, Belaunzarán-Zamudio PF, Crabtree-Ramirez B, Galindo-Fraga A, Pérez-Aguinaga ME, Sierra-Madero JG. Impact of the immune reconstitution inflammatory syndrome (IRIS) on mortality and morbidity in HIV-infected patients in Mexico. Int J Infect Dis. 2011;15(6):e408–14.
44. Bicanic T, Meintjes G, Rebe K. Immune reconstitution inflammatory syndrome in HIV-associated cryptococcal meningitis: a prospective study. J Acquir Immune Defic Syndr. 2009;51(2):130–4.
45. Kambugu A, Meya DB, Rhein J. Outcomes of cryptococcal meningitis in Uganda before and after the availability of high active antiretroviral therapy. CID. 2008;46(11):1694–701.
46. Crum-Cianfone N, Grandits G, Echols S. Trends and causes of hospitalizations among HIV-infected persons during the late HAART Era: what is the impact of CD4 Counts and HAART use? J Acquir Immune Defic Syndr. 2010;54(3):248–57.
47. Crowell T, Gebo K, Blankson J. Hospitalization rates and reasons among HIV elite controllers and persons with medically controlled HIV infection. J Infect Dis. 2015;211(11):1692–702.
48. Office of statewide health planning and development. Trends in the hospitalization of persons living with HIV/AIDS in California, 1988 to 2008. http://www.library.illinois.edu/learn/research/citation/ama.html. Published 2011.
49. Health, United States, 2015: With special feature on racial and ethnic health disparities. National Center for Health Statistics. 2016. https://www.cdc.gov/nchs/data/hus/hus15.pdf. Accessed 7 Dec 2016
50. Bachhuber M, Southern W. Hospitalization rates of people living with HIV in the United States, 2009. Public Health Rep. 2014;129(2):178–86.

14

Determinants to antiretroviral treatment non-adherence among adult HIV/AIDS patients

Berhe Beyene Gebrezgabher[1], Yigzaw Kebede[2], Melaku Kindie[2], Desalegn Tetemke[1], Mebrahtu Abay[1] and Yalemzewod Assefa Gelaw[2*]

Abstract

Background: Adhering 95% and above of antiretroviral therapy reduces the rate of disease progression and death among people's living human immunodeficiency virus. Though manifold factors have reported as determinant factors of antiretroviral therapy adherence status, perhaps determinants of non-adherence differ up on the activities of patients in the study setting.

Methods: An institution based unmatched case–control study was conducted in Aksum town. Individuals who had a 6-month follow-up with complete individual information were included in the study. Document review and interviewer based techniques were used to collect the data. Binary logistic regression analysis was used to identify the determinant factors of non-adherence.

Results: A total of 411 (137 cases and 274 control) study participants were included in the study. The majority of them were male in sex. Having 2 years and above duration on ART [AOR = 7, 95% CI (2.2, 22.6)], history of adverse effect [AOR = 6.9, 95% CI (1.4, 32.9)], substance use [AOR = 5.3, 95% CI (1.4, 20.0)], living with parents [AOR = 3.4, 95% CI (1.2, 10.3)], having depression symptom [AOR = 3.3, 95% CI (1.4, 7.5)], <350 cells/mm^3 cluster of differentiation 4 count [AOR = 3.2, 95% CI (1.8, 5.8)] and low dietary diversity [AOR = 2, 95% CI (1.1, 3.7)] were found significant determinants of non-adherence to antiretroviral drug.

Conclusion: Program, social and individual related factors showed a statistically significant associated with non-adherence to antiretroviral therapy. Managing lifestyle by developing self-efficacy of individuals and treating related threat to improve adherence status of antiretroviral therapy is recommended in this study.

Keywords: Antiretroviral therapy, Case–control study, Non-adherence, Northern Ethiopia

Background

In 2013 globally, 35 million people living with Human Immunodeficiency Virus (HIV). Worthily, sub-Saharan Africa (23.5–26.1 million) people living with HIV which is 71% of the global prevalence UNAIDS [1]. Ethiopia, an estimated 793,700 (716,300–893,200) people living with HIV/AIDS [2].

Antiretroviral therapy (ART) is a proven treatment for HIV/ADS patients in improving the health status and quality of life of HIV/AIDS patients by reducing the rate of disease progression [3]. Appropriately taking of the treatment is the advisable option in order to obtain full benefits of ART; durable suppression of viral replication, reduced destruction of CD4 cells, prevention of viral resistance, promotion of immune reconstitution, and slowed disease progression [4]. Poor ART adherence is a notable public health problem in developing countries [5].

An individual considered as non-adherence for ART if he/she had a history of taking doses 2 or more hours

*Correspondence: yalassefa@gmail.com
[2] Department of Epidemiology and Biostatistics, Institute of Public Health, College of Medicine and Health Science, University of Gondar, 196 Gondar, Ethiopia

before, and/or 2 or more hours after the time of a doctor's advice to take doses or missing doses completely (i.e., <95% adherence = missing >2 doses of 30 doses or >3 doses of 60 doses) [5, 6]. In 2012, over 9.7 million people living with HIV in low- and middle-income countries were receiving ART, however, ensuring adherence to HIV treatment remains challenging in all countries [7].

Adherence of ART is a complex behavior, which is influenced by several determinants, majorly patient loss to follow-up and ensuring adherence to ART regimens remain major challenges in Ethiopia [2, 5].

Variables such as; availability of reminder, substance use, malnutrition, dietary diversity, CD4 count, depression symptom, adverse effect of ART and duration on ART were reported as a determinant factor for non-adherence to ART [5, 6, 8–12]. Duration on ART [13, 14] and CD4 count in [11, 15] were associated with non-adherence to ART. Determinant factors for non-adherence are multiple and have different effects. This study was aimed to identify determinants of non-adherence to ART among HIV-infected adults in Aksum town health facilities, northern Ethiopia.

Methods

An institution based unmatched case–control study was carried out from March 20 to May 15, 2015, in Aksum Health Center and Aksum Hospital, Aksum, Ethiopia. Aksum town is located 1067 km away in Northeast Ethiopia of Addis Ababa, the capital city of Ethiopia.

Sample size and sampling procedure

The sample size of the study was calculated by Epi-Info™ 7 software Statcalc program using the following assumptions; proportion of non-adherence among not exposed (controls) 12.1%, proportion of non-adherence among exposed (cases) 21.7%, odds ratio 2.18 [16], 5% level of significance, 80% power of the study and 1:2 case to control ratio.

All HIV/AIDS positive adults (18+ years old) who had at least three consecutive visits before a data collection period were considered as a study population of this study. The baseline data was collected from two health facilities using clinical record review. For the present study, study groups based on ART adherence status was defined as cases; patients who had a history of greater 5% (missing >2 doses out of 30 doses or >3 doses out of 60 doses) all of scheduled regimens which supposed to take in a month and controls were near-perfect (>95%) take to dose of all regimens which supposed to take in a month [17, 18]. All cases who had to follow-up during the data collection period were included in the study whereas controls were included by systematic random sampling techniques in every other four appointees.

Data collection and data analysis

The data were collected using chart review and interviewer administered techniques by two diploma nurses and three case managers working in ART clinics supervised by two bachelor nurse professionals. The structured questionnaire consisted of socio-demographic, socio-economic, nutritional, medical and psychological were used for the data collection tool. A 1-day training on the objective of the study, confidentiality of information and interviewing techniques were given. Baseline information was filled out from ART registration and follow-up forms.

Dietary diversity was assessed by asking the number of reported different foods and food groups consumed in a household over a 24-h period of the data collection time, does not include food group consumed outside the home. It was categorized into three groups; low if ≤3 food items consumed, medium if 4–6 food items consumed and high if ≥6 food items consumed [19].

Patient Health Questionnaire (PHQ) with 9-items on which score ranges from 0 to 27 were used to assess the depression of the study participants. Individuals up on their response categorized into five categories as (no depression, mild depression, moderate depression, moderately severe depression and severe depression) [20].

Precoding and manual checking of the questionnaire were done by the principal investigator before the data entry. Data was entered using Epi-Info and exported to SPSS version 20 for further cleaning and analysis purpose. Binary logistic regression model used to identify the determinant factors. Collinearity diagnostic test was conducted using tolerance to check for co-linearity between independent variables and interaction effect. Variables in the bivariable analysis having a p value <0.2 were considered for multivariate analysis to adjust the confounders. The strength and presence of statistical association were assessed by OR, p value and 95% confidence interval (95% CI). Variables with a p value ≤0.05 were considered as statistically significant determinant factors of non-adherence to ART. Hosmer–Lemeshow goodness-of-fit test (p = 0.9289) was used to assess the fitness of the model.

Results

A total of 411 HIV-positive individuals (137 cases and 274 controls) who had at least 6 months ART follow-up participated in the study. More than half (58.2%) of the study participants were male. The mean age ± (SD) at the time of data collection for cases and controls were 37.21 (±9.95) and 35 (±8.85) years, respectively (Table 1).

Table 1 Socio-demographic characteristics at the time of presentation and during data collection time of cases and controls, Aksum town, northern Ethiopia 2015

Variables	Frequency of adherence status	
	Case, n (%)	Control, n (%)
Sex		
Male	69 (50.4)	170 (62)
Female	68 (49.6)	104 (38)
Age		
15–29	23 (16.8)	54 (19.7)
30–39	60 (43.8)	127 (46.4)
40–49	35 (25.5)	74 (27.0)
≥50	19 (13.9)	19 (6.9)
Marital status		
Single	25 (18.2)	47 (17.2)
Married	64 (46.7)	128 (46.7)
Widowed	14 (10.2)	32 (11.7)
Divorced/separated	34 (24.8)	67 (24.4)
Residence		
Urban	114 (83.2)	253 (92.3)
Rural	23 (16.8)	21 (7.7)
Educational level (grade)		
No formal education	29 (21.2)	57 (20.8)
Primary education (1–8)	68 (49.6)	128 (46.7)
Secondary education (9–12)	33 (24.1)	69 (25.2)
12+	7 (5.1)	20 (7.3)
Occupation		
No occupation	21 (15.3)	42 (15.3)
Government employed	25 (18.3)	52 (19)
Business/self employed	40 (29.2)	96 (35)
Daily laborer	51 (37.2)	84 (30.7)

Determinants of non-adherence to antiretroviral therapy

In multivariable analysis variables, such as duration of treatment, ART adverse effect, substance use, living condition, depression, CD4 cell count and dietary diversity were found to be independent determinant factors with non-adherence to ART.

Patients who had more than 2 years ART follow-up [AOR = 7, 95% CI (2.2, 22.6)] were 7 times more likely to not adhere as compared to those who had 6–12 months follow-up. Patients who had a history of ART adverse drug effect [AOR = 6.9, 95% CI (1.4, 32.9)] were 6.9 times more likely to be non-adherent as compare to the counterpart. HIV-positive substance user [AOR = 5.3, 95% CI (1.4, 20)] individuals who were 5.3 times more likely to be non-adherence as compared with the counterpart.

Non-adherence were 3.4 times more likely to occur among those who live with their parents [AOR = 3.4, 95% CI (1.2, 10.3)] as compared to those who live alone. This study also showed that depression is associated with non-adherence of ART. The odds of non-adherence were 3.3 times more likely to those who had depression symptom [AOR = 3.3, 95% CI (1.4, 7.5)] as compared to their counterparts.

HIV-positive individuals who had <350 cells/mm^3 CD4 cell count [AOR = 3.2, 95% CI (1.8, 5.8)] were 3.2 times more likely to not adhere as compared to those HIV-positive individuals who had CD4 cell count ≥350 cells/mm^3. Moreover, low dietary diversity [AOR = 2, 95% CI (1.1–3.7)] were two times to not adhere as compared to the counterparts (Table 2).

Discussion

ART has a proven clinical benefit in HIV-infected people by slow downing the progressing to AIDS. Incomplete adherence to the treatment leads to immune suppression and the selection drug resistant HIV [21]. Non-adherence increases HIV-related morbidity and mortality [22]. Numerous studies were conducted on the determinants of ART drug-adherence and/or non-adherence of HIV/AIDS patients in the country. However, studies signify the consequence of non-adherence is one or more factors that may have different effects consequently; the study setting, socio-demographic characteristics of the study participants, and sample size. This study showed that having 2 years and above duration on ART, depression symptoms, history of ART adverse effect, substance use, living with parents, <350 cells/mm^3 CD4 count and low dietary diversity in the household as determinant factors for non-adherence to ART.

Coherent with the previous studies in Ethiopia [13, 23] HIV-positive participants who had more than 2 years ART follow-up were not taken ART drugs appropriately. This finding was also coherent with the Asia study conducted in Vientiane, Lao PDR [24]. Findings of Asia [25, 26] inconsistent with the present study, patients who have been on ART for short period were more likely to be non-adherent. The possible reason for the discrepancy could be these studies were included those patients who had less than 6 months' duration on ART since ART at an early phase of treatment may have severed adverse drug effects. On top of the treatment duration of the patients, the accessibility of health facilities, living conditions, socio-demographic characteristics of the population in Asia is differ from Ethiopia which might have effect on the adherence status of the patient.

Like the report of previous studies conducted in Ethiopia [11] and in Nepal [26] in the present study, participants that had experience of adverse drug effect during their medication were more likely to non-adherence to ART. But, this study is not consistent with a systematic review of Asian developing countries in 2012 reported [27]. The possible explanation will be they already

Table 2 Binary and multiple logistic regression model showing determinants of non-adherence to antiretroviral therapy, among adults on ART Aksum town, northern Ethiopia 2015

Explanatory variables	Adherence status to ART		COR (95% CI)	AOR (95% CI)
	Non-adherent number (%)	Adherent number (%)		
Sex				
Male	69 (50.4)	170 (62)	1	1
Female	68 (49.6)	104 (38)	1.6 (1.1–2.4)	1.4 (0.8–2.4)
Age				
18–29	23 (16.8)	54 (19.7)	1	1
30–39	60 (43.8)	127 (46.4)	1.1 (0.6–2.0)	1.1 (0.5–2.4)
40–49	35 (25.5)	74 (27)	1.1 (0.6–2.1)	0.7 (0.3–1.7)
≥50	19 (13.9)	19 (6.9)	2.3 (1.1–5.2)	1.7 (0.6–5.0)
Residence				
Urban	114 (83.2)	253 (92.3)	1	1
Rural	23 (16.8)	21 (76.7)	2.4 (1.3–4.6)	1.4 (0.5–4.0
Occupation				
No occupation	21 (15.3)	42 (15.3)	1	1
Employed	25 (18.3)	52 (19)	0.9 (0.5–2)	1.4 (0.5–4.2)
Business	40 (29.2)	96 (35)	0.8 (0.4–1.6)	1.8 (0.7–4.0)
Farmer	14 (10.2)	10 (3.7)	2.8 (1.1–7.4)	2.3 (0.5–10.3)
Daily laborer	37 (27)	74 (27)	1 (0.5–1.9)	1.9 (0.8–4.7)
Duration on ART (months)				
6–12	7 (5.1)	38 (13.9)	1	1
13–24	14 (10.2)	38 (13.9)	2.0 (0.7–5.5)	2 (0.5–8.8)
≥25	116 (84.7)	198 (72.2)	3.2 (1.4 7.4)	7 (2.2,22.6)**
ART adverse effect				
Yes	26 (19)	3 (1.1)	21.2 (6.3–71.3)	6.9 (1.4,32.9)**
No	111 (81)	271 (98.9)	1	1
Substance use				
Yes	21 (15.3)	5 (1.8)	9.7 (3.6–26.5)	5.3 (1.4–20.0)*
No	116 (84.7)	269 (98.2)	1	1
Live with				
Alone	33 (24.1)	83 (30.3)	1	1
Parents	18 (13.1)	21 (7.7)	2.2 (1.02–4.6)	3.4 (1.2–10.3)*
Family	86 (62.8)	170 (62)	1.3 (0.8–2.1)	1.5 (0.8–2.8)
Depression status				
Depressed	41 (29.9)	19 (6.9)	5.7 (3.2–10.4)	3.3 (1.4–7.5)*
Not depressed	96 (70.1)	255 (93.1)	1	1
CD4 cell count (cells/mm^3)				
<350	58 (42.3)	45 (16.4)	3.7 (2.4–6.0)	3.2 (1.8–5.8)*
≥350	79 (57.7)	229 (83.6)	1	1
Dietary diversity				
Low	57 (41.6)	43 (15.7)	3.8 (2.4–6.1)	2 (1.1–3.7)*
Medium and above	80 (58.4)	231 (84.3)	1	1
Daily eating pattern				
≤2 meals	69 (50.4)	103 (37.6)	1.7 (1.1–2.6)	1.01 (0.6–1.8)
≥3 meals	68 (49.6)	171 (62.4)	1	1
Opportunistic infection				
Yes	28 (20.4)	5 (1.8)	13.8 (5.2–36.7)	3.6 (1–13.1)
No	109 (79.6)	269 (98.2)	1	1

Table 2 continued

Explanatory variables	Adherence status to ART		COR (95% CI)	AOR (95% CI)
	Non-adherent number (%)	Adherent number (%)		
Reminder use				
Yes	127 (92.7)	268 (97.8)	0.3 (0.1–0.8)	0.5 (0.–2.0)
No	10 (7.3)	6 (2.2)	1	1
Stigma				
Yes	17 (12.4)	10 (3.6)	3.7 (1.7–8.4)	2.8 (0.9–8.5)
No	120 (87.6)	264 (96.4)	1	1
WHO stage				
Stage I	16 (11.7)	68 (24.8)	1	1
Stage II and above	121 (88.3)	206 (75.2)	2.5 (1.4–4.5)	1.6 (0.8–3.5)
BMI				
Under weight	38 (27.7)	41 (15)	1	1
Normal	97 (70.8)	224 (81.7)	0.5 (0.3–0.8)	0.7 (0.3–1.3)
Over weight	2 (1.5)	9 (3.3)	0.2 (0.1–1.2)	0.4 (0.01–3.0)
Treatment other than ART				
Yes	41 (29.9)	40 (14.6)	2.5 (1.5–4.1)	1.4 (0.7–3.0)
No	96 (70.1)	234 (85.4)	1	1

* $p < 0.05$

** $p < 0.001$

counselled on the possible side effects of the drug during their medication follow-up time.

Substance uses among patients during ART medication was also found to be the independent determinant factors of non-adherence, a finding consistent with a study done in southern Ethiopia [16], Tanzania [28] and Nepal [26].

In the present study, the living conditions are a determinant factor of non-adherence. Patients living with their families were more likely to non-adherence of ART drug as compared to those living independent from their families, consistent with previous study done in southern Ethiopia [29] inconsistent with a study done in Canada [30] and Cambodia [31]. The difference may be due to clients' self-efficacy and attitude towards ART medication is stumpy in the study setting, even at a country level.

The presence of depressive symptoms during medication is also reported as one of determinant factor for ART drug adherence, supported with studies done in South-west Ethiopia [14, 29], South Africa [32] and Netherlands [33]. Possibly depressed patients could easily forget to take their dose while they managed the depression symptoms.

Similar to other studies conducted in Ethiopia [15, 34, 35], and in Africa [32, 36] the level of CD4 count during initiation of treatment have independent effect for adherence status. Non-adherence was higher among patients with a CD4 count <350 cells/mm^3 compared to their counterparts. The finding is supported by studies in Ethiopia [15, 34, 35] however, a finding reported in Yirgalem Hospital, southern Ethiopia [23] was not consistent with the present study. This may be due to the previous study controlling for both WHO stages and CD4 cell count for the initiation criteria of ART.

Moreover, low dietary habits of the patient are reported as the independent determinant factors of non-adherence. This finding is supported by reports in South and North Ethiopia [15, 16] and Zambia [37].

Unlike previous studies, socio-demographic factors such as sex, age, residence, occupation, eating pattern and patient level factors; didn't show statistically significant association with non-adherence of ART. This may be because of in this locales the barriers of non-adherence were beyond the listed variables.

Since identifications of case and controls were done based on the registration log book and individual chart review, this paper may be prone to misclassification bias. Because of the adherence status of the patient were assessed by patient self-report, the non-adherence status may underestimate. Moreover, information bias was also a problem while assessing dietary diversity, substance use and depression symptom.

Conclusion

Having more than 2-year duration on ART follow-up, experiencing, adverse ART drug effect, substance use, living with parents, having depression symptom, CD4 cell count <350 cells/mm^3 and low dietary diversity were all found independent determinant factors of non-adherence of ART drug. Defining the adherence status with viral load suppression and/or measured by detectable viral load during chronic care and identifying the treatment outcome of non-adherence patient is recommended for future researcher.

Authors' contributions

BBG, YK, YAG, MKY, DT and MA equally participated in this study. All authors read and approved the final manuscript.

Author details

[1] Department of Public Health, Health Science College, Axum University, Axum, Ethiopia. [2] Department of Epidemiology and Biostatistics, Institute of Public Health, College of Medicine and Health Science, University of Gondar, 196 Gondar, Ethiopia.

Acknowledgements

Aksum Hospital and Health Center staff, study participants, data collectors and supervisors deserve acknowledgement for their unreserved support.

Competing interests

BBG, YK, and YAG participated from objective formulation to manuscript drafting. MK, DT and MA are participated during data analysis and manuscript drafting. All authors shared professional contribution for this study.

References

1. UNAIDS. The Gap Report Switzerland Geneva updated Sept 2014. July 2014.
2. HIV AIDS Prevention and Control Organization. Federal Democratic Republic of Ethiopia country progress report on the HIV response. Addis Ababa:MOH; 2014.
3. Joint United Nations Programme on HIV/AIDS. United Nation AIDS world AIDS day report 2011 (Faster, Smarter, Better). Geneva:UNAIDS; 2011.
4. Steel G, Nwokike J, Joshi MP. Development of a multi-method tool to measure ART adherence in resource-constrained settings: the South Africa experience. RPM Plus. Arlington, VA: Management Sciences for Health; 2007.
5. Asmare M, Aychiluhem M, Ayana M, Jara D. Level of ART adherence and associated factors among HIV sero-positive adult on highly active antiretroviral therapy in Debre Markos Referral Hospital, Northwest Ethiopia. J Antivir Antiretrovir. 2014;6:120–6. doi:10.4172/jaa.10000107.
6. Sarna A, Kellerman S. Access to antiretroviral therapy for adults and children with HIV infection in developing countries: horizons studies, 2002–2008. Public Health Rep. 2010;125(2):305–15.
7. The World Health Organization. Global update on HIV treatment: results, impact and opportunities. 2013.
8. Mills EJ, et al. Adherence to antiretroviral therapy in sub-Saharan Africa and North America: a meta-analysis. JAMA. 2006;296(6):679–90.
9. Stein MD, et al. Adherence to antiretroviral therapy among HIV-infected methadone patients: effect of ongoing illicit drug use. Am J Drug Alcohol Abuse. 2000;26(2):195–205.
10. Ortego C, et al. Adherence to highly active antiretroviral therapy (HAART): a meta-analysis. AIDS Behav. 2011;15(7):1381–96.
11. Tessema B, et al. Magnitude and determinants of non-adherence and nonreadiness to highly active antiretroviral therapy among people living with HIV/AIDS in Northwest Ethiopia: a cross-sectional study. AIDS Res Ther. 2010;7(1):1.
12. Ethiopian Federal Minstry of Health. National Guidelines for Comprehensive HIV Prevention, Care and Treatment. Addis Ababa: Ethiopian Federal Minstry of Health; 2014.
13. Mitiku H, Abdosh T, Teklemariam Z. Factors affecting adherence to antiretroviral treatment in Harari National Regional State, eastern Ethiopia. ISRN AIDS. 2013;. doi:10.1155/2013/960954.
14. Amberbir A, et al. Predictors of adherence to antiretroviral therapy among HIV-infected persons: a prospective study in Southwest Ethiopia. BMC Public Health. 2008;8(1):1.
15. Berhe N, Tegabu D, Alemayehu M. Effect of nutritional factors on adherence to antiretroviral therapy among HIV-infected adults: a case control study in northern Ethiopia. BMC Infect Dis. 2013;13(1):1.
16. Bitew BD, et al. Determinants of none-adherence to antiretroviral therapy among HIV-infected adults in Arba Minch General Hospital, Gamo Gofa Zone, southern Ethiopia: a case control study. Am J Health Res. 2014;5(2):234–40.
17. Kaplan JE, Benson C, Holmes KK, Brooks JT, Pau A, Masur H, Centers for Disease Control and Prevention (CDC), National Institutes of Health, HIV Medicine Association of the Infectious Diseases Society of America. Guidelines for prevention and treatment of opportunistic infections in HIV-infected adults and adolescents. MMWR Recomm Rep. 2009;58(RR-4):1–207.
18. Machtinger EL, Bangsberg DR. Adherence to HIV antiretroviral therapy HIV InSite Knowledge Base chapter. 2006.
19. De Matteis A, et al. Baseline survey of food security and nutrition in Mozambique. Maputo: Technical Secretariat for Food Security and Nutrition: Vulnerability Analysis Group; 2006.
20. Kroenke K, Spitzer RL. The PHQ-9: a new depression diagnostic and severity measure. Psychiatr Ann. 2002;32(9):1–7.
21. Bangsberg DR, Moss AR, Deeks SG. Paradoxes of adherence and drug resistance to HIV antiretroviral therapy. J Antimicrob Chemother. 2004;53(5):696–9.
22. Haddad PM, Brain C, Scott J. Nonadherence with antipsychotic medication in schizophrenia: challenges and management strategies. Patient Relat Outcome Meas. 2014;5:43–62.
23. Irano ZA, et al. Determinants of non-adherence to antiretroviral therapy and modeling progression of adherence level: at Yirgalem Regional Hospital, Ethiopia; January, 2012. Int J Med Health Sci Res. 2015;2(1):1–14.
24. Hansana V, et al. Adherence to antiretroviral therapy (ART) among people living with HIV (PLHIV): a cross-sectional survey to measure in Lao PDR. BMC Public Health. 2013;13:617.
25. Jiamsakul A, Kumarasamy N, Ditangco R, Li PC, Phanuphak P, Sirisanthana T, Sungkanuparph S, Kantipong P, Lee CK, Mustafa M, Merati T. Factors associated with suboptimal adherence to antiretroviral therapy in Asia. J Int AIDS Soc. 2014;17(1):18911. doi:10.7448/IAS.17.1.18911.
26. Wasti SP, et al. Factors influencing adherence to antiretroviral treatment in Nepal: a mixed-methods study. PLoS ONE. 2012;7(5):e35547.
27. Wasti SP, et al. Factors influencing adherence to antiretroviral treatment in Asian developing countries: a systematic review. Tropl Med Int Health. 2012;17(1):71–81.
28. Idindili B, Jullu B, Mugusi F, Tanner M. A case-control study of factors associated with non-adherent to antiretroviral therapy among HIV infected people in Pwani Region, eastern Tanzania. Tanzania J Health Res. 2012;14(3):194–203.
29. Alagaw A, et al. Factors associated with antiretroviral treatment adherence among adult patients in Wolaita Soddo Hospital, Wolaita Zone, southern Ethiopia. Sci J Public Health. 2014;2:69–77.
30. Godin G, et al. Prediction of adherence to antiretroviral therapy: a one-year longitudinal study. AIDS care. 2005;17(4):493–504.
31. Spire B, et al. Adherence to antiretroviral therapy in patients enrolled in a comprehensive care program in Cambodia: a 24-month follow-up assessment. Antivir Ther. 2008;13(5):697–703.
32. Peltzer K, et al. Antiretroviral treatment adherence among HIV patients in KwaZulu-Natal, South Africa. BMC Public Health. 2010;10(1):1.
33. Langebeek N, et al. Predictors and correlates of adherence to combination antiretroviral therapy (ART) for chronic HIV infection: a meta-analysis. BMC Med. 2014;12(1):142.
34. Biressaw S, et al. Adherence to antiretroviral therapy and associated factors among HIV infected children in Ethiopia: unannounced home-based pill count versus caregivers' report. BMC Pediatr. 2013;13(1):132.
35. Amberbir A, et al. Predictors of adherence to antiretroviral therapy among HIV-infected persons: a prospective study in Southwest Ethiopia. BMC Public Health. 2008;8(1):265.
36. Mbuagbaw L, et al. Trends and determining factors associated with adher ence to antiretroviral therapy (ART) in Cameroon: a systematic review and analysis of the CAMPS trial. AIDS Res Ther. 2012;9(1):1.
37. Sasaki Y, et al. Adherence to antiretroviral therapy (ART) during the early months of treatment in rural Zambia: influence of demographic characteristics and social surroundings of patients. Ann Clin Microbiol Antimicrob. 2012;11(1):1.

15

The dynamic changes of interferon lambdas related genes and proteins in JAK/STAT pathway in both acute and chronic HIV-1 infected patients

Guoxian Zhao[1,2†], Lifeng Liu[1,2†], Bin Su[1,2], Tong Zhang[1,2], Peng Chen[1,2], Wei Li[1,2,3*] and Hao Wu[1,2*]

Abstract

Background: Host immune responses during acute HIV-1 infection can influence the viral setpoint, which is a predictor of disease progression. Interferon (IFN)-lambdas are newly classified type III interferons, which use JAK-STAT pathway. Currently, the dynamics of IFN-lambdas related genes and proteins expression in the signaling pathway have not been well elaborated, especially in acute HIV-1-infected patients.

Objectives: To evaluate the dynamic changes of IFN-lambdas related genes and proteins in JAK/STAT pathway in acute HIV-1-infected patients, and analyze their correlation with CD4 T cell counts and HIV-1 viral loads.

Study design: Real-time PCR and flow cytometry methods were used to evaluate the dynamic changes of IFN-lambdas related genes and proteins in JAK/STAT pathway in both acute and chronic HIV-1-infected patients.

Results: The IFN-alpha receptors (R), IFN-gamma R, IFN-lambdas R and STAT1 mRNA and protein levels increased in acute HIV-1-infected patients ($p < 0.01$), in addition, Mx1 mRNA levels in acute HIV-1-infected patients are higher than those in HIV-negative subjects. IFN-lambdas R and IFN-alpha R mRNA levels are inversely correlated with $CD4^+$ T-cell counts, but are positively correlated with viral loads.

Conclusions: The dynamic changes of IFNs related genes in JAK-STAT pathway in acute HIV-1 infection will deepen our understanding of the roles of IFN-lambdas in HIV pathogenesis.

Keywords: Acute HIV-1 infection, IFN-lambdas, Signaling pathway, STAT1, Mx1

Background

Host immune responses during acute HIV-1 infection can influence the establishment of the viral setpoint, which is a predictor of disease progression, therefore, it is of importance to characterize the immune responses during acute HIV-1 infection. Viral infection can induce the production of interferons, which use JAK-STAT pathway [1]. Interferons (IFN)-lambdas are newly classified type III interferons [2, 3], until now, the dynamics of IFN-lambdas related genes and proteins expression in the signaling pathway have not been well elaborated, especially in acute HIV-1-infected patients.

IFN-α and IFN-β are main type I interferons, 12 closely related genes encode IFN-α. IFN-γ is the sole type II interferon. In 2003, type III IFNs which include three IFN-lambdas genes were newly identified by two independent groups. The receptor (R) of the type III IFNs is composed of a short chain (IL-10R2) and a long chain (IL28AR), IL28AR is utilized only by IFN-λ [2, 3]. IL28AR was shown to be expressed on some blood cells including B cells, T cells, dendritic cells (DCs) and macrophages [4]. Type III IFNs trigger responses through the JAK/STAT pathway, after binding to their receptors, JAK and STAT proteins are activated. There are six types of STAT

*Correspondence: vision988@126.com; whdoc@ccmu.edu.cn
†Guoxian Zhao and Lifeng Liu contributed equally to this work
[1] Center for Infectious Diseases, Beijing You'an Hospital, Capital Medical University, Beijing 100069, China

proteins in the pathway: STAT1, STAT2, STAT3, STAT4, STAT5a, STAT5b, STAT6. Activated STAT1, STAT2, and interferon regulatory factor 9 (IRF-9) form a complex called IFN-stimulated gene factor 3 (ISGF3), once assembled, ISGF3 is then translocated into nucleus where it binds to the IFN-stimulated response elements (ISRE), ISRE is located in the promoter of numerous IFN stimulated genes (ISGs). Some ISG-encode proteins mediate a variety of antiviral activities, such as myxovirus resistance protein A (MxA) and 2′,5′-oligoadenylate synthetase (OAS) [5].

IFNs are generally considered as cytokines with strong antiviral activities. The dynamics of type I and II IFNs in acute and chronic HIV-1-infected patients have been reported by previous studies. IFN-alpha is transiently expressed in acute HIV-1 infection (AHI), type I IFNs consist of several subtypes, only IFN-alpha is significantly elevated in chronic HIV-1 infection [6, 7]. IFN-gamma is detected as early as the acute phase and continually detected throughout the course of infection. In chronic, clinical progression or non-progression patients, IFN-gamma persistently elevated [8, 9]. IFN-lambdas can induce type-1 IFN-like antiviral response and blocks HCV infection in human primary hepatocyte and HUH7 cell lines [10]. IFN-lambdas can induce IFN-α/β-like antiviral response and inhibition of HBV replication in murine heptocyte cell lines [11]. IFN-lambda3 can inhibit HIV infection of macrophage through the JAK-STAT pathway and induce antiviral state in culture primary T-cells. When macrophages were pretreated once with IFN-lambdas, a nearly complete inhibition of HIV-1 replication in macrophages was observed [12].

Based on the ongoing burden of HIV infection among men who have sex with men (MSM) in China, we established an open Beijing Primo Cohort study in 2007 to identify acute HIV-1 infections [13]. This cohort study, with carefully estimated dates of seroconversion, has afforded us the great opportunity to investigate the dynamic changes of IFN-lambdas related genes and proteins expression in JAK/STAT pathway in acute HIV-1-infected patients. Moreover, phenotypic and functional perturbations of monocyte subsets in acute and chronic HIV-1 infected patients were characterized using this Beijing Primo Cohort [14]. Until now, the dynamics of IFN-lambdas related genes and proteins expression in the signaling pathway have not been well elaborated, especially in acute HIV-1-infected patients.

In the study, real-time PCR and flow cytometry methods were used to evaluate the dynamic changes of IFN-lambdas related genes and proteins in JAK/STAT pathway in acute HIV-1-infected patients, and then we analyzed their correlation with $CD4^+$ T-cell counts and HIV-1 viral loads.

Objectives

The aim of this study was to evaluate the dynamic changes of IFN-lambdas related genes and proteins in JAK/STAT pathway in AHI patients, and evaluate their correlation with $CD4^+$ T cell counts and viral loads.

Study design

Study subjects

Twenty MSM with acute HIV-1 infection (AHI) were enrolled from an open Beijing Primo Cohort study in 2007 to identify acute HIV-1 infections. The progression of early HIV-1 infection can be depicted as six discrete stages as proposed by Fiebig et al. [15, 16]. These 20 AHI patients were at Fiebig stage III–V. Twenty-four HIV-1-infected treatment-naïve patients were randomly enrolled from HIV/AIDS clinic of Beijing You'an Hospital, these cART-naïve patients with chronic HIV infection (CHI) were diagnosed at least 1.2 years (median 1.8 years, range from 1.2 to 2.3 years) before enrollment. The patients who have accepted antiretroviral therapy (ART) or were the intravenous drug users or co-infected with HBV/HCV were excluded from this study. Twenty-two male MSM HIV-negative controls (HC) were included as controls, the ages of all groups were matched.

The protocol for this study was approved by the Beijing You'an Hospital Ethics Committee and written informed consent was provided according to the declaration of Helsinki. The guidelines for Human Experimentation (PR China) were followed throughout. Upon admission, all patients provided written informed consent for their information, clinical samples (blood and plasma) were stored and used for research. The methods were carried out in accordance with approved guidelines and regulations. 5800 men who have sex with men (MSM) were screened by our team and were followed up every 2–3 months. Once acute HIV-1-infected cases were identified, blood samples were collected, and then PBMCs were isolated and cryopreserved.

RNA extraction and quantitative RT-PCR

Viral RNA was purified from peripheral blood mononuclear cell (PBMC) samples using the QIAamp Viral RNA Mini Kit (Qiagen, Duesseldorf, Germany) according to the manufacturer's protocol. Total cDNA was synthesized by reverse transcription using First Strand cDNA Synthesis Kit (Invitrogen, USA) with random primers. The real-time RT-PCR for the quantification of IFN, IFN R, β-actin and other genes were performed with the Power SYBR® Green PCR Master Mix (Invitrogen, USA). The primers used in this study were listed in Table 1.

The reaction mixture was first denatured at 95 °C for 4 min and then 40 cycles of PCR were performed using the following protocol: 95 °C 30 s; 60 °C 30 s; 72 °C 30 s.

Table 1 Nucleotide sequences of the primers used for real-time PCR

Target gene	Accession number	Type	Primer sequence	Productamplicon size (bp)
IFN lambda 1	NM_172140	F R	GTGCTGGTGACTTTGGTGCTA GAGAAGCCTCAGGTCCCAAT	225
IFN alpha R2	NM_207584.2	F R	GTCAGGCCTCTGCCACCTCT GGGTCCTGGAGTGGACTCTTTCT	172
IFN gamma R1	NM_000416.2	F R	GCCAGGGTTGGACAAAAAGA GACTTCCTGCTCGTCTCCATTTA	168
IFN lambda R1	NM_170743.3	F R	CCTCAGTGCCAGAACCATCTACA CCATGAGGGTCTTCCAGATCACA	152
STAT1	NM_007315.3	F R	CCCTTCTGGCTTTGGATTGAA CTTCCCGGGAGCTCTCACTGA	172
STAT2	NM_198332.1	F R	GAGAGCCCTCCTGGCAAGTTA GACGATTCACTGAAGCGCAGT	185
STAT3	NM_003150.3	F R	TTGCCAGTTGTGGTGATCTCC GCTGCTCGATGCTCAGTCCTC	199
STAT4	NM_003151.3	F R	TCAGGAAGGGCAAGCACTGGT GGAAGGGATGGGTAGCCAGGA	150
STAT5A	NM_003152.3	F R	GGATCCTGGTTGACGCCATGT GCTTGGATCCTCAGGCTCTCC	122
STAT5B	NM_012448.3	F R	GCTGGAAGCCTTGCTGATGCC CTGAGCTTGGATCCTCAGGCTCT	114
STAT6	NM_003153.4	F R	GCCCACTCACTCCAGAGGACCT GGTGTTGGGGAAAGTCGACAT	121
IRF9	NM_006084.4	F R	GAGCAAGTGGAGAGTGGGCAGTT CCAGACAGCTGGACCTCCTGTGT	189
OAS1	NM_016816.2	F R	CAGTTAAATCGCCGGGGAGAGT GCTGGAGCGAACTCAGTACGAA	101
MX1	NM_002462.4	F R	GGTGGTGGTCCCCAGTAATG CCGGCACTTGACAATCATGT	150
Beta actin	NM_001101.3	F R	GCACGGCATCGTCACCAACT GCTGGGGTGTTGAAGGTCTCA	177

F forward primer, *R* reverse primer, *bp* base pair, *STAT* signal transducer and activator of transcription, *IRF9* IFN regulatory factor 9, *OAS1* 2′,5′-oligoadenylate synthetase 1, *MX1* myxovirus resistance 1

The mRNA level of each selected gene was normalized with β-actin to obtain mRNA relative expression level.

The quantification of PCR data was achieved using the comparative Ct method. We calculated the $2^{-\Delta\Delta Ct}$, where $\Delta\Delta Ct = \Delta Ct_{sample} - \Delta Ct_{reference}$. The ΔCt_{sample} was calculated as Ct value for any sample normalized to the endogenous housekeeping gene and $\Delta Ct_{reference}$ was the Ct value for the control also normalized to the endogenous housekeeping gene. The mean value of $2^{-\Delta\Delta Ct}$ from control group was considered equal to 1; the fold change over the mean $2^{-\Delta\Delta Ct}$ of controls was calculated for all samples.

Antibodies and flow cytometry

Antibodies (Abs) used in this study were as follows: mouse phycoerythin (PE)-conjugated anti-human IFN-alpha/beta R2 Ab (clone MMHAR-2, R&D Systems), mouse PE-conjugated anti-human IFN-lambdas R1 Ab (clone 601106, R&D Systems), mouse PE-conjugated anti-human IFN-gamma Receptor 1 (clone GIR-208, Thermo Fisher Scientific), Mouse eFluor® 450-conjugated anti-human STAT1 (KIKSI0803, Thermo Fisher Scientific), Rabbit FITC anti-Human STAT2 (Thermo Fisher Scientific), Mouse PE-Cyanine7-conjugated anti-human STAT3 (clone LUVNKLA, Thermo Fisher Scientific), mouse APC-conjugated anti-human STAT4 (clone 4LURPLE, Thermo Fisher Scientific), mouse FITC-conjugated anti-human STAT5 (clone SRBCZX, Thermo Fisher Scientific), mouse PerCP-eFluor® 710-conjugated anti-human STAT6 (clone CHI2S4N, Thermo Fisher Scientific). All STATs Abs were used in phosphorylated state, phosphorylation of STATs occur in response to IFN, and is essential for normal transcriptional activity of the IFN stimulated gene factor 3 complex. Rabbit Alexa Fluor® 488 conjugated anti-human IRF9(clone EPR3939, Abcam), purified rabbit anti-human MxA Ab (Abcam) purified mouse anti-human OAS1Ab (Abcam), goat DyLight® 488 conjugated anti-mouse IgG (H+L)

(Abcam). The isotype control antibodies were purchased from the corresponding company, respectively.

Cryopreserved peripheral blood mononuclear cells (PBMCs) were used, and cells were stained with appropriate target Abs and isotype Abs using conventional surface and/or intracellular staining methods. Cryopreserved PBMCs were thawed in RPMI 1640 medium (Invitrogen, Carlsbad, CA, USA), washed with PBS, and then incubated at room temperature for 20 min with the cells viability marker fixable viability stain 510 (BD Biosciences, San Jose, CA, USA). When intracellular staining was required, cells were first fixed and permeabilized using BD Cytofix/Cytoperm Fixation and Permeabilization Solution (BD biosciences), followed by staining for intracellular proteins. Forward scatter (FSC) and side scatter (SSC) light gating were used to exclude cell debris from the analysis. Forward height and forward area were used to exclude doublet cells, and cell viability were evaluated. All expression analysis was performed by flow cytometry using BD FACSCanto™ II with Diva software (BD, Franklin Lakes, NJ), and the data were analyzed using FlowJo 10.0.7 software (Tree Star, Ashland, OR, USA).

$CD4^+$ T-cell count and viral loads measurement

$CD4^+$ T cells were determined by three-color flow cytometry using CD3-APC, CD4-FITC, and CD8-PE monoclonal antibodies (BD Biosciences). Analysis was then carried out by a BD FACSCanto™ II Flow cytometry.

HIV-1 Viral loads tests were done by using an automated real-time PCR-based *m*2000 system (Abbott Molecular Inc. Des Plaines, IL) as manufacturers' instruction and the sensitivity of detection was 40 copies/ml.

Statistical analyses

Statistical analysis was performed using Student's *t*-test or Non parametric tests. All reported *p* values were two-sided and considered significant at $p < 0.05$. The association was evaluated by Spearman's correlation test. All data were analyzed using SPSS 21.0 statistical software (Chicago, IL, USA).

Results

Patients' characteristics

Twenty MSM with acute HIV infection, twenty-four chronic HIV infection and twenty-two HIV-negative controls were enrolled in the study. Basic information of these patients and 22 controls is presented in Table 2. The age between HIV-1-infected patients and HIV-negative controls is matched. The viral loads of HIV-negative controls are not available. Mean $CD4^+$ T cell counts of acute HIV infected patients are lower than those of chronic HIV-1-infected patients and HIV-negative controls ($p = 0.006$).

The mRNA levels of IFN receptors and related genes during acute and chronic HIV-1 infection

In the study, the mRNA levels of the following genes were evaluated by real time PCR: IFN-alpha/beta R2, IFN-gamma R1, IFN-lambdas R1, STAT1, STAT2, STAT3, STAT4, STAT5a, STAT5b, STAT6, IRF9, Mx1, OAS1. As is shown in Fig. 1, IFN-alpha R, IFN-gamma R, IFN-lambdas R, STAT1 and Mx1mRNA levels in acute HIV infected patients were significant higher than those in HIV-negative controls ($p < 0.01$). The IFN-alpha R, IFN-gamma R, IFN-lambdas R, STAT1 and Mx1 R mRNA levels of acute infected patients are 6.03, 9.89, 8.20, 7.03 and 5.89 times higher than those of HIV-negative controls accordingly. In addition, the IFN-gamma R level in chronic HIV infected patients was significant higher than those in HIV-negative controls ($p < 0.01$).

The protein levels of IFN receptors and related genes during acute HIV-1 infection

In the study, the following protein levels were evaluated by flow cytometry: IFN-alpha/beta R2, IFN gamma R1, IFN-lambdas R1, STAT1, STAT2, STAT3, STAT4, STAT5a, STAT5b, STAT6, IRF9, MxA, OAS1. It can be seen from Fig. 2 that the mean fluorescence intensity (MFI) of IFN-gamma R, IFN-lambdas R, IFN-alpha R and STAT1 in acute HIV infected patients were significant higher than those in HIV-negative controls ($p < 0.01$). The IFN-gamma R level in chronic HIV infected patients was significant higher than those in HIV-negative controls ($p < 0.01$).

Table 2 Characteristics of HIV-1-infected patients and HIV-negative controls

	Chronic HIV infected patients	Acute HIV infected patients	HIV-negative control	p value
Cases, no	24	20	22	
Age (years)	33.8 (20–45)	33.2 (18–46)	34.6 (20–49)	0.738
HIV-RNA (copies/ml)	9955 (861–16,483)	22,438 (2029–189,695)	NA	NA
CD4 (cells/μl)	538 (476–789)	363 (164–692)	687 (401–1209)	0.0028

Data are presented as the means with ranges

NA not available

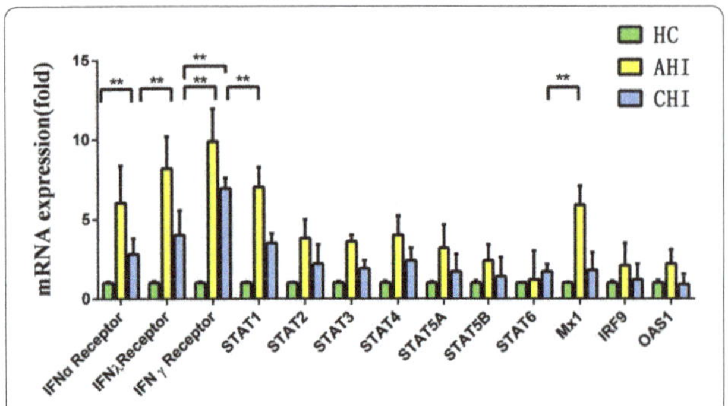

Fig. 1 The IFNs related genes of mRNA levels in HIV-negative controls (HC), acute HIV-1-infected (AHI) patients and chronic HIV-1-infected (CHI) patients. Total RNA extracted from PBMC was subjected to the real-time PCR. The data are expressed as mRNA levels relative (fold) to the control (which defined as 1). The results are shown mean ± standard deviation, the *asterisks* denote $p < 0.01$

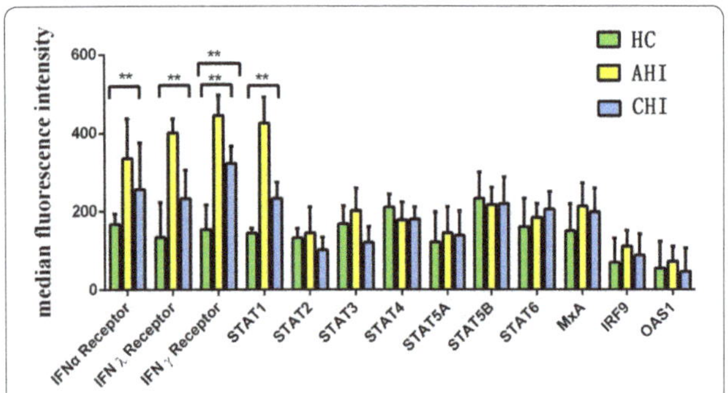

Fig. 2 The mean fluorescence intensity (MFI) of IFNs related proteins in HIV-negative controls (HC), acute HIV-1-infected (AHI) patients and chronic HIV-1-infected (CHI) patients. The flow cytometry was used to evaluate the protein levels. All expression analysis was performed by flow cytometry using BD FACSCanto™ II with Diva software. The results are shown mean ± standard deviation, the *asterisks* denote $p < 0.01$

The correlation between $CD4^+$ T cells, viral loads and mRNA levels of IFN receptors in HIV-1-infected patients

The correlation between IFNs receptors and $CD4^+$ T cell counts and viral loads was evaluated (Fig. 3). IFN-alpha R mRNA levels are inversely correlated with $CD4^+$ T cell counts (Fig. 3a), but are positively correlated with viral loads (Fig. 3b). IFN- lambdas R mRNA levels are inversely correlated with $CD4^+$ T cell counts (Fig. 3e) whereas positively correlated with viral loads (Fig. 3f).

Discussion

IFN-lambdas are newly classified type III interferons, which use JAK-STAT pathway. Currently, the dynamics of IFN-lambdas related genes and proteins expression in the signaling pathway have not been well elaborated, especially in acute HIV-1-infected patients. In the study, we found that in acute HIV-1-infected patients, IFN- alpha R, IFN-gamma R, IFN-lambdas R, STAT1 mRNA and protein levels increased ($p < 0.01$), in addition, Mx1 mRNA levels in AHI are higher than those in HIV-negative subjects. In chronic HIV infected patients, IFN-gamma R levels were significant higher than those in HIV-negative controls ($p < 0.01$). IFN-lambdas R and IFN-alpha R mRNA levels are positively correlated with viral loads, whereas negatively correlated with $CD4^+$ T-cell numbers.

Previous studies have showed that type I and III IFNs can activate similar intracellular signaling pathway and biological activities [17, 18]. In our study, IFN-alpha receptor and IFN-lambdas receptor production were up-regulated in acute HIV-1 infection. Stacey et al. [8, 9] reported that throughout the acute stage of HIV-1 infection, IFN-gamma receptor levels in infected adults steadily increase, with a peak about 20–24 days post-infection. In chronic non-progression or progression HIV-1-infected patients, IFN-gamma receptor persistently elevated. In the study, we found that the IFN-gamma R levels in both acute and chronic HIV infected patients were significant higher than those in HIV-negative controls ($p < 0.01$), our findings were consistent with previous study. The difference between IFN-lambdas and IFN-gamma expression may be caused by different receptor systems which activate different transcription factors and IFN regulatory factors [19]. Viral infection induced a number of genes and proteins in the signaling pathway upon viral infections, we found that Mx1 and STAT1 mRNA levels can be induced in acute HIV-1 infection. In the study, Mx1 mRNA levels are significantly higher than those of HIV-negative controls, but the MxA protein levels are similar between two groups. Several factors are responsible for the differences. Firstly, due to the deletion of three exons or the presence of a nonsense mutation, Mx1 gene becomes inactive and the translation is terminated in most mouse strains [20]. Secondly, the MxA protein will be hydrolyzed rapidly after its secretion in vitro, so there are fewer MxA protein left in cells. It has been reported that STAT1 protein can be up-regulated by IFN-alpha, gamma and lambdas in human hepatoma cells, melanoma cell lines and Raji cells, respectively [21–23].

In the study, the gene and protein expression target on PBMC rather than $CD4^+$ T cells, DCs or other immune cells. In the further studies, we should sort cells and analyze the gene and protein expression on specific cell type. IFN-lambdas was discovered only a decade ago and showed great potentials in antiviral therapy with much fewer side effects because of limited receptor distribution [24, 25]. In the study, we demonstrated the dynamics of IFN lambdas and the related genes and proteins in

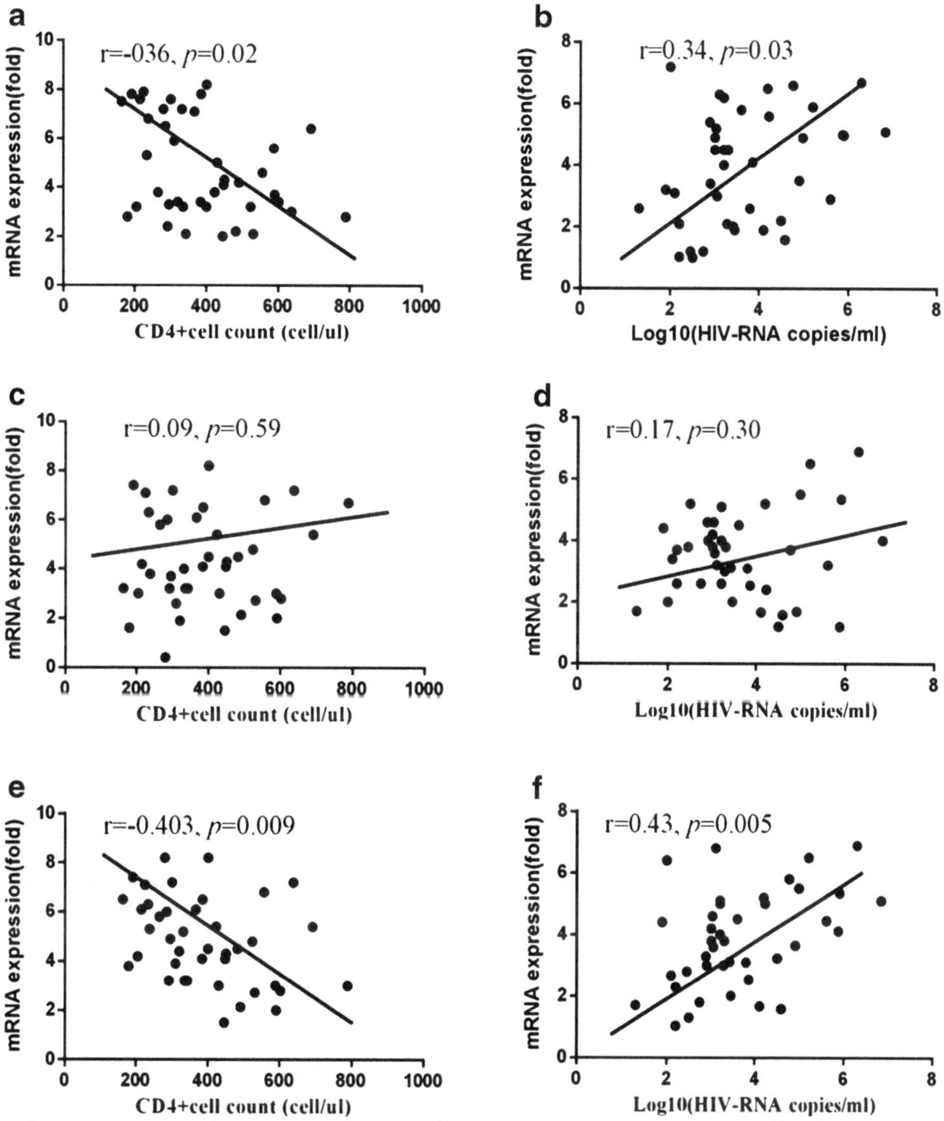

Fig. 3 Correlation between the CD4$^+$ T cells and mRNA levels of IFN-alpha receptor (**a**), IFN-gamma receptor (**c**), and IFN-lambdas receptor (**e**). Correlation between the viral loads and mRNA levels of IFN-alpha receptor (**b**), IFN-gamma receptor (**d**), and IFN-lambdas receptor (**f**). The results were performed Spearman's rank correlation, where coefficients "r" and corresponding *p* values are indicated on each panel

JAK-STAT pathway in acute and chronic HIV-1 infection, and we analyzed their association with CD4$^+$ T-cell counts and HIV-1 viral loads. The dynamic changes of IFNs related genes in JAK-STAT pathway in acute HIV-1 infection will deepen our understanding of the roles of IFN-lambdas in HIV pathogenesis, and our findings may provide valuable information on IFN-lambdas potential applications in clinical settings.

Authors' contributions

WL, LL, BS, and HW conceived the study, designed the experiments, and analyzed the data. GZ, LL, and PC performed the experiments; BS, TZ, and WL contributed to reagents and materials; and GZ, LL, BS, WL, and HW wrote the article. All authors read and approved the final manuscript.

Author details

[1] Center for Infectious Diseases, Beijing You'an Hospital, Capital Medical University, Beijing 100069, China. [2] Beijing Key Laboratory for HIV/AIDS Research, Beijing 100069, China. [3] Center of Interventional Oncology and Liver Diseases, Beijing You'an Hospital, Capital Medical University, Beijing 100069, China.

Acknowledgements

We would like to thank all the workers in the Beijing Key Laboratory for HIV/AIDS Research and physicians at infectious disease department.

Competing interests

The authors declare that they have no competing interests.

Funding

This work was supported by Beijing Municipal of Science and Technology Major Project (D141100000314005, D141100000314002, D161100000416003), National Natural Science Foundation of China (81571973), Beijing Municipal Administration of Hospitals Clinical Medicine Development of Special Funding Support (ZYLX201401), the Beijing Key Laboratory for HIV/AIDS Research (BZ0089), and the Funding for Chinese overseas talents returning to China in 2016 (B.S.).

References

1. Lasfar Ahmed, Lewis-Antes Anita, Smirnov Sergey V, et al. Characterization of the mouse IFN-λ ligand-receptor system: IFN-λs exhibit antitumor activity against B16 melanoma. Cancer Res. 2006;66:4468–77.
2. Sheppard P, Kindsvogel W, Xu W, Henderson K, Schlutsmeyer S, Whitmore TE, et al. IL-28, IL-29 and their class II cytokine receptor IL-28R. Nat Immunol. 2003;4:63–8.
3. Kotenko SV, Gallagher G, Baurin VV, Lewis-Anters A, Shen M, Shah NK, et al. IFN-lambdas mediate antiviral protection through a distinct class II cytokine receptor complex. Nat Immunol. 2003;4:69–77.
4. Witte K, Gruetz G, Volk HD, Looman AC, Asadullah K, Sterry W, et al. Despite IFN-lambda receptor expression, blood immune cells, but not keratinocytes or melanocytes, have an impaired response to type III interferons: implications for therapeutic applications of these cytokines. Genes Immun. 2009;10:702–14.
5. Brand S, Zitzmann K, Dambacher J, Beigel F, Olszak T, Vlotides G, et al. SOCS-1 inhibits expression of the antiviral proteins 2′,5′-OAS and MxA induced by the novel interferon-lambdas IL-28A and IL-29. Biochem Biophys Res Commun. 2005;331:543–8.
6. Hardy GA, Sieg S, Rodriguez B, Anthony D, Asaad R, Jiang W, et al. Interferon-alpha is the primary plasma type-I IFN in HIV-1 infection and correlates with immune activation and disease markers. PLoS ONE. 2013;8:565–72.
7. Chang JJ, Altfeld M. Innate immune activation in primary HIV-1 infection. J Infect Dis. 2010;202:297–301.
8. Stacey AR, Norris PJ, Qin L, Haygreen EA, Taylor E, Heitman J, et al. Induction of a striking systemic cytokine cascade prior to peak viremia in acute human immunodeficiency virus type 1 infection, in contrast to more modest and delayed responses in acute hepatitis B and C virus infections. J Virol. 2009;83:3719–33.
9. Zanussi S, D'Andrea M, Simonelli C, Tirelli U, De Paoli P. Serum levels of RANTES and MIP-1 alpha in HIV-positive long-term survivors and progressor patients. AIDS. 1996;10:1431–2.
10. Diegelmann J, Beigel F, Zitzmann K, Kaul A, Goke B, Auernhammer CJ, et al. Comparative analysis of the lambda-interferons IL-28A and IL-29 regarding their transcriptome and their antiviral properties against hepatitis C virus. PLoS ONE. 2010;5:e15200.
11. Robek MD, Boyd BS, Chisari FV. Lambda interferon inhibits hepatitis B and C virus replication. J Virol. 2005;79:3851–4.
12. Liu Man-qing, Dun-Jin Zhou Xu, Wang Wang Zhou, Ye Li, Li Jie-Liang, et al. IFN-l3 Inhibits HIV infection of macrophages through the JAK-STAT Pathway. PLoS ONE. 2012;7:e35902.
13. Jia Z, Huang X, Wu H, Zhang T, Li N, Ding P, et al. HIV burden in men who have sex with men: a prospective cohort study 2007–2012. 2014; 5: 1–9.
14. Chen Peng, Bin Su, Zhang Tong, Zhu Xiaojing, Xia Wei, Yan Fu, et al. Perturbations of monocyte subsets and their association with T helper cell differentiation in acute and chronic hiV-1-infected Patients. Front Immuno. 2017;8:1–10.
15. Fiebig EW, Wright DJ, Rawal BD, Garrett PE, Schumacher RT, Peddada L, et al. Dynamics of HIV viremia and antibody seroconversion in plasma donors: implications for diagnosis and staging of primary HIV infection. AIDS. 2003;17:1871–9.
16. Cohen MS, Gay CL, Busch MP, Hecht FM. The detection of acute HIV infection. J Infect Dis. 2010;202:270–7.
17. Pagliaccetti NE, Robek MD. Interferon-lambda in HCV Infection and Therapy. Viruses. 2010;2:1589–602.
18. Hermant P, Michiels T. Interferon-lambda in the context of viral infections: production, response and therapeutic implications. J Innate Immun. 2014;6:563–74.
19. Iversen MB, Paludan SR. Mechanisms of type III interferon expression. J Interferon Cytokine Res. 2010;30:573–8.
20. Verhelst J, Hulpiau P, Saelens X. Mx proteins: antiviral gatekeepers that restrain the uninvited. Microbiol Mol Biol Rev. 2013;77:551–66.
21. Zhao LJ, Hua X, He SF, Ren H, Qi ZT. Interferon alpha regulates MAPK and STAT1 pathways in human hepatoma cells. J Virol. 2011;8:157–62.
22. Schmitt MJ, Philippidou D, Reinsbach SE, Margue C, Wienecke-Baldacchino A, Nashan D, et al. Interferon-gamma-induced activation of signal transducer and activator of transcription 1 (STAT1) up-regulates the tumor suppressing microRNA-29 family in melanoma cells. Cell Commun Signal. 2012;10:41–6.
23. Zhou Z, Hamming OJ, Ank N, Paludan SR, Nielsen AL, Hartmann R. Type III interferon (IFN) induces a type I IFN-like response in a restricted subset of cells through signaling pathways involving both the Jak-STAT pathway and the mitogen-activated protein kinases. J Virol. 2007;81:7749–58.
24. Kotenko SV. IFN-lambdas. Curr Opin Immunol. 2011;23:583–90.
25. Lazear HM, Nice TJ, Diamond MS. Interferon-lambda: immune Functions at barrier surfaces and beyond. Immunity. 2015;43:15–28.

16

Impaired human immunodeficiency virus type 1 replicative fitness in atypical viremic non-progressor individuals

Jan Weber[1*], Richard M. Gibson[2], Lenka Sácká[1], Dmytro Strunin[1], Jan Hodek[1], Jitka Weberová[1], Marcela Pávová[1], David J. Alouani[2], Robert Asaad[3], Benigno Rodriguez[3], Michael M. Lederman[3] and Miguel E. Quiñones-Mateu[2,3,4*]

Abstract

Background: Progression rates from initial HIV-1 infection to advanced AIDS vary significantly among infected individuals. A distinct subgroup of HIV-1-infected individuals—termed viremic non-progressors (VNP) or controllers—do not seem to progress to AIDS, maintaining high $CD4^+$ T cell counts despite high levels of viremia for many years. Several studies have evaluated multiple host factors, including immune activation, trying to elucidate the atypical HIV-1 disease progression in these patients; however, limited work has been done to characterize viral factors in viremic controllers.

Methods: We analyzed HIV-1 isolates from three VNP individuals and compared the replicative fitness, near full-length HIV-1 genomes and intra-patient HIV-1 genetic diversity with viruses from three typical (TP) and one rapid (RP) progressor individuals.

Results: Viremic non-progressors and typical patients were infected for >10 years (range 10–17 years), with a mean $CD4^+$ T-cell count of 472 cells/mm^3 (442–529) and 400 cells/mm^3 (126–789), respectively. VNP individuals had a less marked decline in $CD4^+$ cells (mean −0.56, range −0.4 to −0.7 $CD4^+$/month) than TP patients (mean −10.3, −8.2 to −13.1 $CD4^+$/month). Interestingly, VNP individuals carried viruses with impaired replicative fitness, compared to HIV-1 isolates from the TP and RP patients ($p < 0.05$, 95% CI). Although analyses of the near full-length HIV-1 genomes showed no clear patterns of single-nucleotide polymorphisms (SNP) that could explain the decrease in replicative fitness, both the number of SNPs and HIV-1 population diversity correlated inversely with the replication capacity of the viruses ($r = -0.956$ and $r = -0.878$, $p < 0.01$, respectively).

Conclusion: It is likely that complex multifactorial parameters govern HIV-1 disease progression in each individual, starting with the infecting virus (phenotype, load, and quasispecies diversity) and the intrinsic ability of the host to respond to the infection. Here we analyzed a subset of viremic controller patients and demonstrated that similar to the phenomenon observed in patients with a discordant response to antiretroviral therapy (i.e., high $CD4^+$ cell counts with detectable plasma HIV-1 RNA load), reduced viral replicative fitness seems to be linked to slow disease progression in these antiretroviral-naïve individuals.

Keywords: HIV-1, Replicative fitness, Disease progression, Viremic non-progressors

*Correspondence: jan.weber@uochb.cas.cz; weber@uochb.cas.cz; meq@case.edu

[1] Institute of Organic Chemistry and Biochemistry v.v.i., Academy of Sciences of the Czech Republic, Flemingovo n. 2, 166 10 Prague 6, Czech Republic

[3] Department of Medicine, Case Western Reserve University/University Hospitals Cleveland Medical Center, 10900 Euclid Avenue, Cleveland, OH 44106-7288, USA

Background

Infection with human immunodeficiency virus type 1 (HIV-1)—in the absence of antiretroviral therapy—usually follows a well-defined path of virological and immunological changes; however, progression rates to advanced AIDS vary significantly among infected individuals [1, 2]. Based on plasma HIV-1 RNA (viral) load, $CD4^+$ T-cell counts, and symptomatic or asymptomatic HIV-1 infection adult patients have been classified into four groups: (i) rapid progressors (RP), (ii) typical progressors (TP), and two groups of long-term non-progressors (LTNP) namely (iii) elite controllers and (iv) viremic controllers [3, 4]. Among the latter, a rare subgroup of HIV-1-infected individuals has been described who do not seem to progress to AIDS, maintaining high $CD4^+$ T-cell counts despite high levels of viremia (i.e., over 2000 HIV-1 copies RNA/ml of plasma) for many years, also called viremic non-progressors (VNPs) [5–8].

Multiple studies have tried to associate these differences in HIV-1 disease progression with a multitude of host (HIV-1-specific immune response and genetic markers) and viral factors [9–13]. Among the immunological factors, strong HIV-1-specific cytotoxic T cell (CTL) responses have been shown to control HIV-1 infection right after transmission, perhaps determining viral set point in chronic stages of infection, which may help reduce the rate of HIV-1 disease progression [14, 15]. Similarly, a series of host genetic factors that seem to influence HIV-1 progression rates have been well described, including human leukocyte antigen (HLA) class I alleles such as HLA-B*27 and HLA-B*57 [16, 17] and a 32 bp deletion in the CCR5 chemokine receptor gene [18–22]. On the other hand, the impact of restriction cellular factors like APOBEC3, TRIM5α, tetherin, and SAMHD1 on HIV-1 progression is still debated [10, 23]. Altogether, it has been long recognized that immune activation is one of the major contributors to HIV-1 disease and pathogenesis [6, 24–27].

Viral factors—such as impaired HIV-1 replicative fitness—have been associated with slow or limited HIV-1 disease progression [11, 28–31], particularly in patients infected with heavily mutated drug resistant viruses [28, 30, 32–35]. High fitness of transmitted HIV-1 has been related to rapid disease progression [36], while some individuals carrying viruses with decreased replication capacity during acute/early infection have been classified as HIV controllers [37]. Although isolating replication competent HIV-1 strains from elite controllers has been difficult, two studies failed to identify any major defect on the replication ability of these viruses [38, 39]. In contrast, recombinant viruses constructed with HIV-1 *gag*, *pol*, and/or *env* genes from elite controllers exhibited reduced replication capacity compared to recombinant viruses constructed from typical progressors [40–42]. On the other hand, very limited information about the replicative fitness of viruses infecting viremic non-progressor individuals is currently available [6, 43]. If a decrease in HIV-1 replicative fitness is associated with slower/no disease progression, what is causing the virus to have this reduced replication capacity—in the absence of drug resistance mutations—in a certain number of non-progressor patients?

To date, no common pattern or polymorphism(s) shared among HIV-1 variants infecting non-progressor individuals have been clearly defined. Several studies have described changes in the LTR, e.g., in the Sp1 binding site [44] or large deletions [11, 45] that could be associated with slow disease progression. Detrimental mutations in Gag have been associated with viral attenuation [46, 47], which seem to play an important role in HIV-1 disease [48, 49]. Significant replicative fitness loss was observed in recombinant viruses encoding *pol* genes with mutations affecting HLA-A, but surprisingly not HLA-B, binding [50], although the most attenuated viruses were those constructed from HIV-1 elite controllers expressing HLA-B*57 and HLA-B*51 [40]. Changes in the V2 region of gp120 [51, 52] and a single amino acid deletion in gp41 [53] in the *env* gene have also been associated with slow disease progression. However, most of the changes in the HIV-1 genome linked to altered pathogenesis have been identified in accessory genes. Single amino acid substitutions [54, 55] and large deletions [56, 57] in Nef have been associated with a decrease in replicative fitness and slow disease progression. Mutations at positions 72 and 77 in Vpr, disrupting the viral protein function, were frequently detected in non-progressors [58, 59]. Finally, single or large insertions in Vpu [60] and amino acid substitutions in Vif [61, 62] have also been associated with non-progression in HIV-1 disease.

In this pilot study we quantified the replicative fitness of HIV-1 isolates obtained from extremely rare viremic non-progressor HIV-infected individuals and compared them to the fitness of those from patients with typical or rapid disease progression. Using deep sequencing we analyzed the full-length HIV-1 genomes and determined intrapatient HIV-1 diversity to investigate if these viral factors could be contributing to the maintenance of stable $CD4^+$ T-cell counts despite persistence viremia for more than 10 years, in the absence of antiretroviral treatment.

Methods

Clinical samples

Blood samples were obtained during routine patient monitoring from a well-characterized cohort of HIV-infected individuals at the Special Immunology Unite (SIU) at Case Western Reserve University/University

Hospitals Cleveland Medical Center (CWRU/UHCMC), with the written informed consent. Seven subjects were selected and grouped based on the following definitions: (i) *viremic non-progressors* (VNP, n = 3) corresponding to patients serologically proven to be HIV-1-infected for at least 10 years, $CD4^+$ T-cell decline of <45 cells/mm^3 per year and repeated plasma HIV-1 RNA load >1000 copies/ml in the absence of antiretroviral therapy; (ii) *typical progressors* (TP, n = 3) corresponding to patients serologically proven to be HIV-1-infected for at least 10 years, $CD4^+$ T-cell decline of >75 cells/mm^3 per year and repeated plasma HIV-1 RNA load >1000 copies/ml in the absence of antiretroviral therapy; and (iii) *rapid progressor* (RP, n = 1) corresponding to a patient serologically proven to be HIV-1-infected for at least 5 years, $CD4^+$ T-cell decline of >77 cells/mm^3 per year and repeated plasma HIV-1 RNA load >10,000 copies/ml in the absence of antiretroviral therapy. In the case of the VNP and TP patients, $CD4^+$ T-cell numbers and plasma HIV-1 load levels were monitored for a minimum of 30 months (18 months for the RP patient) with at least 10 determinations over this period. Demographics, clinical and virological characteristics are summarized in Table 1.

Cells and viruses

Peripheral blood mononuclear cells (PBMC), obtained from HIV-seronegative donors, were stimulated with 2.5 μg/ml of phytohemagglutinin (PHA; Gibco BRL) and maintained in RPMI 1640/2 mM L-glutamine media (Cellgro; Mediatech, Herndon, VA) supplemented with 10% fetal bovine serum (Cellgro), 10 mM HEPES buffer (N-2-hydroxyethylpiperazine-N-2-ethanesulfonic acid; Cellgro), 1 ng/ml of interleukin-2 (IL-2) (Gibco, BRL), 100 U of penicillin/m (Cellgro) and 100 μg of

Table 1 Demographic, clinical and virological parameters

Patient ID	Viremic non-progressors (VNP)			Typical progressors (TP)			Rapid progressor (RP)
	VNP-1	VNP-2	VNP-3	TP-1	TP-2	TP-3	RP
Demographics							
Age[a]	44	50	42	40	43	38	30
Sex[b]	M	M	M	M	M	M	M
Race	Black	Caucasian	Black	Caucasian	Black	Black	Black
Risk Factor[c]	MSM	Unknown	MSM	MSM	MSM	MSM	MSM
Years HIV+[d]	14	17	10	14	15	12	5
Follow up (months)[e]	84	37	123	35	19	31	18
$CD4^+$ (cells/mm^3)							
$CD4^+$ count[f]	563	443	479	386	361	126	11
Mean $CD4^+$ count[g]	529	445	442	483	457	293	57
Range $CD4^+$ count[g]	372–711	316–608	280–814	220–789	361–645	126–511	11–124
Slope $CD4^+$ count[h]	−0.6	−0.7	−0.4	−9.6	−8.2	−13.1	−4.7
HIV-1 RNA (log 10 copies/ml)							
HIV-1 RNA[f]	5.46	4.90	4.70	4.41	4.27	4.49	4.64
Mean HIV-1 RNA[g]	4.68	4.91	4.31	4.23	4.45	4.67	4.49
Range HIV-1 RNA[g]	3.61–5.45	4.27–5.08	3.62–4.71	3.89–4.62	4.28–4.62	3.90–4.90	4.09–4.66
Virus characteristics							
HIV-1 subtype[i]	B	B	B	B	B	B	B
HIV-1 coreceptor tropism[j]	R5	R5	R5	R5	R5	R5	D/M

R5 CCR5-tropic virus, *D/M* dual- or mixed-tropic virus

[a] Age at the time of sampling

[b] *M* male

[c] *MSM* men who have sex with men

[d] Years since first HIV-seropositive test to time of blood sample collection for this study

[e] Number of months that the patient had been monitored up to the blood sample collection date

[f] $CD4^+$ T-cell count (cells/mm^3) and HIV-1 RNA plasma load (log10 copies/ml) at the time the blood sample was obtained

[g] Mean and range $CD4^+$ T-cell count and HIV-1 RNA plasma load values determined during the clinical follow up time, to the time of blood sample collection for this study and prior to the initiation of antiretroviral treatment

[h] Rate of $CD4^+$ T-cell count decline (slope) calculated as cells/mm^3 per month, using all $CD4^+$ cell measurements available at the time the blood sample was obtained

[i] HIV-1 subtype determined using the near full-length HIV-1 genome consensus sequences with the Recombinant Identification Program (RIP) from the Los Alamos HIV Sequence Database (https://www.hiv.lanl.gov/content/sequence/RIP/RIP.html) [76]

[j] HIV-1 coreceptor tropism determined using sequencing reads corresponding to the V3 region of gp120, *env* gene with the DEEPGEN™HIV Software Tool Suite [70]

streptomycin/ml (Cellgro), for three days before infection with HIV-1 [28]. HIV-1 isolates were obtained from all seven patients by co-cultivating their PBMCs with PBMCs from HIV-seronegative donors as described [28]. Three primary HIV-1 isolates (HIV-$1_{A\text{-}92UG029}$, HIV-$1_{B\text{-}92US076}$, and HIV-$1_{AE\text{-}CMU06}$) were obtained from the AIDS Research and Reference Reagent Program and propagated in PHA-stimulated, IL-2-treated PBMCs. Tissue culture dose for 50% infectivity ($TCID_{50}$) was determined for each virus in PBMCs in triplicate with serially diluted stocks, based on the reverse transcriptase (RT) activity in culture supernatants on day 7 of culture, using the Reed and Muench method [63]. Viral titers were expressed as infectious units per milliliter (IU/ml).

HIV-1 replicative fitness determination using viral growth kinetics analysis

The ability of the seven patient-derived HIV-1 isolates, plus the primary wild-type HIV-$1_{B\text{-}92US076}$ isolate used as control, to replicate in the absence of drug pressure was determined by measuring viral growth kinetics as described [64, 65]. Briefly, 1×10^6 PHA-stimulated, IL-2-treated PBMCs were infected at a multiplicity of infection (MOI) of 0.001 IU/cell in 1 ml of RPMI 1640 medium and incubated for 2 h at 37 °C in 5% CO_2. HIV-infected cells were then washed twice with 1x PBS and split to be cultured in triplicate wells of a 96-well plate (1×10^5 cells/well). Fresh PHA-stimulated, IL-2–treated PBMCs (5×10^4 cells) were added to each well at days 5 and 10 post-infection. Reverse transcriptase activity in the culture supernatant was assayed on days 0, 4, 6, 8, 11, and 14 post-infection as described [28]. Viral replication was quantified using the slope of the growth curves and performing linear regression analysis derived from the equation $log(y) = mt + log(h)$, where y is virus quantity (cpm), t is time in days, and h is the y-intercept (day 0). All slope values for each virus were used to calculate means and standard deviations. Differences in the mean values were evaluated using a one way analysis of variance test and the significance difference from the control HIV-$1_{B\text{-}92US076}$ calculated using the Bonferroni's Multiple Comparison Test (GraphPad Prism v.6.0b, GraphPad Software).

HIV-1 replicative fitness determination using growth competition experiments

Dual infection/competition experiments were carried out as previously described [28, 35, 66, 67]. Briefly, each query virus (patient-derived subtype B HIV-1 isolates and the HIV-$1_{B\text{-}92US076}$ control) was competed against two different non-subtype B HIV-1 control strains (HIV-$1_{A\text{-}92UG029}$ and HIV-$1_{AE\text{-}CMU06}$) in a 1:1 initial proportion using an MOI of 0.001 IU/cell to infected 1×10^6 PBMCs for 2 h at 37 °C and 5% CO_2. Cells were subsequently washed twice with 1× PBS and cultured in a 24-well plate. Cell-free supernatant and cells were harvested at day 10 and stored at −80 °C for subsequent analysis. The final proportions of the two viruses in each competition were quantified using a TaqMan Real-Time PCR assay after normalizing to viral production in the HIV-1 mono-infections as described [28, 35, 67]. Replicative fitness for each patient-derived HIV-1 isolate was calculated and expressed as a percentage of the replicative fitness of the HIV-$1_{B\text{-}92US076}$ control, set as 100%.

Reverse transcription (RT)-PCR amplification of nearly full-length HIV-1 genome

Plasma viral RNA was purified from pelleted virus particles by centrifuging one milliliter of plasma at 20,000g × 60 min at 4 °C, removing 860 μl of cell-free supernatant and resuspending the pellet in the remaining 140 μl, to finally extract viral RNA using QIAamp Viral RNA Mini kit (Qiagen; Valencia, CA). Viral RNA was reverse-transcribed using AccuScript High Fidelity Reverse Transcriptase (Stratagene Agilent; Santa Clara, CA) and five previously described antisense external primers (Pan-HIV-1-1R [68], 1R, 2R, 3R, and 4R [69]) in 20 μl reaction mixtures containing 1 mM dNTPs, 10 mM DTT and 10 units of RNAse inhibitor. Six overlapping fragments, covering almost the entire HIV-1 genome, were amplified using a series of external and nested primers and Phusion High-Fidelity DNA Polymerase (NEB, Ipswich, MA) with defined cycling conditions as previously described [68, 69], i.e., 5′LTR (675 bp; HXB2 coordinates 120 to 794), 5′LTR-*gag*/p7 (1269 bp; 658 to 1924), *gag*/p24-*pol*/RT (2327 bp; 1137 to 3463), *pol*/RT-*vif* (2259 bp; 2976 to 5234), *pol*/int-*env*/gp120 (2921 bp; 4602 to 7522), and *env*/gp120-3′LTR (2587 bp; 6858 to 9444).

Population (Sanger) sequence analysis

Nested PCR products were purified with the QIAquick PCR Purification kit (Qiagen) and sequenced by Sanger (population) sequence (GATC Biotech, Constance, Germany). Nucleotide sequences were analyzed using DNASTAR Lasergene Software Suite v.12.3.1.4 (Madison, WI).

Deep sequencing of nearly full-length HIV-1 genome

All six overlapping HIV-1 fragments, from the seven patient-derived plasma samples, were deep sequenced using a variation of the DEEPGEN™HIV assay [70]. Briefly, the six amplicons were purified (Agencourt AMPure XP, Beckman Coulter) and quantified (2100 Bioanalyzer DNA 7500, Agilent Technologies) prior to using the Ion Xpress Fragment Library Kit (Life Technologies, Carlsbad CA) to construct a multiplexed library for shotgun sequencing on the Ion Personal Genome Machine (PGM, Life Technologies). For that, a mixture of all six purified DNA amplicons (16 ng each) was randomly fragmented and blunt-ends repaired using the Ion Shear Plus Reagent (Life Technologies) followed by DNA purification (Agencourt AMPure XP, Beckman Coulter). The P1 adapter and one of seven barcodes were ligated to the repaired fragment ends prior to DNA purification (Agencourt AMPure XP, Beckman Coulter). DNA fragments were then selected by size (i.e., 280–320 bp; Pippin Prep, Life Technologies) and each barcoded library, i.e., a mixture of all six amplicons per sample, was purified (Agencourt AMPure XP, Beckman Coulter) and normalized using the Ion Library Equalizer Kit (Life Technologies). All seven barcoded DNA libraries, corresponding to seven patient-derived amplicons, were pooled in equimolar concentrations and templates prepared and enriched for sequencing on the Ion Sphere Particles (ISPs) using the Ion OneTouch 200 Template Kit v2 (Life Technologies) in the Ion OneTouch 2 System (Life Technologies). Templated ISPs were quantified (Qubit 2.0, Life Technologies) and loaded into an Ion 318 Chip (Life Technologies) to be sequenced on the Ion PGM using the Ion PGM Sequencing 200 Kit v2 (Life Technologies). Sequencing run, signal processing and base calling was performed with Torrent Analysis Suite version 5.0.4. All deep sequencing experiments were performed in the CLIA/CAP-accredited University Hospitals Translational Laboratory under a good laboratory practice framework.

Read mapping, variant calling, phylogenetic and viral diversity analysis

Reads were mapped and aligned (assembled) against the HIV-1_{HXB2} (GenBank: K03455) reference sequence using SeqMan NGen (DNASTAR Lasergene Software Suite v.12.3.1.4), and the assemblies analyzed using SeqMan Pro (DNASTAR Lasergene Software Suite v.12.3.1.4). Full-length HIV-1 consensus sequences were generated for each patient-derived virus, compared to the corresponding population sequences obtained by Sanger sequencing, aligned using ClustalW [71] and their phylogeny reconstructed using the neighbor-joining statistical method as implemented within MEGA 6.06 [72]. Variant calling (i.e., single nucleotide polymorphisms, including substitutions, deletions and insertions) and their frequencies in the virus population relative to the HIV-1_{HXB2} reference sequence were quantified using a proprietary pipeline (Alouani and Quiñones-Mateu, unpublished results). Intra-patient HIV-1 quasispecies diversity was determined using near full-length HIV-1 genome (or individual genes and coding region sequences) based on the p-distance model as described for deep sequencing [73].

Statistical analyses

Descriptive results are expressed as mean values, standard deviations, range, and confidence intervals. As described above, differences in the mean of the slope values for the viral growth kinetics curves were determined using a One Way Analysis of Variance test and the difference from the reference HIV-1_{NL4-3} virus calculated using the Bonferroni's Multiple Comparison Test. All differences with a P value of <0.05 were considered statistically significant. All statistical analyses were performed using GraphPad Prism v.6.0b (GraphPad Software, La Jolla, CA) unless otherwise specified. Nucleotide sequences of the nearly full-length HIV-1 genomes, both consensus and individual reads, obtained by deep sequencing in this study have been submitted to the Los Alamos National Laboratory HIV-DB Next Generation Sequence Archive (http://www.hiv.lanl.gov/content/sequence/HIV/NextGenArchive/Weber2017).

Results

Clinical, virologic, and immunologic characteristics of viremic non-progressors, typical and rapid progressor patients

As described above, for this study we identified three treatment-naïve HIV-infected individuals classified as VNPs. At the time of the study, these patients were infected with HIV-1 for over 10 years (range 10–17 years), maintaining relatively high CD4$^+$ T-cell counts (mean 472, range 280–814 cells/mm^3) with limited decline in CD4$^+$ T-cell count (mean slope −0.56, range −0.4 to −0.7 CD4$^+$ T-cells/month) despite sustained plasma HIV-1 RNA loads above 4000 copies/ml (mean 5.02 $\log_{10}$, range 3.61–5.45 copies/ml) during the time these patients were monitored prior to this study (range 37–123 months) (Table 1; Additional file 1: Figure S1). For comparison, we selected three patients classified as typical progressors (each infected for at least 10 years, range 12–15 years), and one rapid progressor infected for 5 years. Overall, the CD4$^+$ T-cell counts for the TPs were similar to that of the VNPs (mean 400, range 126–789 cells/mm^3) albeit with a more marked decline in CD4$^+$ T-cells over time (mean slope −10.3, range −8.2 to −13.1 CD4$^+$ T-cells/month). Plasma HIV-1 RNA levels for the TPs were similarly high (mean 4.45 $\log_{10}$, range 3.89–4.9 copies/ml). As expected, the CD4$^+$ T-cell counts from the RP patient were significantly lower than those for the VNP and TP individuals (mean 57, range 11–124 cells/mm^3), declining at a rate of −4.7 CD4$^+$ T-cells/month with high plasma HIV-1 RNA loads (mean 4.49 $\log_{10}$, range 4.09–4.66 copies/ml) (Table 1; Additional file 1: Figure S1). The rest of the clinical baseline characteristics showed no significant differences regarding age, gender distribution, ethnicity, and mode of transmission of HIV-1.

Replicative fitness of HIV-1 isolates from VNP, TP, and RP patients

We used two different but complementary approaches to quantify the ability of all seven patient-derived HIV-1 isolates (i.e., 3 VNPs, 3 TPs, and 1 RP) to replicate in vitro in the absence of any host selective pressure, including antiretroviral drugs. A first glimpse of the replicative fitness of these viruses was obtained using classical viral growth kinetics in PBMCs from HIV-seronegative donors (Fig. 1a). Statistical analysis of the slope of the growth curves showed that the replicative fitness of all three VNP viruses was significantly reduced compared to the replicative fitness of the three TP and RP viruses ($p < 0.05$, 95% CI, Fig. 1b). Since in vitro dual infection/growth competition experiments are considered the gold standard method to measure viral fitness [30, 74] we competed each one of the seven HIV-1 isolates against two different non-subtype B HIV-1 control strains (HIV-$1_{A\text{-}92UG029}$

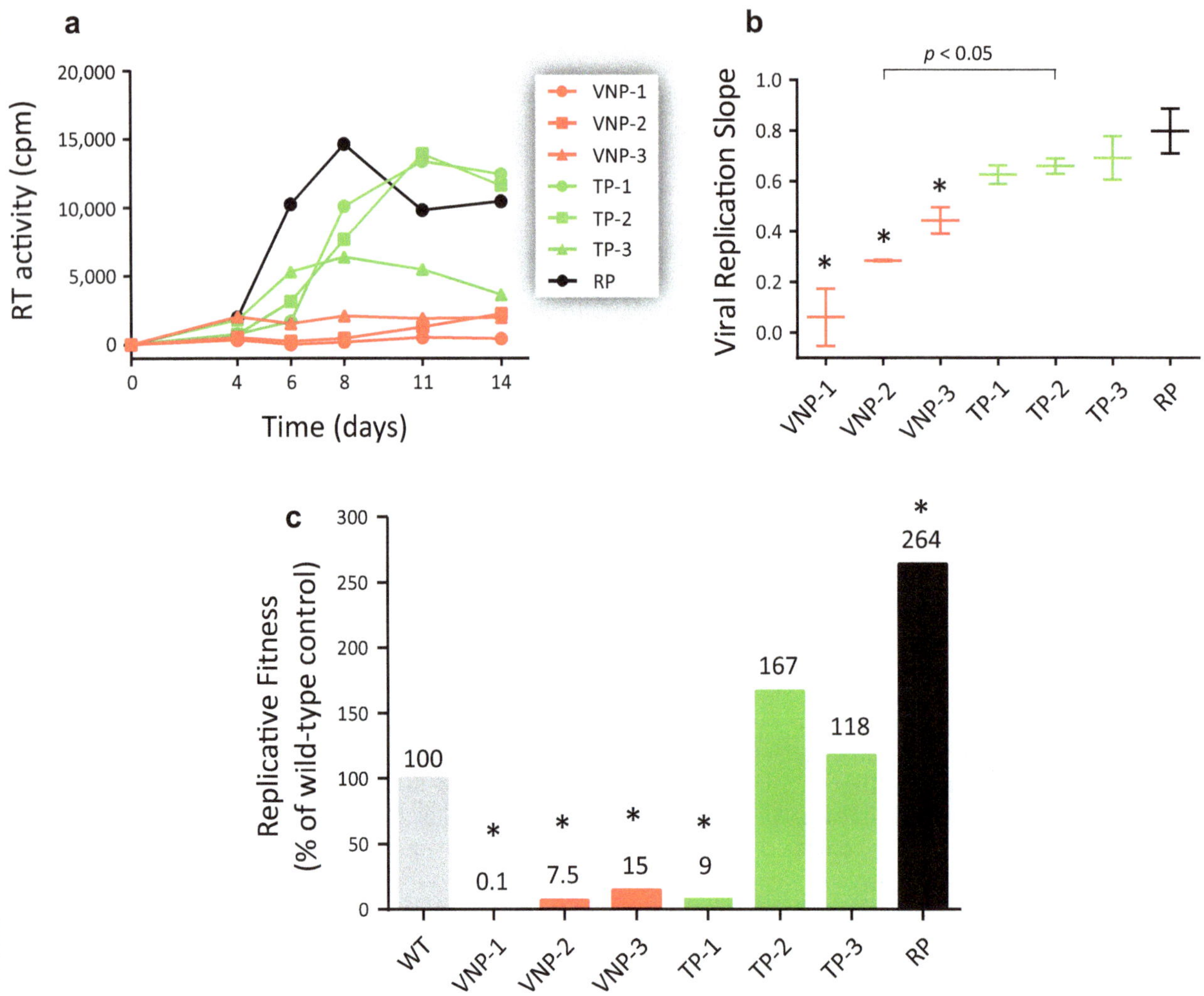

Fig. 1 Replicative fitness of seven patient-derived HIV-1 isolates in the absence of any host selective pressure, including antiretroviral drugs. **a** Seven HIV-1 isolates from 3 viremic non-progressor (VNP), 3 typical (TP) and one rapid (RP) progressor patients were evaluated for their ability to replicate in peripheral blood mononuclear cells (PBMC). Virus replication was quantified by measuring reverse transcriptase (RT) activity in the cell-free supernatant. **b** Viral replication slopes were calculated using the slopes between cpm values at days 0 and 4, 0 and 6, 0 and 8, 0 and 11, and 0 and 14. All five slope values for each virus were used to calculate the mean, standard deviation, and 10th and 90th percentiles. Differences in the mean values were calculated using a One Way Analysis of Variance test and the significance difference from the primary wild-type HIV-$1_{B\text{-}92US076}$ control isolate calculated using the Bonferroni's Multiple Comparison Test. **c** Each patient-derived HIV-1 isolate was competed against two different non-subtype B HIV-1 control strains (HIV-$1_{A\text{-}92UG029}$ and HIV-$1_{AE\text{-}CMU06}$) in PBMCs and their replicative fitness calculated and expressed as a percentage of the replicative fitness of the reference virus HIV-$1_{B\text{-}92US076}$ (set as 100%) as described [28, 35, 66, 67]. Values represent results obtained from single growth competition experiments. Viral replication kinetics and growth competitions marked with an *asterisk* were significantly different to the HIV-$1_{B\text{-}92US076}$ control ($p < 0.05$, 95% CI)

and HIV-$1_{AE\text{-}CMU06}$). Interestingly, all three VNP viruses showed a marked decrease in replicative fitness, i.e., 0.1, 7.5, and 15% relative to that of the primary HIV-$1_{B\text{-}92US076}$ isolate used as control (Fig. 1c). With the exception of the TP-1 virus (9%), the replicative fitness of the other two TP viruses was not impaired relative to the fitness of the HIV-$1_{B\text{-}92US076}$ control (167 and 118% for TP-2 and TP-3, respectively). Finally, the RP virus had a 2.6-fold higher replicative fitness than the HIV-$1_{B\text{-}92US076}$ control and, in average, was 35-fold more fit to replicate in PBMCs than the VNP viruses (Fig. 1c).

Characterization of HIV-1 isolates from VNP, TP, and RP individuals: subtyping, drug resistance, and coreceptor tropism

To further characterize the HIV-1 isolates, viral RNA was used to amplify and sequence near full-length HIV-1 genomes (HXB2 coordinates 157–99,428) using both Sanger and deep sequencing. For deep sequencing, amplicons corresponding to all 7 viruses were multiplexed into a single 318c chip (78% loading efficiency of Ion Sphere Particles), generating 3,856,115 total quality reads with a mean read length of 131 bp (mean range 130–133 bp). Although the average sequencing coverage at each nucleotide position varied with each sample and HIV-1 genomic region analyzed ($p < 0.0001$, one-way ANOVA), the mean coverage for each viral sequence ranged from 2079 reads for the RP virus to 8500 for VNP-3 (Fig. 2a). These metrics ensured the minimum coverage of 1000 per nucleotide position sequenced required to guarantee the detection of a minor variant present at least at 1% of the population [75]. As expected, coverage decreases abruptly at the ends of the amplicons (e.g., 5′LTR and 3′LTR in Fig. 2a); however, we observed an inexplicable decrease in coverage around positions 6655–6719 (corresponding to variables regions V1 and V2 in gp120, *env* gene) that do not correspond with the end of any of the overlapping PCR products covering this genomic region.

The entire HIV-1 genome from all seven viruses was classified as subtype B using the Recombinant Identification Program from the Los Alamos HIV Sequence Database [76] (Table 1; Additional file 2: Figure S2). We used our proprietary DEEPGEN™HIV Software Tool Suite [70] to confirm the absence of mutations (at >1% frequency in the HIV-1 population) associated with drug resistance in the protease (PR), reverse transcriptase (RT), and/or integrase (INT) coding regions. The same tool was used to determine HIV-1 coreceptor tropism based on sequencing reads corresponding to the V3 region of gp120. HIV-1 isolates from VNP and TP patients were all CCR5-tropic viruses, while the RP individual was infected with a dual- or mixed-tropic virus (Table 1).

HIV-1 genetic polymorphisms in VNP, TP, and RP viruses

HIV-1 isolates from viremic non-progressor individuals showed a clear impairment on their ability to replicate in PBMCs in vitro. Since the fitness decrease was not associated with drug resistance mutations, we decided to analyze the entire HIV-1 genomes to try to identify any particular signature(s) that could be responsible for the decrease in replication capacity. First, we scanned all seven near full-length HIV-1 genomes searching for patterns in single-nucleotide polymorphisms (SNPs) among the three groups of patients. As described in Fig. 2b, we observed a higher concentration of SNPs in the variable regions of gp120; however, no clear clustering of the VNP or TP groups was evident when the SNP patterns of the near full-length genomes were analyzed. For example, VNP-1 and VNP-3 clustered with TP-3, while VNP-2 was closer to TP-1 and TP-2. Similar results were observed when SNP patterns were analyzed in each individual HIV-1 genomic region, with the exception of gp41 where significant clustering of VNP-1 with VNP-3 and all three TNP viruses was evident (Additional file 3: Figure S3).

Next, we focused on HIV-1 genetic polymorphisms that have been associated with impaired HIV-1 replicative fitness and/or disease progression [11, 31, 32, 40, 42, 44–62, 77, 78]. We identified a series of SNPs in LTR and amino acid substitutions—at different frequencies in

(See figure on next page.)
Fig. 2 **a** Coverage, i.e., number of reads per nucleotide position, obtained by deep sequencing the seven patient-derived HIV-1 isolates. Near full-length HIV-1 genomes were RT-PCR amplified and deep sequenced as described in "Methods". The position relative to the HIV-1 genome of the six overlapping amplicons used to amplify and sequence the near full-length HIV-1 genomes (HXB2 position 157 to 9428, not counting primer sequences) is indicated. **b** Hierarchical clustering analysis of the single nucleotides polymorphisms (SNPs) was used to group the seven patient-derived HIV-1 isolates by similarity. Dendrograms were calculated using the Euclidean distance and Complete cluster methods with 1000 bootstrap iterations as described (http://www.hiv.lanl.gov/content/sequence/HEATMAP/heatmap.html) Bootstrap values >60% are indicated by an *asterisk*. *Green and grey blocks* indicate the presence or absence of SNPs, respectively, in each HIV-1 isolate relative to the HIV-1_{HXB2} reference. **c** A Neighbor-joining phylogenetic tree was constructed using the near full-length HIV-1 consensus sequences generated for each patient-derived virus (obtained from deep sequencing reads) and rooted using the HIV-1_{HXB2} sequence (GenBank accession number AF033819). Bootstrap resampling (1000 data sets) of the multiple alignment tested the statistical robustness of the tree, with percentage values above 75% indicated by an *asterisk*. *s/site* substitutions per nucleotide site

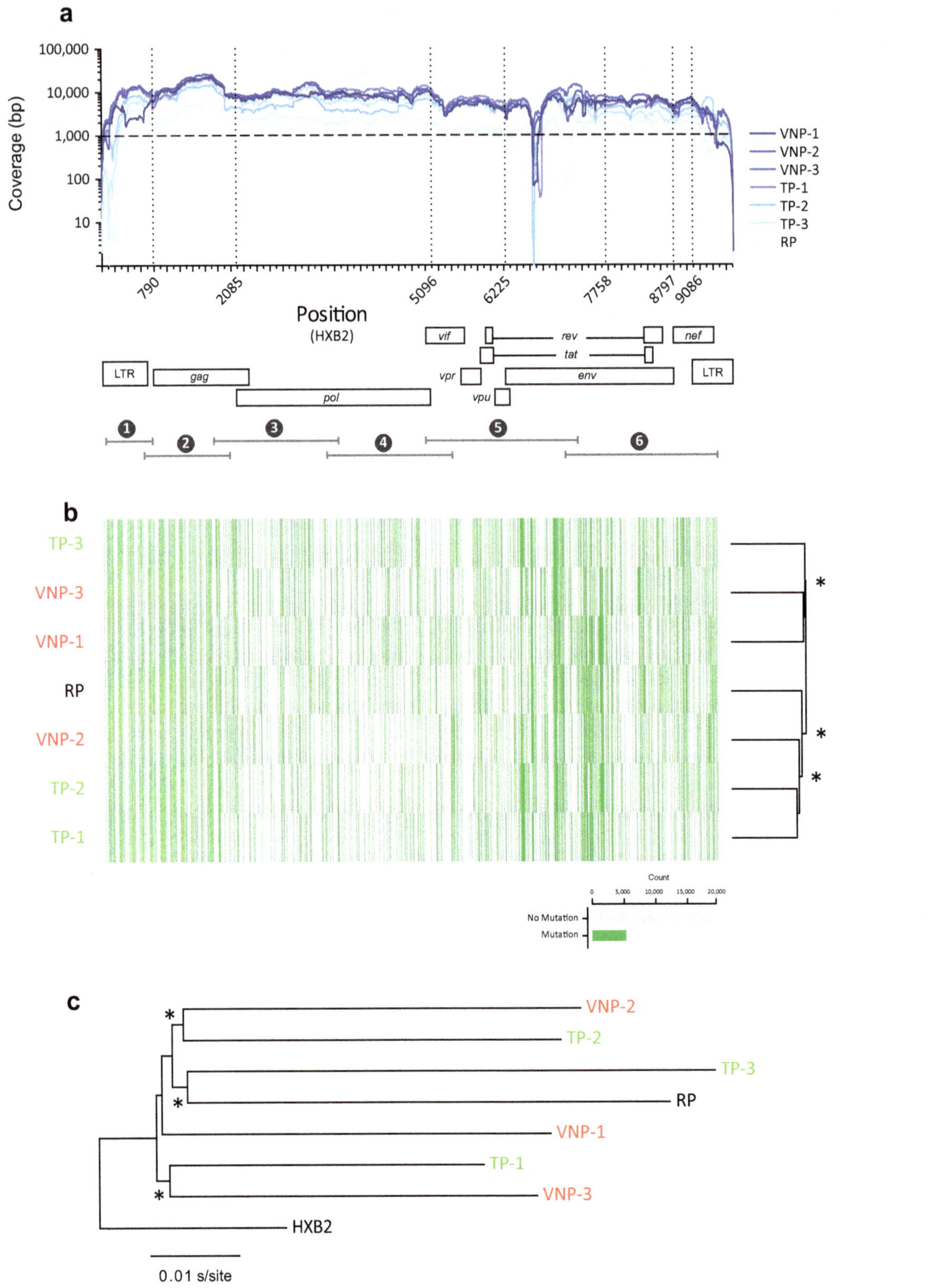
a
Coverage (bp)
100,000
10,000
1,000
100
10
790
2085
5096
6225
7758
8797
9086
Position
(HXB2)
VNP-1
VNP-2
VNP-3
TP-1
TP-2
TP-3
RP
vif
rev
nef
tat
LTR
gag
vpr
env
LTR
pol
vpu
1
2
3
4
5
6
b
TP-3
VNP-3
VNP-1
RP
VNP-2
TP-2
TP-1
Count
No Mutation
Mutation
c
VNP-2
TP-2
TP-3
RP
VNP-1
TP-1
VNP-3
HXB2
0.01 s/site

Table 2 HIV-1 genetic polymorphisms identified in this study, which have previously been associated with disease progression and/or impaired replicative fitness

Position[a]	Viremic non-progressors (VNP)			Typical progressors (TP)			Rapid progressor (RP)
	VNP-1	VNP-2	VNP-3	TP-1	TP-2	TP-3	RP
LTR							
287–292	A219G (18%)	A292ins (1%)	C290T (2%)		A219G (3%) A219ins (3%)	T287C (11%) T292A (99%)	
319–324	T319A (99%)	T319A (100%) A324G (100%)	T319A (99%) A324G (27%)	T319A (99%) A324G (99%)	T319A (99%) 320ins (11–57%) A324G (72%)	T319A (99%)	T319A (100%)
325–333	329ins (39%) C333T (11%)	332del (3%)	328ins (1%)		G331A (1%)		
346–356	G350A (1%)		A348T (11%) 355del (2%)	G350A (3%)			
361–371	G363A (6%) G364A (7%)					G366A (1%)	T32C (9%) G363A (10%)
374–385	A374G (74%) A378G (1%) G379A (1%) G385A (97%)	G377A (3%) 381ins (1%)	A374G (7%)	381ins (1%)	A378G (2%) 380ins (1%) C381T (99%) G384A (1%)	374ins (91%) G384A (100%) G385A (100%)	A374G (9%) 374ins (52%) G384A (99%)
386–397	C386T (97%) C387G (2%) G389A (30%)	G395A (2%)	380del (1%)	G389A (2%)		396ins (99%)	387G (3%) G393A (2%)
398–409	G399A (7%)		398ins (2%)	403ins (1%) 405ins (3%)	T398A (90%)	G409A (8%)	G400A (18%)
427–431	430del (1%), 431del (1%)	430del (2%)	430del (9%), 431del (1%)	430del (2%)	431del (2%)		
455–515	11SNPs (>1%), 13 indels (>1%)	8 SNPS, 11 indels	3 SNPs (>1%), 12 indels (>1%)	3 SNPs (>1%), 5 indels (>1%)	2 SNPs (>1%), 6 indels (>1%)	4 SNPs (>1%), 2 indels (>1%)	5 SNPs (>1%), 3 indels (>1%)
gag							
823–825	E12Q (99%)						
988–990		S67A (16%)			S67A (3%)	S67A (100%)	
1093–1095	D102E (98%)	D102E (9%)			D102E (73%)		D102E (100%)
1225–1227		A146P (86%)					
1513–1515			T242N (99%)				
1531–1533	G284A (99%)					G284A (99%)	G284A (99%)
1954–1956			T389I (99%)				T389I (100%)
2233–2235		E482D (99%)					
vif							
5434–5436	R132S (92%)						
vpr							
5773–5775	F72S (4%)						
5788–5790		R77Q (99%)	R77Q (99%)	R77Q (99%)	R77Q (99%)	R77Q (99%)	R77Q (99%)
5806–5826	Ins (7%)						
rev							
8522–8524	Q74H (99%)	Q74P (99%)			Q74P (75%)		
8612–8614		V104G (99%)				V104L (33%)	
nef							
9208–9210		T138C (99%)					
8839–8841		T15A (99%)	T15A (98%)	T15N (100%)			
8950–8952							
9100–9102	H102Y (99%)	H102Y (99%)	H102W (99%)	H102W (99%)	H102Y (99%)	H102Y (99%)	H102Y (100%)
9340–9342	E182Q (99%)		E182V (99%)	E182V (99%)			

[a] Positions in the HIV-1 genome relative to the HIV-1_{HXB2} (GenBank: K03455) strain reference. Single-nucleotide polymorphisms (SNPs) in the LTR or amino substitutions in the HIV-1 coding regions are indicated, including their frequency in the virus population (%) quantified by deep sequencing. For example: A219G (18%) in the LTR of the VNP-1 HIV-1 isolate or R77Q (99%) in the *vpr* gene of the VNP-2 HIV-1 isolate. Indels, insertions and/or deletions

the virus population—in *gag*, *vif*, *vpr*, *rev*, and *nef* genes (Table 2). Although no clear pattern of signature mutations was shared among the individual viruses from each group, some of the mutations were present only in VNP and not in TP or RP sequences, e.g., in the LTR (insertion at position 329, G364A, C386T, or G399A), *gag* (E12Q, A146P, T242 N, or E482D), *vif* (R132S), *vpr* (F72S), and *nef* (T138C). Interestingly, most of these mutations were identified in the VNP-1 isolate, which had the most impaired replicative fitness of the group (Fig. 1). In fact, the number of HIV-1 genetic polymorphisms previously associated with fitness decrease and/or disease progression was significantly higher in the VNP group compared with the TP and RP viruses (mean 39.3, 21.6, and 22, respectively, $p = 0.036$) (Table 2; Fig. 3a). Moreover, a strong significant inversed correlation was observed between the number of HIV-1 genetic polymorphisms in each viral isolate and the HIV-1 replicative fitness values determined by the slopes of the viral growth curves ($r = -0.956$, $p = 0.0007$, Pearson coefficient correlation) (Fig. 3b). Although not significant, most likely perhaps due to the low fitness calculated for the TP-1 virus, a similar trend was observed using the replicative fitness values from the growth competition experiments ($r = -0.547$, $p = 0.203$, Pearson coefficient correlation).

Genetic diversity of VNP, TP, and RP viruses

We used the consensus sequences of the near full-length HIV-1 genomes generated by deep sequencing to construct a neighbor-joining phylogenetic tree. As observed in Fig. 2c, the HIV-1 sequences did not cluster together according to their group, i.e., VNP, TP, and RP. Identical results were obtained using the population sequences generated by Sanger sequencing (data not shown). Based on the consensus near full-length HIV-1 sequences, intra-group genetic distances were not significantly different between VNP and TP viruses (0.089 and 0.096 substitutions/site, respectively, $p = 0.345$; Maximum Composite Likelihood model). Next we used the myriad of reads obtained by deep sequencing to calculate intra-patient HIV-1 population diversity based on the p-distance model [73]. Interestingly, the VNP viruses showed significantly higher genetic diversity than the TP and RP viruses (mean 3.07, 2.52, and 1.93 substitutions/site, $p = 0.009$) when the near full-length HIV-1 genomes were analyzed (Fig. 4a). Although this trend was consistent across individual HIV-1 genomic regions and genes (data not shown), the higher genetic diversity in VNP viruses was significant in two regions of the *gag* gene: p2 (4.82, 3.09, and 2.76 substitutions/site, $p = 0.008$) and p6 (2.9, 1.62, and 1.59 substitutions/site, $p = 0.02$), and the V4 region of gp120 (13.4, 1.54, and 6.39 substitutions/site, $p = 0.018$) (Fig. 4a). More importantly, we observed a strongly significant negative correlation between genetic diversity of the near full-length HIV-1 genomes and the replicative fitness values determined by the slopes of the viral growth curves ($r = -0.878$, $p = 0.009$, Pearson coefficient correlation) (Fig. 4b). The same significant inverse associations were observed for the two regions of the *gag* gene: p2 ($r = -0.833$, $p = 0.019$, Pearson coefficient correlation) and p6 ($r = -0.856$, $p = 0.013$, Pearson coefficient correlation), and the V4 region of gp120 ($r = -0.825$, $p = 0.022$, Pearson coefficient correlation) (Fig. 4b) but not for those regions with no significant differences in HIV-1 diversity between the three groups of patients. Similar results, i.e., more heterogeneous virus population (VNPs) having lower viral replicative fitness values, were obtained when replicative fitness was determined using growth competition experiments (regression values ranging from -0.791 to -0.867, $p < 0.05$, Pearson coefficient correlation; data not shown).

Discussion

Since the discovery of HIV-1 as the etiological agent of AIDS [79, 80], multitude of studies have attempted to understand the differences on HIV-1 disease progression, particularly host and/or viral factors that could be associated with HIV-1 pathogenesis [11, 12, 81]. The common ("normal") inverse correlation between $CD4^+$ T-cell count and plasma HIV RNA load usually governs HIV-1 pathogenesis, i.e., elevated plasma viremia is typically accompanied by a decrease in $CD4^+$ T-cells, leading to disease progression [2]. Some HIV-infected individuals have shown uncommon rates of disease progression (slow, non-progressor or elite controllers) but all of them have reduced or undetected plasma HIV RNA loads [3, 4, 42, 82]. On the other hand, a rare group of patients termed viremic non-progressors (VNP) seem to resemble Simian Immunodeficiency Virus (SIV) infection in sooty mangabeys, i.e., active viral replication without (or very limited) disease progression [26, 82–84]. Here we identified three atypically VNP HIV-infected individuals and proceeded to study their HIV-1 isolates, focusing on replicative fitness and viral genomic analysis to try to understand the maintenance of stable $CD4^+$ T-cell counts despite persistence viremia for more than 10 years, in the absence of antiretroviral treatment.

As described above, viremic non-progressor (controller) patients do not progress to AIDS, maintaining high $CD4^+$ T-cell counts with HIV-1 replication for many years [5–7, 85]. The three VNP individuals described in this study had been infected with HIV-1 for at least 10 years at the time the blood sample was taken, with stable $CD4^+$ T-cell counts and high plasma HIV RNA loads. When compared with three typical (TP) and one rapid progressor (RP) patients, the number of $CD4^+$ T-cells

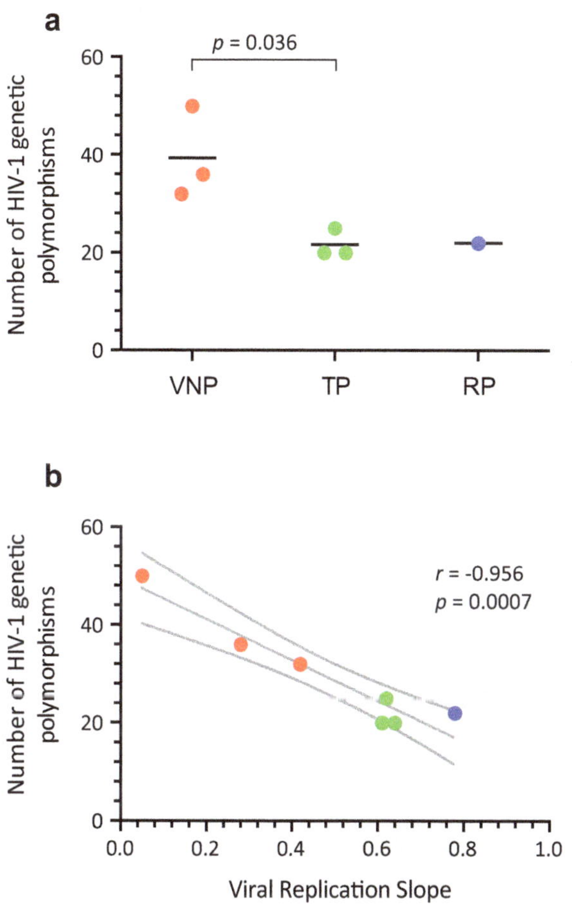

Fig. 3 **a** Comparison of the number of HIV-1 genetic polymorphisms in the near full-length HIV-1 genome that have been associated with impaired HIV-1 replicative fitness and/or disease progression [11, 31, 32, 40, 42, 44–62, 77, 78] among the three groups of patients, i.e., VNP, RP, and TP. Unpaired t test was used to assess the statistical significance between VNP and TP patients. A detailed list of the mutations is included in Table 2. **b** Pearson correlation coefficient was used to determine the strength of association between the number of HIV-1 genetic polymorphisms and the HIV-1 replicative fitness calculated by viral growth kinetics analysis (viral replication slope) described in Fig. 1. *r* correlation coefficient, *p* two-tailed p value. *Dotted lines* represent 95% confidence intervals

barely declined in the VNPs over this period of time, similar to what have been described for other adult and children VNPs [43, 82–84, 86]. No other significant differences were observed among the VNP and TP patients, including plasma viral load levels and basic virus characteristics such as HIV-1 subtype (all clade B) and coreceptor tropism (all CCR5-tropic viruses).

Most studies involving the characterization of viremic non-progressor (controller) patients have focused in host factors to try to understand their odd HIV-1 disease progression profile. For example, the presence of the HLA-B*27 allele was associated with the VNP phenotype [43], while a higher frequency of the protective single nucleotide polymorphism −35 CC in the HLA-C gene was found in VNP patients [5]. Preferential Gag-specific CD8^{+} T cell responses have also been observed in viremic controllers [84] and limited infection of CD4^{+} central memory cells [8], perhaps related to low CCR5 expression on these cells [86], seem to be associated with lack of disease progression in VNPs. Limited deregulation of a series of interferon-stimulated genes correlating with time to disease progression was also identified in VNPs [85]. However, and similar to the absence of immune activation during natural SIV infection in sooty mangabeys [27, 87, 88], healthy CD4^{+} T cell counts despite detectable viremia seem to be common in most viremic non-progressor patients [86]. Yet, just a limited number of studies have analyzed HIV-1 strains infecting VNPs [6, 43].

Here we showed that the replicative fitness of all three VNP-derived HIV-1 isolates was impaired compared to the fitness of the viruses obtained from the TP and RP patients. We and others have reported that HIV-1 replicative fitness is associated with disease progression [28–30, 42], that is, viruses with decreased replication capacity influence the natural history of HIV-1 infection, correlating with diminished viral burden and HIV-1 pathogenesis. Viruses from long-term non-progressor [28], slow progressor [41, 42] and elite controller [37, 40, 42] patients have been shown to have impaired replication capacity; however, the fitness of viruses from VNP individuals have not been extensively described. Choudhary et al. [6] showed that HIV-1 isolates derived from VNP were as cytopathic as viruses isolated from typical progressor patients. On the other hand, O'Connell et al. [43] observed a slight decrease in the fitness of a virus from a VNP patient, transmitted from a chronic progressor partner, but failed to identify any amino acid substitution(s) potentially responsible for this phenotype.

Reduced HIV-1 replicative fitness is usually the consequence of changes in the viral quasispecies following the evasion of key selective pressures, e.g., host immune response and/or antiretroviral treatment [30, 31]. These changes are accompanied by single or multiple mutations in the targeted HIV-1 genomic region, deviating the virus population from the wild-type quasispecies distribution and impairing their ability to replicate efficiently compared to the original virus [89, 90]. The effect of a multitude of drug resistance mutations (in the *pol* gene) in viral replicative fitness have been amply described [30, 74]. A number of CTL escape mutations have been identified in HIV and SIV that carry a concomitant replicative fitness cost [46, 91, 92], including HIV-1 mutant variants escaping Gag-specific CD8^{+} T cell responses—like those identified in viremic controllers [84]—that had reduced

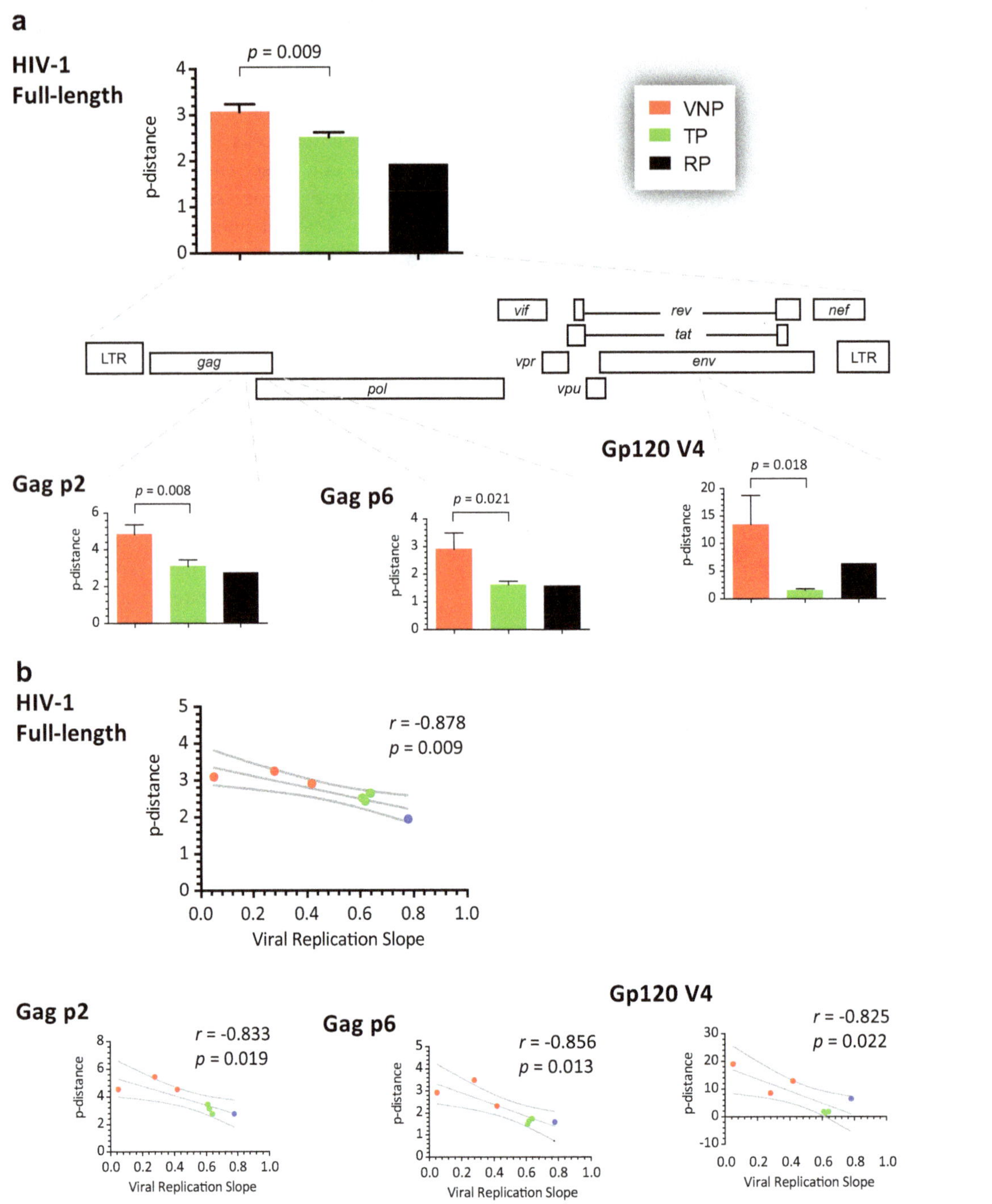

Fig. 4 **a** Comparison of intra-patient HIV-1 population diversity, based on the p-distance model [73], among the three groups of patients, i.e., VNP, RP, and TP. Unpaired t test was used to assess the statistical significance between VNP and TP patients. Only those HIV-1 regions significantly different, i.e., near full-length HIV-1 genome, Gag p2, Gag p6, and Gp120 V4, are included. **b** Pearson correlation coefficient was used to determine the strength of association between intra-patient HIV-1 population diversity values (p-distance) and the HIV-1 replicative fitness calculated by viral growth kinetics analysis (viral replication slope) described in Fig. 1. *r* correlation coefficient, *p* two-tailed p value. *Dotted lines* represent 95% confidence intervals

replicative fitness [40]. Other studies have shown how multiple mutations and/or deletions in the LTR and all HIV-1 coding regions have a range of effects on the ability of the virus to replicate (virus attenuation) [11, 31, 32, 40, 42, 44–62, 78]. Here we used deep sequencing to analyze near full-length HIV-1 genomes from all VNP-derived viruses, and compared them with the sequences from the TP- and RP-derived viral genomes. Despite identifying a series of SNPs in different genomic regions, some of them previously associated with a reduction in replicative fitness and/or disease progression [11, 31, 32, 40, 42, 44–62, 77, 78], no clear pattern of signature mutations was detected in the viruses from the VNPs that could explain the impairment in replication capacity. Interestingly, it was the number of these HIV-1 genetic polymorphisms that correlated significantly with the replicative fitness of each HIV-1 isolate. In fact, it is reasonable to think that viruses with a higher number of critical SNPs have a more marked decrease in replicative fitness, similar to what has been described for multidrug-resistant HIV-1 variants carrying multiple mutations in the protease, reverse transcriptase and/or integrase coding regions [30, 74]. These results were corroborated by calculating intra-patient HIV-1 population diversity, i.e., the highly replication impaired VNP viruses had a more complex virus quasispecies population, most likely as a consequence of trying to evade the host immune response [93], which was highlighted by the significant correlation between replicative fitness and HIV-1 genetic diversity in highly immunogenic regions such as Gag and Gp120 [31, 42, 92]. We and others have described similar results where drug resistant HIV-1 variants with more heterogeneous virus population had lower viral replicative fitness [94, 95]. It is possible that impaired (less replication competent) HIV-1 strains are capable to ascertain a limited host immune response in VNPs, enough to maintain high levels of viremia, resulting in viral evolution but limiting host immune activation that could exacerbate HIV disease, i.e., decrease $CD4^+$ T-cell counts. It is also possible that the preferential replication of HIV-1 in effector memory T cells, and preservation of central memory T cells, in VNPs [8] could result in greater virus production per HIV-infected cell. All interesting possibilities to be addressed in further studies.

Although prevalence of elite controllers seems to be less than 1% of the HIV-infected population [96, 97], a recent study involving over 13,000 HIV-infected individuals identified 271 viremic controllers for a 2.03% prevalence [82]. Interestingly, viremic pediatric nonprogressor patients with high $CD4^+$ T cell counts seem to be more common than adults VNP individuals [86]. Is it possible that VNP patients are more common than what we originally thought? If so, what can we learn from these individuals that could help monitor and control HIV-1 infection in less fortunate patients? Several studies have pointed to high levels of immune activation as the major cause of HIV-1 pathogenesis [24, 98] and low immune activation seems to be—at least in part- responsible for the lack of disease progression in VNP individuals [86]. Moreover, the VNP-like phenotype during natural SIV infections in sooty mangabeys is definitely not related to a low rate of viral production nor an impairment on replicative fitness of the virus [25, 87]. However, we cannot rule out that original infection with less replication-competent viruses (therefore seeding HIV-1 reservoirs with replication impaired variants) could contribute to the decrease in immune activation, leading to the viremic non-progressor phenotype in these patients. Here we observed that all three VNP patients carried HIV-1 isolates with decreased replicative fitness compared to typical and rapid progressor individuals, and that accumulation of single-nucleotide polymorphisms (mutations) across the HIV-1 genome may be contributing to the overall fitness impairment. Therefore, it is possible that similar to the phenomenon observed in patients with a discordant response to antiretroviral therapy, i.e., high $CD4^+$ cell counts with detectable plasma HIV-1 RNA load [99, 100], reduced viral replicative fitness could be contributing to late disease progression in untreated viremic controller individuals. Additional studies involving host immunology and genetics, together with more detailed analysis of the HIV-1 strains infecting VNP patients, are necessary to better understand HIV-1 pathogenesis, including approaches to prevent HIV-1 disease and potentially eliminate HIV reservoirs.

Additional files

Additional file 1: Figure S1. $CD4^+$ T-cell counts and plasma HIV-1 RNA load values available for all seven patients described in this study. Vertical dashed lines indicate the time of sampling. Grey arrows depict the number of years since primary HIV-1 infection. The period of time the patients were under antiretroviral treatment (ART) is indicated by black boxes.

Additional file 2: Figure S2. Subtyping of the near full-length HIV-1 consensus sequences, obtained by deep sequencing, was performed using the Recombination Identification Program (RIP 3.0) from the Los Alamos HIV Sequence Database as described (1). The similarity plots show distance measurements between the query sequence (patient-derived HIV-1) and the reference HIV-1 sequences from different subtypes.

Additional file 3: Figure S3. Hierarchical clustering analysis of single nucleotide polymorphisms (SNPs) in all HIV-1 coding regions plus the long-terminal regions (LTRs). Dendograms were calculated using the Euclidian distance and Complete cluster methods with 1000 bootstrap iterations as described in Los Alamos HIV Sequence Database (http://www.hiv.lanl.gov.content/sequence/HEATMAP/heatmap.html). Bootstrap values >60% are indicated by an asterisk. Green and grey blocks indicate the presence and absence of SNPs, respectively.

Abbreviations

HIV-1: human immunodeficiency virus type 1; VNP: viremic non-progressors; TP: typical progressor; RP: rapid progressor; LTNP: long-term non-progressors; SNP: single-nucleotide polymorphism; HLA: human leukocyte antigen; CTL: cytotoxic T cell; PBMC: peripheral blood mononuclear cells; MOI: multiplicity of infection.

Authors' contributions

JW and MEQM designed the study, collected and assembled the data, wrote and drafted the manuscript. RMG, LS, DS, JH, JW, and MP performed all cell culture, molecular, and sequencing experiments. JW, MML, BR and MEQM contributed to the overall analysis of the data. All authors read and approved the final manuscript.

Author details

[1] Institute of Organic Chemistry and Biochemistry v.v.i., Academy of Sciences of the Czech Republic, Flemingovo n. 2, 166 10 Prague 6, Czech Republic. [2] University Hospital Translational Laboratory, University Hospitals Cleveland Medical Center, Cleveland, OH, USA. [3] Department of Medicine, Case Western Reserve University/University Hospitals Cleveland Medical Center, 10900 Euclid Avenue, Cleveland, OH 44106-7288, USA. [4] Department of Pathology, Case Western Reserve University, Cleveland, OH, USA.

Acknowledgements

We thank Michelle Gallagher and the Case Western Reserve University/University Hospitals Center for AIDS Research (NIH P30 AI036219) for providing access to critical clinical information.

Competing interests

The authors declare that they have no competing interests.

Funding

J.W. was supported by a research grant from the Ministry of Education, Youth and Sports of the Czech Republic (LK11207). M.E.Q-M was partially supported by research Grant NIH-AI-71747, the CWRU/UH Center for AIDS Research (P30 AI036219) and funding from University Hospitals Cleveland Medical Center (UHCMC) for the University Hospitals Translational Laboratory (UHTL).

References

1. Poorolajal J, Hooshmand E, Mahjub H, Esmailnasab N, Jenabi E. Survival rate of AIDS disease and mortality in HIV-infected patients: a meta-analysis. Public Health. 2016;139:3–12.
2. Lackner AA, Lederman MM, Rodriguez B. HIV pathogenesis: the host. Cold Spring Harb Perspect Med. 2012;2(9):a007005.
3. Casado C, Colombo S, Rauch A, Martinez R, Gunthard HF, Garcia S, Rodriguez C, Del Romero J, Telenti A, Lopez-Galindez C. Host and viral genetic correlates of clinical definitions of HIV-1 disease progression. PLoS ONE. 2010;5(6):e11079.
4. Okulicz JF, Marconi VC, Landrum ML, Wegner S, Weintrob A, Ganesan A, Hale B, Crum-Cianflone N, Delmar J, Barthel V, et al. Clinical outcomes of elite controllers, viremic controllers, and long-term nonprogressors in the US Department of Defense HIV natural history study. J Infect Dis. 2009;200(11):1714–23.
5. Ballana E, Ruiz-de Andres A, Mothe B, de Arellano ER, Aguilar F, Badia R, Grau E, Clotet B, del Val M, Brander C, et al. Differential prevalence of the HLA-C −35 CC genotype among viremic long term non-progressor and elite controller HIV+ individuals. Immunobiology. 2012;217(9):889–94.
6. Choudhary SK, Vrisekoop N, Jansen CA, Otto SA, Schuitemaker H, Miedema F, Camerini D. Low immune activation despite high levels of pathogenic human immunodeficiency virus type 1 results in long-term asymptomatic disease. J Virol. 2007;81(16):8838–42.
7. Curriu M, Fausther-Bovendo H, Pernas M, Massanella M, Carrillo J, Cabrera C, Lopez-Galindez C, Clotet B, Debre P, Vieillard V, et al. Viremic HIV infected individuals with high CD4 T cells and functional envelope proteins show anti-gp41 antibodies with unique specificity and function. PLoS ONE. 2012;7(2):e30330.
8. Klatt NR, Bosinger SE, Peck M, Richert-Spuhler LE, Heigele A, Gile JP, Patel N, Taaffe J, Julg B, Camerini D, et al. Limited HIV infection of central memory and stem cell memory $CD4^+$ T cells is associated with lack of progression in viremic individuals. PLoS Pathog. 2014;10(8):e1004345.
9. Mothe B, Ibarrondo J, Llano A, Brander C. Virological, immune and host genetics markers in the control of HIV infection. Dis Markers. 2009;27(3):105–20.
10. Santa-Marta M, de Brito PM, Godinho-Santos A, Goncalves J. Host factors and HIV-1 replication: clinical evidence and potential therapeutic approaches. Front Immunol. 2013;4:343.
11. Wang B. Viral factors in non-progression. Front Immunol. 2013;4:355.
12. Cohen OJ, Kinter A, Fauci AS. Host factors in the pathogenesis of HIV disease. ImmunolRev. 1997;159:31–48.
13. O'Brien SJ, Moore JP. The effect of genetic variation in chemokines and their receptors on HIV transmission and progression to AIDS. Immunol Rev. 2000;177:99–111.
14. Pantaleo G, Demarest JF, Schacker T, Vaccarezza M, Cohen OJ, Daucher M, Graziosi C, Schnittman SS, Quinn TC, Shaw GM, et al. The qualitative nature of the primary immune response to HIV infection is a prognosticator of disease progression independent of the initial level of plasma viremia. Proc Natl Acad Sci USA. 1997;94(1):254–8.
15. Saez-Cirion A, Lacabaratz C, Lambotte O, Versmisse P, Urrutia A, Boufassa F, Barre-Sinoussi F, Delfraissy JF, Sinet M, Pancino G, et al. HIV controllers exhibit potent CD8 T cell capacity to suppress HIV infection ex vivo and peculiar cytotoxic T lymphocyte activation phenotype. Proc Natl Acad Sci USA. 2007;104(16):6776–81.
16. Goulder PJ, Bunce M, Krausa P, McIntyre K, Crowley S, Morgan B, Edwards A, Giangrande P, Phillips RE, McMichael AJ. Novel, cross-restricted, conserved, and immunodominant cytotoxic T lymphocyte epitopes in slow progressors in HIV type 1 infection. AIDS Res Hum Retrovir. 1996;12(18):1691–8.
17. Migueles SA, Sabbaghian MS, Shupert WL, Bettinotti MP, Marincola FM, Martino L, Hallahan CW, Selig SM, Schwartz D, Sullivan J, et al. HLA B*5701 is highly associated with restriction of virus replication in a subgroup of HIV-infected long term nonprogressors. Proc Natl Acad Sci USA. 2000;97(6):2709–14.
18. Balotta C, Bagnarelli P, Violin M, Ridolfo AL, Zhou D, Berlusconi A, Corvasce S, Corbellino M, Clementi M, Clerici M, et al. Homozygous delta 32 deletion of the CCR-5 chemokine receptor gene in an HIV-1-infected patient. AIDS. 1997;11(10):F67–71.
19. Dean M, Carrington M, Winkler C, Huttley GA, Smith MW, Allikmets R, Goedert JJ, Buchbinder SP, Vittinghoff E, Gomperts E, et al. Genetic restriction of HIV-1 infection and progression to AIDS by a deletion allele of the CKR5 structural gene. Hemophilia Growth and Development Study, Multicenter AIDS Cohort Study, Multicenter Hemophilia Cohort Study, San Francisco City Cohort, ALIVE Study. Science. 1996;273(5283):1856–62.
20. Eugen-Olsen J, Iversen AK, Garred P, Koppelhus U, Pedersen C, Benfield TL, Sorensen AM, Katzenstein T, Dickmeiss E, Gerstoft J, et al. Heterozygosity for a deletion in the CKR-5 gene leads to prolonged AIDS-free survival and slower CD4 T-cell decline in a cohort of HIV-seropositive individuals. AIDS. 1997;11(3):305–10.
21. Huang Y, Paxton WA, Wolinsky SM, Neumann AU, Zhang L, He T, Kang S, Ceradini D, Jin Z, Yazdanbakhsh K, et al. The role of a mutant CCR5 allele in HIV-1 transmission and disease progression. Nat Med. 1996;2(11):1240–3.
22. Zimmerman PA, Buckler-White A, Alkhatib G, Spalding T, Kubofcik J, Combadiere C, Weissman D, Cohen O, Rubbert A, Lam G, et al. Inherited resistance to HIV-1 conferred by an inactivating mutation in CC chemokine receptor 5: studies in populations with contrasting clinical phenotypes, defined racial background, and quantified risk. Mol Med. 1997;3(1):23–36.
23. Merindol N, Berthoux L. Restriction factors in HIV-1 disease progression. Curr HIV Res. 2015;13(6):448–61.
24. Deeks SG, Kitchen CM, Liu L, Guo H, Gascon R, Narvaez AB, Hunt P, Martin JN, Kahn JO, Levy J, et al. Immune activation set point during early HIV infection predicts subsequent $CD4^+$ T-cell changes independent of viral load. Blood. 2004;104(4):942–7.

25. Silvestri G, Paiardini M, Pandrea I, Lederman MM, Sodora DL. Understanding the benign nature of SIV infection in natural hosts. J Clin Invest. 2007;117(11):3148–54.
26. Chahroudi A, Bosinger SE, Vanderford TH, Paiardini M, Silvestri G. Natural SIV hosts: showing AIDS the door. Science. 2012;335(6073):1188–93.
27. Hirsch VM. What can natural infection of African monkeys with simian immunodeficiency virus tell us about the pathogenesis of AIDS? AIDS Rev. 2004;6(1):40–53.
28. Quinones-Mateu ME, Ball SC, Marozsan AJ, Torre VS, Albright JL, Vanham G, van der Groen G, Colebunders RL, Arts EJ. A dual infection/competition assay shows a correlation between ex vivo human immunodeficiency virus type 1 fitness and disease progression. J Virol. 2000;74(19):9222–33.
29. Troyer RM, Collins KR, Abraha A, Fraundorf E, Moore DM, Krizan RW, Toossi Z, Colebunders RL, Jensen MA, Mullins JI, et al. Changes in human immunodeficiency virus type 1 fitness and genetic diversity during disease progression. J Virol. 2005;79(14):9006–18.
30. Quinones-Mateu ME, Arts EJ. HIV-1 fitness: implications for drug resistance, disease progression, and global epidemic evolution. In: Kuiken C, Foley B, Hahn B, Marx P, McCutchan F, Mellors J, Wolinsky S, Korber B, Los Alamos NM, editors. HIV Sequence Compendium 2001. Los Alamos: Theoretical Biology and Biophysics Group, Los Alamos National Laboratory; 2001. p. 134–70.
31. Quinones-Mateu ME, Arts EJ. Virus fitness: concept, quantification, and application to HIV population dynamics. Curr Top Microbiol Immunol. 2006;299:83–140.
32. Armand-Ugon M, Quinones-Mateu ME, Gutierrez A, Barretina J, Blanco J, Schols D, De Clercq E, Clotet B, Este JA. Reduced fitness of HIV-1 resistant to CXCR4 antagonists. Antivir Ther. 2003;8:1–8.
33. Quinones-Mateu ME, Tadele M, Parera M, Mas A, Weber J, Rangel HR, Chakraborty B, Clotet B, Domingo E, Menendez-Arias L, et al. Insertions in the reverse transcriptase increase both drug resistance and viral fitness in a human immunodeficiency virus type 1 isolate harboring the multi-nucleoside reverse transcriptase inhibitor resistance 69 insertion complex mutation. J Virol. 2002;76(20):10546–52.
34. Weber J, Chakraborty B, Weberova J, Miller MD, Quinones-Mateu ME. Diminished replicative fitness of primary human immunodeficiency virus type 1 isolates harboring the K65R mutation. J Clin Microbiol. 2005;43(3):1395–400.
35. Weber J, Rangel HR, Chakraborty B, Tadele M, Martinez MA, Martinez-Picado J, Marotta ML, Mirza M, Ruiz L, Clotet B, et al. A novel TaqMan real-time PCR assay to estimate ex vivo human immunodeficiency virus type 1 fitness in the era of multi-target (pol and env) antiretroviral therapy. J Gen Virol. 2003;84:2217–28.
36. Claiborne DT, Prince JL, Scully E, Macharia G, Micci L, Lawson B, Kopycinski J, Deymier MJ, Vanderford TH, Nganou-Makamdop K, et al. Replicative fitness of transmitted HIV-1 drives acute immune activation, proviral load in memory CD4+ T cells, and disease progression. Proc Natl Acad Sci USA. 2015;112(12):E1480–9.
37. Miura T, Brumme ZL, Brockman MA, Rosato P, Sela J, Brumme CJ, Pereyra F, Kaufmann DE, Trocha A, Block BL, et al. Impaired replication capacity of acute/early viruses in persons who become HIV controllers. J Virol. 2010;84(15):7581–91.
38. Blankson JN, Bailey JR, Thayil S, Yang HC, Lassen K, Lai J, Gandhi SK, Siliciano JD, Williams TM, Siliciano RF. Isolation and characterization of replication-competent human immunodeficiency virus type 1 from a subset of elite suppressors. J Virol. 2007;81(5):2508–18.
39. Julg B, Pereyra F, Buzon MJ, Piechocka-Trocha A, Clark MJ, Baker BM, Lian J, Miura T, Martinez-Picado J, Addo MM, et al. Infrequent recovery of HIV from but robust exogenous infection of activated CD4(+) T cells in HIV elite controllers. Clin Infect Dis. 2010;51(2):233–8.
40. Brumme ZL, Li C, Miura T, Sela J, Rosato PC, Brumme CJ, Markle TJ, Martin E, Block BL, Trocha A, et al. Reduced replication capacity of NL4-3 recombinant viruses encoding reverse transcriptase-integrase sequences from HIV-1 elite controllers. J Acquir Immune Defic Syndr. 2011;56(2):100–8.
41. Lassen KG, Lobritz MA, Bailey JR, Johnston S, Nguyen S, Lee B, Chou T, Siliciano RF, Markowitz M, Arts EJ. Elite suppressor-derived HIV-1 envelope glycoproteins exhibit reduced entry efficiency and kinetics. PLoS Pathog. 2009;5(4):e1000377.
42. Lobritz MA, Lassen KG, Arts EJ. HIV-1 replicative fitness in elite controllers. Curr Opin HIV AIDS. 2011;6(3):214–20.
43. O'Connell KA, Pelz RK, Dinoso JB, Dunlop E, Paik-Tesch J, Williams TM, Blankson JN. Prolonged control of an HIV type 1 escape variant following treatment interruption in an HLA-B*27-positive patient. AIDS Res Hum Retroviruses. 2010;26(12):1307–11.
44. de Arellano RE, Martin C, Soriano V, Alcami J, Holguin A. Genetic analysis of the long terminal repeat (LTR) promoter region in HIV-1-infected individuals with different rates of disease progression. Virus Genes. 2007;34(2):111–6.
45. Kondo M, Shima T, Nishizawa M, Sudo K, Iwamuro S, Okabe T, Takebe Y, Imai M. Identification of attenuated variants of HIV-1 circulating recombinant form 01_AE that are associated with slow disease progression due to gross genetic alterations in the nef/long terminal repeat sequences. J Infect Dis. 2005;192(1):56–61.
46. Martinez-Picado J, Prado JG, Fry EE, Pfafferott K, Leslie A, Chetty S, Thobakgale C, Honeyborne I, Crawford H, Matthews P, et al. Fitness cost of escape mutations in p24 Gag in association with control of human immunodeficiency virus type 1. J Virol. 2006;80(7):3617–23.
47. Miura T, Brockman MA, Schneidewind A, Lobritz M, Pereyra F, Rathod A, Block BL, Brumme ZL, Brumme CJ, Baker B, et al. HLA-B57/B*5801 human immunodeficiency virus type 1 elite controllers select for rare gag variants associated with reduced viral replication capacity and strong cytotoxic T-lymphocyte [corrected] recognition. J Virol. 2009;83(6):2743–55.
48. Prince JL, Claiborne DT, Carlson JM, Schaefer M, Yu T, Lahki S, Prentice HA, Yue L, Vishwanathan SA, Kilembe W, et al. Role of transmitted Gag CTL polymorphisms in defining replicative capacity and early HIV-1 pathogenesis. PLoS Pathog. 2012;8(11):e1003041.
49. Wright JK, Novitsky V, Brockman MA, Brumme ZL, Brumme CJ, Carlson JM, Heckerman D, Wang B, Losina E, Leshwedi M, et al. Influence of Gag-protease-mediated replication capacity on disease progression in individuals recently infected with HIV-1 subtype C. J Virol. 2011;85(8):3996–4006.
50. Mostowy R, Kouyos RD, Hoof I, Hinkley T, Haddad M, Whitcomb JM, Petropoulos CJ, Kesmir C, Bonhoeffer S. Estimating the fitness cost of escape from HLA presentation in HIV-1 protease and reverse transcriptase. PLoS Comput Biol. 2012;8(5):e1002525.
51. Shioda T, Oka S, Xin X, Liu H, Harukuni R, Kurotani A, Fukushima M, Hasan MK, Shiino T, Takebe Y, et al. In vivo sequence variability of human immunodeficiency virus type 1 envelope gp120: association of V2 extension with slow disease progression. J Virol. 1997;71(7):4871–81.
52. Wang B, Mikhail M, Dyer WB, Zaunders JJ, Kelleher AD, Saksena NK. First demonstration of a lack of viral sequence evolution in a nonprogressor, defining replication-incompetent HIV-1 infection. Virology. 2003;312(1):135–50.
53. Alexander L, Weiskopf E, Greenough TC, Gaddis NC, Auerbach MR, Malim MH, O'Brien SJ, Walker BD, Sullivan JL, Desrosiers RC. Unusual polymorphisms in human immunodeficiency virus type 1 associated with nonprogressive infection. J Virol. 2000;74(9):4361–76.
54. Kirchhoff F, Easterbrook PJ, Douglas N, Troop M, Greenough TC, Weber J, Carl S, Sullivan JL, Daniels RS. Sequence variations in human immunodeficiency virus type 1 Nef are associated with different stages of disease. J Virol. 1999;73(7):5497–508.
55. Premkumar DRD, Ma XZ, Maitra RK, Chakrabarti BK, Salkowitz J, Yen-Lieberman B, Hirsch MS, Kestler HW. The nef gene from a long-term HIV type 1 nonprogressor. AIDS Res Hum Retrovir. 1996;12:337–45.
56. Deacon NJ, Tsykin A, Solomon A, Smith K, Ludford-Menting M, Hooker DJ, McPhee DA, Greenway AL, Ellet A, Chatfield C, et al. Genomic structure of an attenuated quasispecies of HIV-1 from a blood transfusion donor and recipients. Science. 1995;270:988–91.
57. Salvi R, Garbuglia AR, Di Caro A, Pulciani S, Montella F, Benedetto A. Grossly defective nef gene sequences in a human immunodeficiency virus type 1-seropositive long-term nonprogressor. J Virol. 1998;72(5):3646–57.
58. Caly L, Saksena NK, Piller SC, Jans DA. Impaired nuclear import and viral incorporation of Vpr derived from a HIV long-term non-progressor. Retrovirology. 2008;5:67.
59. Lum JJ, Cohen OJ, Nie Z, Weaver JG, Gomez TS, Yao XJ, Lynch D, Pilon AA, Hawley N, Kim JE, et al. Vpr R77Q is associated with long-term

nonprogressive HIV infection and impaired induction of apoptosis. J Clin Invest. 2003;111(10):1547–54.
60. Rangel HR, Garzaro D, Rodriguez AK, Ramirez AH, Ameli G, Del Rosario Gutierrez C, Pujol FH. Deletion, insertion and stop codon mutations in vif genes of HIV-1 infecting slow progressor patients. J Infect Dev Ctries. 2009;3(7):531–8.
61. De Maio FA, Rocco CA, Aulicino PC, Bologna R, Mangano A, Sen L. Unusual substitutions in HIV-1 vif from children infected perinatally without progression to AIDS for more than 8 years without therapy. J Med Virol. 2012;84(12):1844–52.
62. Hassaine G, Agostini I, Candotti D, Bessou G, Caballero M, Agut H, Autran B, Barthalay Y, Vigne R. Characterization of human immunodeficiency virus type 1 vif gene in long-term asymptomatic individuals. Virology. 2000;276(1):169–80.
63. Reed LJ, Muench H. A simple method of estimating fifty percent endpoints. Am J Hyg. 1938;27:493–7.
64. Weber J, Vazquez AC, Winner D, Rose JD, Wylie D, Rhea AM, Henry K, Pappas J, Wright A, Mohamed N, et al. Novel method for simultaneous quantification of phenotypic resistance to maturation, protease, reverse transcriptase, and integrase HIV inhibitors based on 3'Gag(p2/p7/p1/p6)/PR/RT/INT-recombinant viruses: a useful tool in the multitarget era of antiretroviral therapy. Antimicrob Agents Chemother. 2011;55(8):3729–42.
65. Weber J, Rose JD, Vazquez AC, Winner D, Margot N, McColl DJ, Miller MD, Quinones-Mateu ME. Resistance mutations outside the integrase coding region have an effect on human immunodeficiency virus replicative fitness but do not affect its susceptibility to integrase strand transfer inhibitors. PLoS ONE. 2013;8(6):e65631.
66. Selhorst P, Vazquez AC, Terrazas-Aranda K, Michiels J, Vereecken K, Heyndrickx L, Weber J, Quinones-Mateu ME, Arien KK, Vanham G. Human immunodeficiency virus type 1 resistance or cross-resistance to nonnucleoside reverse transcriptase inhibitors currently under development as microbicides. Antimicrob Agents Chemother. 2011;55(4):1403–13.
67. Weber J, Weberova J, Carobene M, Mirza M, Martinez-Picado J, Kazanjian P, Quinones-Mateu ME. Use of a novel assay based on intact recombinant viruses expressing green (EGFP) or red (DsRed2) fluorescent proteins to examine the contribution of pol and env genes to overall HIV-1 replicative fitness. J Virol Methods. 2006;136(1–2):102–17.
68. Gall A, Ferns B, Morris C, Watson S, Cotten M, Robinson M, Berry N, Pillay D, Kellam P. Universal amplification, next-generation sequencing, and assembly of HIV-1 genomes. J Clin Microbiol. 2012;50(12):3838–44.
69. Henn MR, Boutwell CL, Charlebois P, Lennon NJ, Power KA, Macalalad AR, Berlin AM, Malboeuf CM, Ryan EM, Gnerre S, et al. Whole genome deep sequencing of HIV-1 reveals the impact of early minor variants upon immune recognition during acute infection. PLoS Pathog. 2012;8(3):e1002529.
70. Gibson RM, Meyer AM, Winner D, Archer J, Feyertag F, Ruiz-Mateos E, Leal M, Robertson DL, Schmotzer CL, Quinones-Mateu ME. Sensitive deep sequencing-based HIV-1 genotyping assay to simultaneously determine susceptibility to protease, reverse transcriptase, integrase, and maturation inhibitors, as well as HIV-1 coreceptor tropism. Antimicrob Agents Chemother. 2014;58(4):2167–85.
71. Larkin MA, Blackshields G, Brown NP, Chenna R, McGettigan PA, McWilliam H, Valentin F, Wallace IM, Wilm A, Lopez R, et al. Clustal W and Clustal X version 2.0. Bioinformatics. 2007;23(21):2947–8.
72. Tamura K, Peterson D, Peterson N, Stecher G, Nei M, Kumar S. MEGA5: molecular evolutionary genetics analysis using maximum likelihood, evolutionary distance, and maximum parsimony methods. Mol Biol Evol. 2011;28(10):2731–9.
73. Shao W, Kearney MF, Boltz VF, Spindler JE, Mellors JW, Maldarelli F, Coffin JM. PAPNC, a novel method to calculate nucleotide diversity from large scale next generation sequencing data. J Virol Methods. 2014;203:73–80.
74. Quinones-Mateu ME, Arts EJ. Fitness of drug resistant HIV-1: methodology and clinical implications. Drug Res Updates. 2002;5(6):224–33.
75. Wang C, Mitsuya Y, Gharizadeh B, Ronaghi M, Shafer RW. Characterization of mutation spectra with ultra-deep pyrosequencing: application to HIV-1 drug resistance. Genome Res. 2007;17(8):1195–201.
76. Siepel AC, Halpern AL, Macken C, Korber BTM. A computer program designed to screen rapidly for HIV type 1 intersubtype recombinant sequences. AIDS Res Hum Retrovir. 1995;11(11):1413–6.
77. Hiebenthal-Millow K, Greenough TC, Bretttler DB, Schindler M, Wildum S, Sullivan JL, Kirchhoff F. Alterations in HIV-1 LTR promoter activity during AIDS progression. Virology. 2003;317(1):109–18.
78. Rangel HR, Weber J, Chakraborty B, Gutierrez A, Marotta ML, Mirza M, Kiser P, Martinez MA, Este JA, Quinones-Mateu ME. Role of the human immunodeficiency virus type 1 envelope gene in viral fitness. J Virol. 2003;77(16):9069–73.
79. Klatzmann D, BarrÇ-Sinoussi F, Nugeyre MT, Dauguet C, Vilmer E, Griscelli C, Brun-Vezinet F, Rouzioux C, Gluckman JC, Cherman JC, et al. Selective tropism of lymphadenopathy associated virus (LAV) for helper induced T lymphocytes. Science. 1984;225:59–63.
80. Popovic M, Sarngadharan MG, Read E, Gallo RC. Detection, isolation, and continuous production of cytopathic retroviruses (HTLV-III) from patients with AIDS and pre-AIDS. Science. 1984;224:497–500.
81. Fenyo EM, Fiore J, Karlsson A, Albert J, Scarlatti G. Biological phenotypes of HIV-1 in pathogenesis and transmission. Antibiot Chemother. 1994;46:18–24.
82. Leon A, Perez I, Ruiz-Mateos E, Benito JM, Leal M, Lopez-Galindez C, Rallon N, Alcami J, Lopez-Aldeguer J, Viciana P, et al. Rate and predictors of progression in elite and viremic HIV-1 controllers. Aids. 2016;30(8):1209–20.
83. Groves KC, Bibby DF, Clark DA, Isaksen A, Deayton JR, Anderson J, Orkin C, Stagg AJ, McKnight A. Disease progression in HIV-1-infected viremic controllers. J Acquir Immune Defic Syndr. 2012;61(4):407–16.
84. Tomescu C, Liu Q, Ross BN, Yin X, Lynn K, Mounzer KC, Kostman JR, Montaner LJ. A correlate of HIV-1 control consisting of both innate and adaptive immune parameters best predicts viral load by multivariable analysis in HIV-1 infected viremic controllers and chronically-infected non-controllers. PLoS ONE. 2014;9(7):e103209.
85. Rotger M, Dalmau J, Rauch A, McLaren P, Bosinger SE, Martinez R, Sandler NG, Roque A, Liebner J, Battegay M, et al. Comparative transcriptomics of extreme phenotypes of human HIV-1 infection and SIV infection in sooty mangabey and rhesus macaque. J Clin Invest. 2011;121(6):2391–400.
86. Muenchhoff M, Adland E, Karimanzira O, Crowther C, Pace M, Csala A, Leitman E, Moonsamy A, McGregor C, Hurst J, et al. Nonprogressing HIV-infected children share fundamental immunological features of nonpathogenic SIV infection. Sci Transl Med. 2016;8(358):358ra125.
87. Chakrabarti LA. The paradox of simian immunodeficiency virus infection in sooty mangabeys: active viral replication without disease progression. Front Biosci. 2004;9:521–39.
88. Klatt NR, Silvestri G, Hirsch V. Nonpathogenic simian immunodeficiency virus infections. Cold Spring Harb Perspect Med. 2012;2(1):a007153.
89. Najera I, Holguin A, Quinones-Mateu ME, Munoz-Fernandez MA, Najera R, Lopez-Galindez C, Domingo E. Pol gene quasispecies of human immunodeficiency virus: mutations associated with drug resistance in virus from patients undergoing no drug therapy. J Virol. 1995;69(1):23–31.
90. Domingo E, Escarmis C, Menendez-Arias L, Holland J. Viral quasispecies and fitness variations. In: Domingo E, Webster R, Holland J, editors. Origin and evolution of viruses. San Diego: Academic Press; 1999. p. 141–61.
91. Peyerl FW, Bazick HS, Newberg MH, Barouch DH, Sodroski J, Letvin NL. Fitness costs limit viral escape from cytotoxic T lymphocytes at a structurally constrained epitope. J Virol. 2004;78(24):13901–10.
92. Troyer RM, McNevin J, Liu Y, Zhang SC, Krizan RW, Abraha A, Tebit DM, Zhao H, Avila S, Lobritz MA, et al. Variable fitness impact of HIV-1 escape mutations to cytotoxic T lymphocyte (CTL) response. PLoS Pathog. 2009;5(4):e1000365.
93. Malim MH, Emerman M. HIV-1 sequence variation: drift, shift, and attenuation. Cell. 2001;104(4):469–72.
94. Gibson RM, Weber J, Winner D, Miller MD, Quinones-Mateu ME. Contribution of human immunodeficiency virus type 1 minority variants to reduced drug susceptibility in patients on an integrase strand transfer inhibitor-based therapy. PLoS ONE. 2014;9(8):e104512.
95. Kitrinos KM, Nelson JA, Resch W, Swanstrom R. Effect of a protease inhibitor-induced genetic bottleneck on human immunodeficiency virus type 1 env gene populations. J Virol. 2005;79(16):10627–37.

96. Grabar S, Selinger-Leneman H, Abgrall S, Pialoux G, Weiss L, Costagliola D. Prevalence and comparative characteristics of long-term nonprogressors and HIV controller patients in the French Hospital Database on HIV. Aids. 2009;23(9):1163–9.
97. Lambotte O, Boufassa F, Madec Y, Nguyen A, Goujard C, Meyer L, Rouzioux C, Venet A, Delfraissy JF, Group S-HS. HIV controllers: a homogeneous group of HIV-1-infected patients with spontaneous control of viral replication. Clin Infect Dis. 2005;41(7):1053–6.
98. Finkel TH, Tudor-Williams G, Banda NK, Cotton MF, Curiel T, Monks C, Baba TW, Ruprecht RM, Kupfer A. Apoptosis occurs predominantly in bystander cells and not in productively infected cells of HIV- and SIV-infected lymph nodes. Nat Med. 1995;1(2):129–34.
99. Deeks SG, Barbour JD, Martin JN, Swanson MS, Grant RM. Sustained $CD4^+$ T cell response after virologic failure of protease inhibitor-based regimens in patients with human immunodeficiency virus infection. J Infect Dis. 2000;181(3):946–53.
100. Mezzaroma I, Carlesimo M, Pinter E, Muratori DS, Di Sora F, Chiarotti F, Cunsolo MG, Sacco G, Aiuti F. Clinical and immunologic response without decrease in virus load in patients with AIDS after 24 months of highly active antiretroviral therapy. Clin Infect Dis. 1999;29(6):1423–30.

17

Hospitalization causes and outcomes in HIV patients in the late antiretroviral era in Colombia

María Fernanda Álvarez Barreneche[1*], Carlos Andrés Restrepo Castro[1,2], Alicia Hidrón Botero[1,3,4], Juan Pablo Villa Franco[1], Ivan Mauricio Trompa Romero[2], Laura Restrepo Carvajal[1], Alejandro Eusse García[1], Adriana Ocampo Mesa[5], Lina María Echeverri Toro[5,6], Glenys Patricia Porras Fernández de Castro[7], Jaime Mauricio Ramírez Rivera[5,6] and Carlos Andrés Agudelo Restrepo[1,5,8]

Abstract

Background: Antiretroviral therapy (ART) has modified the natural history of HIV-infection: the incidence of opportunistic infections (OIs) has decreased and mortality associated to HIV has improved dramatically. The reasons for hospitalization have changed; OIs are no longer the most common reason for admission. This study describes the patient population, admission diagnosis and hospital course of HIV patients in Colombia in the ART era.

Methods: Patients admitted with HIV/AIDS at six hospitals in Medellin, Colombia between August 1, 2014 and July 31, 2015 were included. Demographic, laboratory, and clinical data were prospectively collected.

Results: 551 HIV-infected patients were admitted: 76.0% were male, the median age was 37 (30–49). A new diagnosis of HIV was made in 22.0% of patients during the index admission. 56.0% of patients of the entire cohort had been diagnosed with HIV for more than 1 year and 68.9% were diagnosed in an advanced stage of the disease. More than 50.0% of patients had CD4 counts less than 200 CD4 cells/μL and viral loads greater than 100,000 copies. The main reasons for hospital admissions were OIs, tuberculosis, esophageal candidiasis and Toxoplasma encephalitis. The median hospital stay was 14 days (IQR 8–23). Admission to the intensive care unit (ICU) was required in 10.3% of patients and 14.3% were readmitted to the hospital; mortality was 5.4%.

Conclusions: Similar to other countries in the developing world, in Colombia, the leading cause of hospitalization among HIV-infected patients remain opportunistic infections. However, in-hospital mortality was low, similar to those described for high-income countries. Strategies to monitor and optimize the adherence and retention in HIV programs are fundamental to maximize the benefit of ART.

Keywords: Acquired immune deficiency syndrome, Human immunodeficiency virus, Hospitalization, Opportunistic infections, Antiretroviral, Adherence

Background

Life expectancy for patients infected with the human immunodeficiency virus (HIV) has improved significantly in the era of antiretroviral therapy (ART), largely due to the reduction in mortality attributable to diseases related to acquired immunodeficiency syndrome (AIDS) [1]. A recent systematic review and meta-analysis has summarized data on causes of hospital admission among children and adults living with HIV globally: AIDS-related illnesses (including tuberculosis [TB]) and bacterial infections were the second most common cause of adult HIV admissions in all geographical regions and the most common cause of hospital mortality [2]. Studies in high-income countries have shown changes in the main causes of hospitalization and death of HIV patients:

*Correspondence: mariafda_12@hotmail.com
[1] School of Health Sciences, Universidad Pontificia Bolivariana, Carrera 44 # 18-56, Antioquia, Medellín, Colombia

opportunistic diseases have given way to chronic diseases and neoplasms not associated with AIDS [2–5]. On the other hand, in developing countries, high mortality rates persist despite availability of antiretrovirals; AIDS defining events continue to be reported as the main cause of hospitalization and death [6–10].

Although the change in the epidemiological profile of hospitalized patients with HIV has been widely documented in high-income and in developing countries, little is known about the reasons for hospital admission and hospital outcomes in the current era of the HIV epidemic in Colombia [11, 12]. This study describes the clinical characteristics, causes of hospital admission and mortality rates of patients with HIV infection from six high complexity care hospitals in Medellin, Colombia.

Methods

Study design and patient collection

Patients diagnosed with HIV, older than 18 years of age and hospitalized for more than 24 h in any of six reference hospitals in Medellin, Colombia, between August 1, 2014 and July 31, 2015, were included. Patients who were unconscious, pregnant women (who are usually treated in high risk obstetric units in Colombia, not in the infectious disease ward) and patients who did not agree to participate were excluded. The information was prospectively collected using Magpi® software (formerly DataDyne, Washington, WA), and included socio-demographic variables, baseline characteristics at admission, reason for hospital admission and clinical outcomes. Patients that could not be interviewed were excluded from the analysis, but the reason for admission was recorded. The definitions of the variables were based on previous studies and those established by National Institutes of Health [13]. Adherence measurement was given by self-report of the patient: the patient taking more than 95% of total doses in the last month was defined as adherent according with Simoni et al. [14]. Hospital readmission was defined as a new (different) hospitalization for the same cause during the year of the study. Laboratory data and clinical outcomes were extracted from the patient´s medical chart.

Ethics statement

The study was approved by the ethics committee of each of the participating hospitals. All study participants provided a written informed consent for collecting information; the patient´s identity was protected, individual records were coded and accessed only by research staff. None of the enrolled participants were below 18 years of age. A post hoc authorization was given to review the clinical records of all HIV patients hospitalized at participating hospitals during the study period in order to identify patients lost due to care in services other than infectious diseases.

Statistical analysis

Data were exported to SPSS® version 17 (IBM, Armonk, NY) to perform analyses using frequency distribution measures for qualitative variables and measures of central tendency, dispersion and position for quantitative variables. Manual review of medical records was performed to resolve discrepancies found in the database.

Results

901 HIV-positive patients were hospitalized during the year of the study in participating institutions, representing 0.79% of 114.505 admissions. Of those, 551 patients were included. One hundred twenty-six (14%) patients were excluded and 224 (24.9%) patients were missed, mainly because they were cared for by services other than infectious diseases (Fig. 1).

The median age was 37 years (IQR 30–49). Patients mostly belonged to a low socioeconomic class (n = 372, 67.5%) with a basic education level (only elementary and/or high school) in 70.8% (390 patients). HIV diagnosis was made in advanced stage disease (< 200 CD4 cells/μL and/or AIDS defining entities) in 68.9% (380) of the patients. More than 50.0% of patients had CD4 counts less than 200 CD4 cells/μL and viral loads greater than 100,000 copies at admission. Diagnosis of HIV was made during the index admission in 22% (121) of patients and their median CD4 count was 59 cells/μL (interquartile range [IQR] 27–149.5). Of the 430 patients with a previous HIV diagnosis, 42% (181 patients) had already had an opportunistic infection, with tuberculosis being the most common one. In this group, ART had been prescribed to 85.1% (366/430), but only 63.4% (273/430) were receiving it on admission, and only 199 patients (54.1%) reported being adherent to ART. The main reasons for non-adherence were drug dependence, social or occupational instability, psychiatric disorders and lack of family support. Multiple antiretroviral regimens have been received by 48% (175/366) of patients; the average number of previous regimens was 1.5 (SD ± 0.82).

Baseline characteristics were similar for all patients compared to the subsets of patients with a previous HIV diagnosis and a prior AIDS-defining illness, except the median CD4 count was lower and the proportion of patients without antiretroviral therapy was greater in the AIDS-defining illness group (Table 1).

The main reason for hospitalization was an AIDS-defining illness in 54.6% (301/551) of patients, and tuberculosis was the most frequent OI in this group (42.5%, 128/301). The second most frequent reason for admission were non HIV-related affections with bacterial

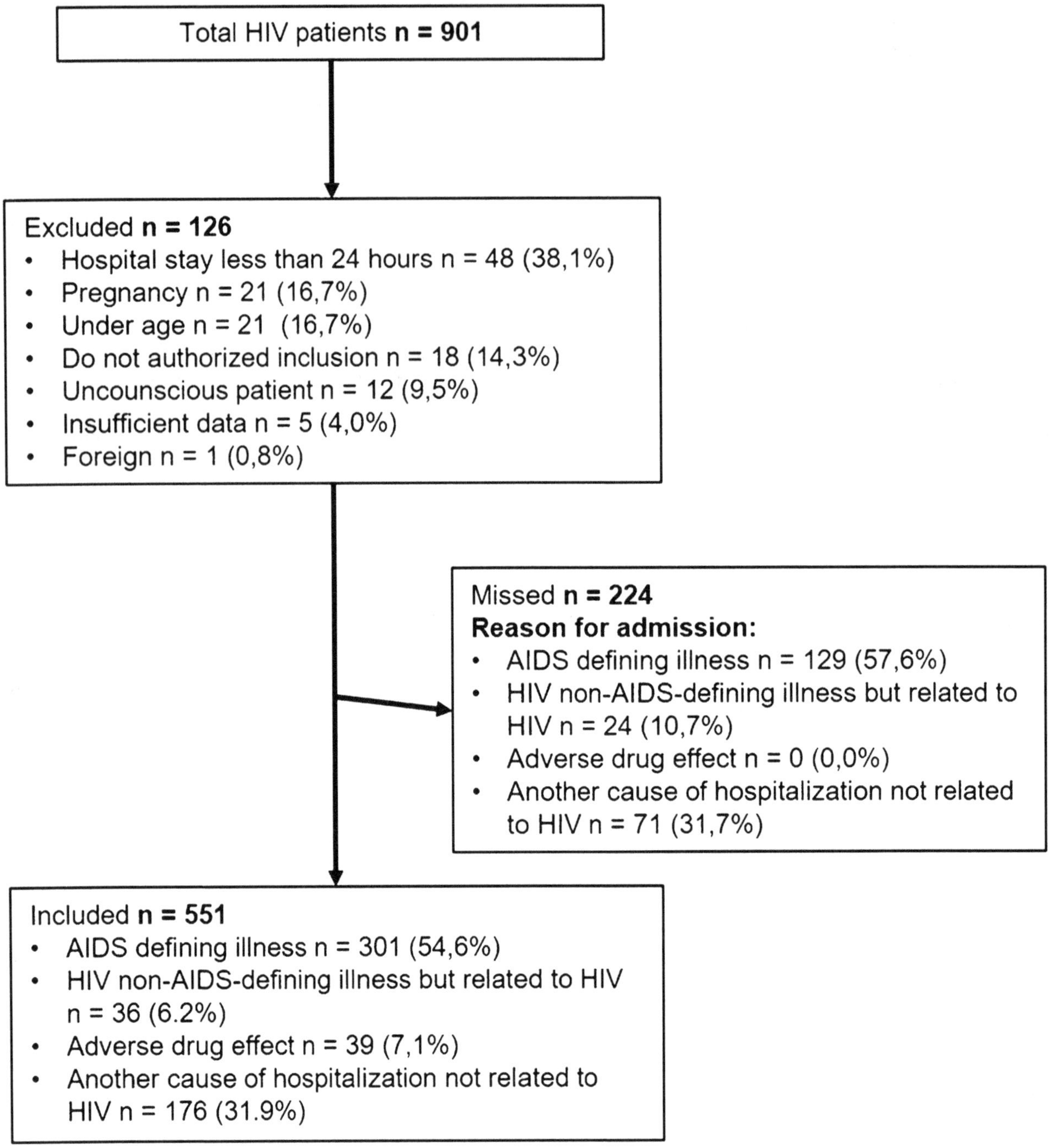

Fig. 1 HIV patients hospitalized in Medellín, Colombia from August 2014 to July 2015

infections predominating (11.0%, 62 of 551 hospitalizations) (Table 2).

Admission to the ICU was required in 57 patients (10.3%); of these, 33.3% (19) had tuberculosis. Median hospital stay was 14 days (IQR 8–23) and 14.3% (79) of patients required re-admission to the hospital. Adverse events to medications received during the hospital stay were reported for 9.6% (n = 57) of the patients. Nosocomial infections were reported for 27 patients (4.9%).

Global mortality was 5.4% (30/551 patients). Of the patients who died, 70% (n = 21) had a previous diagnosis of HIV, 52.4% (n = 11) were receiving ART, and 38.1% (n = 8) were being followed-up in an HIV program. 96.6% (n = 28) of the patients that died had less than 50

Table 1 Baseline characteristics for 551 patients with HIV infection admitted to medical ward

Patient characteristics	All patients, n = 551 (100%)	Previous HIV diagnosis, n = 430 (78%)	AIDS-defining illness, n = 301 (54.6%)
Age, median (IQR)	37 (30–49)	36 (30–48)	37 (30–50)
Male	418 (76)	321 (74.6)	231 (76.7)
Low income	372 (67.5)	289 (67.2)	225 (74.7)
Lower educational attainment	390 (70.8)	188 (43.7)	154 (51.1)
New HIV diagnosis	121 (22)	–	88 (29.2)
ART status			
Receiving ART prior to admission	273 (49.5)	273 (63.4)	131 (43.5)
Not on ART	278 (50.4)	64 (14.9)	111 (36.8)
Abandonment of ART	–	93 (21.6)	59 (19.6)
Adherence to ART[a]	–	199/366 (54.4)	83/190 (43.6)
Attending HIV program	–	258 (60.0)	86 (28.5)
Attending HIV program and receiving ART	–	226/258 (87.6)	72(23.9)
CD4 cell count, cells/µl Median (IQR)	98 (36.2–98)	117 (41–310)	59 (24–131)
HIV viral load, copies/mL Median (IQR)	100.278 (1.505–384.250)	36.381 (77–216.441)	179.000 (26.597–622.022)
Anemia[b]	104 (18.9)	90 (20.9)	76 (25.2)
Past history of TB	88 (20.4)	88 (20.4)	55 (18.2)

[a] Adherence to ART is calculated with patients who had abandoned ART or were receiving ART prior to admission

[b] Anemia was defined using WHO criteria (hemoglobin < 11.0 g/dL for both males and females)

CD4 cells/µL, 80% (n = 24) had been admitted for an AIDS-defining illness, and 36.6% (11 patients) had two or more OIs (Table 3).

Discussion

This study describes the clinical characteristics, main causes of hospitalization and mortality rates in adult patients with HIV in a developing country. Contrary to what has been reported in high-income countries where cardiovascular, hepatic or neoplastic etiologies not associated with AIDS are the main causes of hospitalization [15–18], we found OIs to be the main reason for admission and mortality. Of the 30 patients who died, 80% (24 patients) died due to the opportunistic infection that caused the admission.

In low and middle-income countries the majority of admissions are still due to AIDS-defining events; a significant proportion of patients get diagnosed with HIV during this index admission or die with a recent diagnosis [6, 19]. Differences in opportunities to have access to programs, provision of medication and a timely diagnosis have been shown to influence the outcome of patients [20]. In our study 78% of hospitalized patients had a known diagnosis of HIV, 60% were getting follow-up in an HIV program and close to 60% were on ART. However, 57% (155) of patients on ART did not have adequate immunovirologic control. Our findings parallel national surveillance data in reference to HIV epidemiology [21]. In 2016, of 73,465 HIV-patients, 91.5% had access to ART, and, nonetheless, only 57.5% had accomplished virologic suppression [21]. The reasons for this gap between access to care and immunovirologic control were not directly assessed by our study. Most of our patients had socio-economic conditions that could favor non-adherence to ART [22, 23]. Our findings, in alignment with national data, suggest public health measures focusing on strategies to improve adherence and retention in HIV programs to maximize the benefit of antiretroviral treatment.

Studies from other developing countries report high mortality rates in patients hospitalized with HIV compared to those of industrialized countries (up to 38% vs. 2.6%). Mortality is associated to advanced disease stages, severity of immunologic compromise (low CD4 count), presence of opportunistic infections, and lack of resources for care [6, 15]. Although Colombia is considered a low-middle income country, we found comparable hospital mortality rates (5%) to those of industrialized countries [15, 16, 18] despite opportunistic infections as the primary reason for admission and advanced disease stage. This discrepancy between high frequency of opportunistic infections and low mortality is unexpected and could possibly reflect gaps in the overall quality of acute versus long-term, ambulatory care. Whether the

Table 2 Causes of hospitalization in HIV patients in Medellín, Colombia from August 2014 to July 2015 (N = 551)

Variable	n (%)
AIDS defining illness[a]	301 (54.6)
Tuberculosis	128 (23.3)
Extrapulmonary tuberculosis	84 (15.2)
Pulmonary tuberculosis	44 (8.0)
Esophageal candidiasis	56 (10.1)
Toxoplasma encephalitis	43 (7.8)
Disseminated histoplasmosis	39 (7.1)
CMV infection	36 (6.5)
Extrapulmonary cryptococcosis	32 (5.8)
Pneumonia by *P. jiroveci*	32 (5.8)
Lymphoma[b]	27 (4.9)
Kaposi's sarcoma	11 (2.0)
Herpes simplex > 1 month	10 (1.8)
Cryptosporidiosis > 1 month	10 (1.8)
HIV Encephalopathy	8 (1.4)
Wasting syndrome	7 (1.3)
MAC	4 (0.7)
Recurrent salmonellosis	2 (0.3)
Adverse drug effect	39 (7.1)
Non-AIDS-defining illness but related to HIV	35 (6.2)
Another cause of hospitalization not related to HIV	176 (31.9)
Bacterial infection	61 (11.0)
Others[c]	115 (20.9)

[a] The total percentage exceeds 100% because *some patients had > 1 defining illness*

[b] Burkitt lymphoma, *primary central nervous system lymphoma, immunoblastic lymphoma*

[c] Other: gastrointestinal, neurological, hematological and cardiac alterations, viral infection, pneumopathy, reactive lymphadenopathy

Table 3 Main findings of HIV patients in Medellín, Colombia from August 2014 to July 2015

Variable	Patients who died (n = 30) n (%)	Patients who survived (n = 521) n (%)
Age	41.5	39.3
Male	25/30 (83.3)	393/521 (75.4)
Diagnosis during the index admission	9/30 (30.0)	112/521 (21.5)
Previous HIV diagnosis[a]	21/30 (70.0)	409/521 (78.5)
Diagnosis 1–12 months	6/30 (20.0)	117/521 (22.5)
Diagnosis > 12 months	15/30 (50.0)	292/521 (56.0)
On antiretroviral therapy at admission[b]	11/21 (52.4)	262/409 (64.2)
Adherence[c]	5/18 (27.7)	194/354 (54.8)
CD4 T-cells count < 200 cells/mL[d]	28/29 (96.6)	352/521 (67.4)
AIDS-defining illness on admission	24/30 (80.0)	277/521 (53.2)
Patients with newly diagnosed TB	7/30 (23.3)	121/521 (23.2)
AIDS defining illness no TB	17/30 (56.6)	156/521 (29.9)
Two or more OIs	11/30 (36.6)	96/521 (18.4)
Non-AIDS-defining illness but related to HIV	2/30 (6.6)	33/521 (6.3)

[a] ≥ 1 month previous to hospitalization

[b] In patients diagnosed with HIV before admission

[c] In patients who had abandoned ART or were receiving ART prior to admission

[d] One patient had no CD4 T-cells count

low mortality rate observed is due to the quality of care provided in high-complexity hospitals with highly trained staff and medical resources to care for these patients, remains to be proved. However, previous studies suggest that increased physician experience in caring for patients with AIDS improves survival [24–26].

Strengths of the study include that it is a large, multicenter study with prospective design. Patients that were not included were analyzed retrospectively, finding similar causes of admission to those reported for the entire cohort (Fig. 1). Among the weaknesses, researchers did not have access to outpatient medical records, so information about HIV history was obtained from patient interviews, which could be associated with memory bias. Because of the prospective nature of the study and the requirement for informed consent, patients with CNS involvement who were unable to consent and who lacked a family member capable to do so were excluded. We recognize that this behavior might have generated some selection bias in the study. Additionally, patients were cared for in reference hospitals in Medellín, institutions with highly specialized staff and advanced technological resources. This is not the case for many health institutions in Colombia nor perhaps for health institutions in other developing countries. Our data may not be generalized to smaller cities in developing countries with differ to what happens in other Colombian cities lower complexity care hospitals.

Conclusion

Opportunistic infections continue to be de the leading cause of hospitalization in adult HIV patients in Colombia. The gap between access to care and treatment and treatment goal achievement reflect possible programmatic limitations. Despite this, mortality rates observed were low, similar to those described for high-income countries. Our findings suggest focusing on measures to improve retention in care, ensure adherence and improve the opportunity for diagnosis, could have a long-term positive impact on the incidence of opportunistic infections and hospital admissions.

Abbreviations
AIDS: acquired immunodeficiency syndrome; ART: antiretroviral therapy; HIV: human immunodeficiency virus; ICU: intensive care unit; MAC: Mycobacterium avium complex; OI: opportunistic infections.

Authors' contributions
MFA, CAR and CAA proposed the idea; MFA, CAA, CAR, AIH, JPV and IMT together designed the study. All authors contributed in data collection, analysis and manuscript preparation. MFA, CAR, AIH, CAA drafted the manuscript. All authors read and approved the final manuscript.

Author details
[1] School of Health Sciences, Universidad Pontificia Bolivariana, Carrera 44 # 18-56, Antioquia, Medellín, Colombia. [2] Division of Infectious Diseases, Department of Internal Medicine, IPS Universitaria Clínica León XIII, Antioquia, Medellín, Colombia. [3] Division of Infectious Diseases, Department of Internal Medicine, Hospital Pablo Tobón Uribe, Antioquia, Medellín, Colombia. [4] Division of Infectious Diseases, Department of Internal Medicine, Emory University School of Medicine, Atlanta, GA, USA. [5] Division of Infectious Diseases, Department of Internal Medicine, Centros Especializados San Vicente Fundación, Antioquia, Rionegro, Colombia. [6] Division of Infectious Diseases, Department of Internal Medicine, Hospital Universitario, San Vicente Fundación, Antioquia, Medellín, Colombia. [7] Department of Internal Medicine, Hospital General de Medellín, Antioquia, Medellín, Colombia. [8] Division of Infectious Diseases, Department of Internal Medicine, Clínica Universitaria Bolivariana, Antioquia, Medellín, Colombia.

Acknowledgements
We thank Clínica Bolivariana, IPS Universitaria Clínica León XXIII, Hospital Pablo Tobón Uribe, Hospital San Vicente Fundación, Hospital General de Medellín, for allowing us to carry out the study in each of the institutions.

Competing interests
The authors declare that they have no competing interests.

References
1. Mocroft A, Ledergerber B, Katlama C, Kirk O, Reiss P, d'Arminio Monforte A, et al. Decline in the AIDS and death rates in the EuroSIDA study: an observational study. Lancet. 2003. https://doi.org/10.1016/S0140-6736(03)13802-0.
2. Ford N, Shubber Z, Meintjes G, Grinsztejn B, Eholie S, Mills EJ, et al. Causes of hospital admission among people living with HIV worldwide: a systematic review and meta-analysis. Lancet HIV. 2015. https://doi.org/10.1016/S2352-3018(15)00137-X.
3. May M, Gompels M, Delpech V, Porter K, Post F, Johnson M, et al. Impact of late diagnosis and treatment on life expectancy in people with HIV-1: UK Collaborative HIV Cohort (UK CHIC) Study. BMJ. 2011. https://doi.org/10.1136/bmj.d6016.
4. Ingle SM, May MT, Gill MJ, Mugavero MJ, Lewden C, Abgrall S, et al. Impact of risk factors for specific causes of death in the first and subsequent years of antiretroviral therapy among HIV-infected patients. Clin Infect Dis. 2014. https://doi.org/10.1093/cid/ciu261.
5. Grinsztejn B, Luz PM, Pacheco AG, Santos DVG, Velasque L, Moreira RI, et al. Changing mortality profile among HIV-infected patients in Rio de Janeiro, Brazil: shifting from AIDS to non-AIDS related conditions in the HAART era. PLoS ONE. 2013. https://doi.org/10.1371/journal.pone.0059768.
6. Lewden C, Drabo YJ, Zannou DM, Maiga MY, Minta DK, Sow PS, et al. Disease patterns and causes of death of hospitalized HIV-positive adults in West Africa: a multicountry survey in the antiretroviral treatment era. J Int AIDS Soc. 2014. https://doi.org/10.7448/IAS.17.1.18797.
7. Martín-Onraet A, Piñeirua-Menéndez A, Perales-Martínez D, Ortega-Pérez R, Barrera-García A, Sierra-Madero J, et al. Mortalidad hospitalaria en pacientes con infección por VIH: a diez años del acceso universal a TARAA en México. Salud Pública México. 2015;57(Suppl):163–70.
8. Sharma S, Kadhiravan T, Banga A, Goyal T, Bhatia I, Saha P. Spectrum of clinical disease in a series of 135 hospitalized HIV-infected patients from North India. BMC Infect Dis. 2004.
9. Sharifi-Mood B, Alavi-Naini R, Salehi M, Hashemi M, Rakhshani F. Spectrum of clinical disease in a series of hospitalized HIV-infected patients from southeast of Iran. Saudi Med J. 2006;27:1362–6.
10. Meintjes G, Kerkhoff AD, Burton R, Schutz C, Boulle A, Van Wyk G, et al. HIV-related medical admissions to a South African district hospital remain frequent despite effective antiretroviral therapy scale-up. Medicine (Baltimore). 2015. https://doi.org/10.1097/MD.0000000000002269.
11. Montúfar Andrade F, Quiroga A, Builes C, Saldarriaga C, Aguilar C, Mesa M, et al. Epidemiology of human immunodeficiency virus infection in inpatients in a teaching hospital of high complexity in Medellin. Colomb Infect. 2016. https://doi.org/10.4067/S0716-10182014000600015.
12. Agudelo-Gonzalez S, Murcia-Sanchez F, Salinas D, Osorio J. Infecciones oportunistas en pacientes con VIH en el hospital universitario de Neiva, Colombia 2007–2012. Infect. 2015;19(2):52–9. https://doi.org/10.1016/j.infect.2014.11.008.
13. Guidelines for prevention and treatment of opportunistic infections in HIV-infected adults and adolescents. https://aidsinfo.nih.gov/contentfiles/lvguidelines/adult_oi.pdf. Accessed 1 Jan 2017.
14. Simoni JM, Kurth AE, Pearson CR, Pantalone DW, Merrill JO, Frick PA. Self-report measures of antiretroviral therapy adherence: a review with recommendations for HIV research and clinical management. AIDS Behav. 2006. https://doi.org/10.1007/s10461-006-9078-6.
15. Kim JH, Psevdos G, Gonzalez E, Singh S, Kilayko MC, Sharp V. All-cause mortality in hospitalized HIV-infected patients at an acute tertiary care hospital with a comprehensive outpatient HIV care program in New York City in the era of highly active antiretroviral therapy (HAART). Infection. 2013. https://doi.org/10.1007/s15010-012-0386-7.
16. Weber R, Ruppik M, Rickenbach M, Spoerri A, Furrer H, Battegay M, et al. Decreasing mortality and changing patterns of causes of death in the Swiss HIV Cohort Study. HIV Med. 2013. https://doi.org/10.1111/j.1468-1293.2012.01051.x.
17. Corbett EL, Churchyard GJ, Charalambos S, Samb B, Moloi V, Clayton TC, et al. Morbidity and mortality in South African gold miners: impact of untreated disease due to human immunodeficiency virus. Clin Infect Dis. 2002. https://doi.org/10.1086/339540.
18. Reekie J, Kowalska JD, Karpov I, Rockstroh J, Karlsson A, Rakhmanova A, et al. Regional differences in AIDS and non-AIDS related mortality in HIV-positive individuals across Europe and Argentina: the EuroSIDA Study. PLoS ONE. 2012. https://doi.org/10.1371/journal.pone.0041673.
19. Fisher M. Late diagnosis of HIV infection: major consequences and missed opportunities. Curr Opin Infect Dis. 2008. https://doi.org/10.1097/QCO.0b013e3282f2d8fb.
20. Cesar C, Koethe JR, Giganti MJ, Rebeiro P, Althoff KN, Napravnik S, et al. Health outcomes among HIV-positive Latinos initiating antiretroviral therapy in North America versus Central and South America. J Int AIDS Soc. 2016. https://doi.org/10.7448/IAS.19.1.20684.
21. VIH Cuenta de alto Costo Colombia http://cuentadealtocosto.org/site/index.php/patologias/9-patologias/34-vih1/?template=cuentadealtocostocontenido. Accessed 22 Oct 2017.
22. Negash T, Ehlers V. Personal factors influencing patients' adherence to ART in Addis Ababa. Ethiopia. J Assoc Nurses AIDS Care. 2013;24(6):530–8. https://doi.org/10.1016/j.jana.2012.11.004.
23. Hudelson C, Cluver L. Factors associated with adherence to antiretroviral therapy among adolescents living with HIV/AIDS in low- and middle-income countries: a systematic review. AIDS Care. 2015;27(7):805–16. https://doi.org/10.1080/09540121.2015.1011073.
24. Cunningham WE, Tisnado DM, Lui HH, Nakazono TT, Carlisle DM. The effect of hospital experience on mortality among patients hospitalized with acquired immunodeficiency syndrome in California. Am J Med. 1999. https://doi.org/10.1016/S0002-9343(99)00195-3.
25. Kitahata MM, Van Rompaey SE, Dillingham PW, Koepsell TD, Deyo RA, Dodge W, et al. Primary care delivery is associated with greater physician experience and improved survival among persons with AIDS. J Gen Intern Med. 2003. https://doi.org/10.1046/j.1525-1497.2003.11049.x19.
26. Kitahata MM, Koepsell TD, Deyo RA, Maxwell CL, Dodge WT, Wagner EH. Physicians' experience with the acquired immunodeficiency syndrome as a factor in patients' survival. N Engl J Med. 1996. https://doi.org/10.1056/NEJM199603143341106.

18

Risky sexual behavior among patients on long-term antiretroviral therapy

Stephen Okoboi[1,2,3*], Barbara Castelnuovo[1], David M. Moore[4,5], Joseph Musaazi[1], Andrew Kambugu[1], Josephine Birungi[6], Pontiano Kaleebu[7], Mastula Nanfuka[6], Moses R. Kamya[8] and Annelies Van Rie[2,3]

Abstract

Background: While the effects of initiation of antiretroviral treatment (ART) on risky sexual behavior have been extensively studied, less is known about the long-term changes in risky sexual behavior over time in resource-poor settings.

Methods: We conducted a secondary longitudinal analysis of one rural and one urban cohort of patients who initiated ART in Uganda between April 2004 and July 2007 followed up-to 2016. Data on sexual behavior were collected every 6 months for 3.5 years in individuals on ART $\geq$ 4 years (baseline) when a behavioral questionnaire was introduced. Risky sexual behavior was defined as sexual intercourse with $\geq$ 2 partners or inconsistent or no condom use in previous 6 months. We report characteristics overall, and by cohort. We used multivariable generalized estimating equations logistic regression to assess the effects of time on ART on risky sexual behavior.

Results: Of 1012 participants, 402 (39.8%) were urban and 610 (60.2%) were rural residents. Mean age was 42.8 years (SD 8.5). Mean duration of follow-up was 51.3 months (SD 15.3), but longer for urban than rural participants (64.5 vs 36.4 months). Risky sexual behavior declined from 33.1% at baseline to 9.6% after 3.5 years of follow-up in the rural cohort ($p \leq 0.01$ for the test of trend) and was unchanged from 9.7% at baseline to 9.9% after 3.5 years in the urban cohort ($p = 0.51$). Receiving care at a rural clinic (aOR 4.99, 95% CI 3.64–6.84); male gender (aOR 1.66, 95% CI 1.26–2.19) and being younger (aOR 5.60, 95% CI 3.80–8.25 for 18–34 years and aOR 2.34, 95% CI 1.74–3.14 for 35–44 years) were associated with increased odds of risky sexual behavior. Not being married (aOR 0.25; 95% CI 0.19–0.34), and longer time on ART (aOR 0.71 95% CI 0.67–0.76) were associated with reduced odds of risky sex.

Conclusions: We observed a decline in risky sexual behavior in rural people on long-term ($\geq$ 4 years) ART. Rural, male and young individuals had higher odds of self-reported risky sexual behavior. ART programs should continue to emphasize risk reduction practices, especially among people receiving care in rural health facilities, males, younger individuals and those who are married.

Keywords: HIV, Antiretroviral therapy, Sexual behavior, Longitudinal cohorts, Uganda

*Correspondence: okoboi25@gmail.com; okobois@idi.co.ug; sokoboi@idi.co.ug
[1] Infectious Diseases Institute, College of Health Sciences, Makerere University, P.O BOX 22418, Kampala, Uganda

Background

Antiretroviral therapy (ART) transforms HIV infection from a fatal disease to a chronic, manageable condition, increases the quality of life of people living with HIV, greatly improves survival, and reduces the risk of transmission of HIV to a sexual partner [1–3]. Beginning in 2004, ART use in sub-Saharan Africa was dramatically expanded using a public health approach, which led to a rapid expansion of access to treatment in resource-limited settings [1, 2, 4]. In 2017, an estimated 21.7 million people globally were on ART [1]. In Uganda, the number of people on ART is about 750,000 in 2014 [5]. The number of people on ART is likely to further increase following the "recent 'Treat All' recommendations by the World Health Organization (WHO) [2, 3]. The educational campaigns around reduced HIV transmission risk with suppressed viral load (Undetectable = Untransmittable UNAIDS message) and reduced HIV related morbidity and mortality may change the sexual behaviour of persons receiving ART [6] as well as HIV negative individuals. Whilst the public discussion of ART prevention benefits has intensified in the framework of the WHO 'Treat All' strategy, one of the issues voiced is that this might result in increased sexual risk-taking [6–10].

Prior studies have evaluated the association between ART and risky sexual behavior in the first one to 3 years following ART initiation. Prospective cohort studies in South Africa and Uganda found a decrease in risky sexual behavior. In Uganda, risky sexual behavior in men decreased from 16.2% before ART to 4.3% at 12 months after ART initiation [11]. In South Africa, risky sexual behavior decreased 12 months after ART initiation compared to pre-ART (aOR 0.86, 95% CI 0.78–0.95) [12]. In a randomized clinical trial of three different ART monitoring strategies in rural Uganda, risky sexual activity decreased from 22% at ART initiation to 14% at 36 months of ART follow up [13, 14]. In contrast, cross-sectional studies from Togo, Uganda and Cote d'Ivoire found higher rates of participants practicing risky sexual behavior after short durations on ART [15–19]. These conflicting results highlight the complexity of examining the association of ART and risky sexual behavior and its variations in different settings, study participants and treatment program characteristics. Two meta-analyses summarized the association between ART and sexual risk behavior. A meta-analysis of 8 longitudinal studies and 6 cross-sectional studies of the sexual behavior of patients on ART in Sub Saharan Africa (SSA) found a reduction in risky sexual behavior as compared to pre-ART (pooled effect estimate OR 0.47, 95% CI 0.25–0.89 for multiple sexual partners). Furthermore, people on ART were 55% more likely to have protected sex with a partner who was HIV negative or of unknown HIV status as compared to an HIV infected partner [20]. Another meta-analysis of 55 prospective and cross-sectional studies in SSA also found lower sexual risk-taking (OR 0.7; 95% CI 0.62–0.81) among participants on ART compared with those not on ART [21].

To date, most studies examined the effect of ART on sexual risk behavior in the first year(s) of ART; and mainly compared risky sexual behavior before and after ART initiation. Data on the risky sexual behavior among adults on long-term ($\geq$4 years) ART in sub-Saharan Africa is limited. Using data from two clinical cohorts, we evaluated long-term changes in risky sexual behavior among people receiving ART in urban and rural Uganda.

Methods

Study design

This was a secondary analysis of two longitudinal cohorts of individuals on long-term ART: the ART cohort of The Infectious Diseases Institute (IDI), College of Health Sciences at Makerere University in Kampala, Uganda [22] and the ART cohort of The AIDS Support Organization, (TASO) in Jinja, Uganda [23]. The two cohorts had a 2-year difference in ART initiation timelines and this limited direct comparison.

Study setting

The IDI urban ART cohort in Kampala

The adult clinic of the Infectious Diseases Institute (IDI) is a Centre of excellence for HIV care and treatment located in the Mulago Teaching Hospital in Kampala-Uganda. IDI is a large outpatient clinic with over 30,000 patients ever enrolled and cares for people living in five Kampala municipalities. ART is provided free of charge, initially through the Global Fund and later mainly through the US President's Emergency Plan for AIDS Relief (PEPFAR).

Following written informed consent, adults (age $\geq$ 18 years) starting ART between April 2004 and April 2005 were enrolled and followed up (hereafter referred to as the IDI urban cohort). ART was started in patients with WHO Stage 4 or CD4 count $\leq$ 200 cells/ml, (according to national treatment guidelines implemented at that time), and consisted of stavudine (weight-adjusted and its use discontinued in 2013 in Uganda), lamivudine and nevirapine (fixed-dose combination) or zidovudine, lamivudine (fixed-dose combination) and efavirenz. A study doctor and adherence counsellor evaluated patients at study enrolment and every 6 months thereafter, while they attended the general clinic for monthly ART medication refills [22]. At each study visit, a physical examination was performed and information was recorded about HIV status of the partner(s), social support, and sexual history in the past month including promotion of condom use, adherence using visual analogue scale, and reasons for non-adherence. ART was monitored every 6 months through viral load (VL) testing. Participants with a VL $\geq$ 1000 copies/ml were offered enhanced adherence counselling and support including a face-to-face session to discuss the implications of unsuppressed viral load (VL). Adherence strategies used by the patient were reviewed, and an adherence action plan developed. Patients with two consecutive viral loads $\geq$ 1000 copies/ml were considered eligible for a second-line ART regimen.

The TASO rural ART cohort in Jinja

The AIDS Support Organization is one of the first and largest non-governmental organizations in SSA, providing treatment to over 98,000 patients in Uganda. Since 2004, TASO Jinja, one of 11 TASO care facilities in Uganda, has cared for people living with HIV in the Jinja district within a radius of 75 km and currently provides ART to over 5000 people.

In June 2012, TASO Jinja initiated a prospective longitudinal cohort (Long-term Outcome on ART study) among patients who initiated ART between 2004 and 2007 using the WHO Stage 4 or CD4 count $\leq$ 200 cells/ml, (according to national treatment guidelines implemented at that time), and consisted of stavudine (weight-adjusted and its use discontinued in 2013 in Uganda). The Long-Term Outcomes on ART study recruited patients receiving first-line ART for a minimum of 4 years (hereafter referred to as the TASO rural cohort) [23, 24]. Between July 1, 2012, and December 31, 2013, all individuals receiving first-line ART for at least 4 years were eligible to participate in the cohort study and were included after written informed consent. Participants continued to receive adherence counselling and condom use from TASO counsellors and peer educators mostly in groups as part of routine care. From August 2014 until January 2015, enrollment was restricted to patients already on ART for at least 4 years with CD4 cell count $\leq$ 450 cells/mm^3 in order to over-sample for participants who may have virologic failure. All participants continued to receive routine comprehensive HIV care from the TASO service providers. Routine VL testing was not available at TASO Jinja at the time of the study but all participants received a VL test at enrollment. Participants with a VL $\geq$ 1000 copies/ml were offered enhanced adherence counselling and support including a face-to-face session to discuss the implications of unsuppressed VL, assessment of the adherence strategies used by the patient, and development of an adherence action plan. VL was re-assessed after 3 months.

Patients were followed up for additional 3.5 years. Every 6 months, cohort participants completed an interviewer-administered standardized questionnaire (adapted from the HAARP study) [24] to collect behavioral and treatment outcomes. Laboratory monitoring included CD4 counts and VL every 6 months. CD4 counts were performed at the Jinja referral hospital regional laboratory. Plasma samples were stored in liquid nitrogen and shipped to the MRC/UVRI laboratory in Entebbe, Uganda for VL testing and resistance testing.

Data collection and management

The IDI urban cohort data were directly collected into an electronic behavioral medical record by study counsellors who provided risk reduction counselling including condom use promotion and periodically validated by a senior data manager. The TASO rural cohort, data were collected by the research assistants (counsellors) using an interview administered behavioral questionnaire but they did not provide counselling on condom use promotion. Data were double entered using Epi-Info and imported into Access for data management and storage. Laboratory test results were transmitted electronically from the MRC laboratory to the data Centre in TASO Jinja, manually entered in the study database.

For this study, data extracted from TASO and IDI database included socio-demographic information (age, gender, educational level, employment, and marital status), ART start date and regimen, clinical data collected at enrollment, including WHO clinical stage, CD4 cell counts, viral load and sexual behavior (number of partners in past 6 months and consistency of condom use) and adherence data at enrolment and subsequent clinic visits. Risky sexual behavior was defined as sexual intercourse with $\geq$ 2 partners or sexual intercourse with 1 partner and inconsistent condom use.

Statistical analysis

For this analysis, baseline was defined as the time of enrollment into the cohort which occurred after $\geq$ 4 year on ART (rural cohort) or at the 4-year on ART visit (urban cohort). For all patients included in the cohort, data was extracted for an additional 3.5 years after this baseline visit. All participants were followed until death, loss to follow up, transfer out, withdrawal of consent, or 3.5 years after the "baseline" visit.

We described participants characteristics at baseline overall, by gender and cohort (urban/IDI and rural/TASO) using means and frequencies. Continuous variables were compared using an unpaired t-test or Wilcoxon rank sum test if not normally distributed. Pearson Chi-square was used to compare categorical variables.

The main exposure of interest was time on ART (coded as 6-month periods). Other covariates of interest were the site, age, CD4 cell count, viral load, gender, education level, marital status, occupation, and ART regimen at baseline and calendar year of ART initiation. In order to examine the effect of long-term ART on sexual behaviors, separate analyses were performed. At baseline, we performed multivariable logistic regression and included variables in the initial model based on prior knowledge or association of the selected covariates with risky sexual behavior in bivariable analysis. Using a backwards elimination procedure, we started with all covariates in the model and then stepwise removed the covariate with the largest p-value until all the remaining covariates had a p-value less than 0.10 for the association with the outcome of interest.

To model the association between the binary outcome (risky sexual behavior) and the exposure of time on ART, we used a Generalized Estimating Equations (GEE) logistic regression model, with a logit link function to model the association between the binary outcome (risky sexual behavior) and the exposure of time on ART. Using a GEE logistic regression, odds ratios (ORs) were derived that took into account the repeated measures in individual participants and missing data in response variables, using robust standard errors to account for within-subject correlation. Co-variates with a p-value less than 0.10 for the association with the outcome of interest was included in the final model. Data were analyzed using STATA version 15 (StataCorp, College Station, TX).

Effect modifiers exploratory analysis

We assessed for effect modification by the following variables: gender and sexual partners, marital status and sexual partners, current age group and sexual partners. Interaction terms with a p-value < 0.05 were considered statistically significant.

Results

Overall, 1012 individuals receiving ART for ≥ 4 years were included in the analysis. Of these 402 (39.8%) were from the urban (IDI) cohort and 610 (60.2%) from the rural (TASO) cohort. Most patients were female (69.6% urban vs 75.7% rural cohort) and about half (53.3% urban vs 54.4% rural) of all patients were not married. At baseline, the mean age was 42.8 years (SD = 8.5), with rural patients being older than urban patients (mean age 44.6 vs 39.8 years; p-value 0.05) (Table 1). Slightly over a half (53.5%) of the urban but only 35.3% of the rural participants attained secondary education or higher (p-value < 0.01). At baseline, the most common ART regimen was zidovudine, lamivudine and nevirapine in the rural cohort and a tenofovir-based regimen in the urban cohort. At baseline, almost all participants (~ 90% in both cohorts) had a CD4 > 200 cells/mm^3, but the mean CD4 count was lower in the urban cohort (mean CD4 cell count 426 cells/mm^3 and 564 cells/mm^3 for urban cohorts and rural, respectively).

Table 1 Baseline characteristics of the cohort participants

Variable	N	Urban (IDI) N (%)	N	Rural (TASO) N (%)
Baseline age in years	402		610	
18–34		118 (29.3)		52 (8.5)
35–44		180 (44.8)		274 (44.9)
> 45		104 (25.9)		284 (46.6)
Gender				
Female		280 (69.6)		462 (75.7)
Male		122 (30.4)		148 (24.3)
Marital status				
Married/cohabiting		187 (46.5)		278 (46.6)
Not married		215 (53.5)		332 (54.4)
Educational level				
No formal education		15 (3.7)		110 (18.0)
Primary level		173 (43.0)		285 (46.7)
≥ Secondary level		214 (53.3)		215 (35.3)
Employment				
Formal employment		178 (44.3)		105 (17.6)
No formal employment		224 (55.7)		491 (82.4)
Baseline ART regimen				
ZDV 3TC EFV		123 (33.5)		113 (18.5)
D4T 3TC NVP		66 (18.0)		0
ZDV 3TC NVP		0		356 (58.3)
TDF based regimen		177 (48.5)		141 (23.0)
Mean time on ART		8.7 (SD 1.2)		7.0 (SD 0.3)
Baseline viral load				
Mean log 10 viral load copies/ml		2.65 (SD 0.34)		1.91 (SD 1.27)
< 1000 cells/ml		385 (96)		501 (82.1)
≥ 1000 cells/ml		16 (4.0)		109 (17.9)
Baseline CD4 cell/mm^3				
Mean CD4		426(SD 194.4)		564.3 (284.2)
< 200 cells/mm^3		43 (10.7)		54 (8.85)
200–499 cells/mm^3		237 (60.0)		213 (34.9)
> 499 cells/mm^3		122 (30.4)		340 (55.7)
WHO staging				
Stage 1		2 (0.5)		25 (4.2)
Stage 2		51(12.7)		243 (41.3)
Stage 3		232 (57.7)		205 (34.8)
Stage 4		117 (29.1)		116 (19.7)

Some percentages do not add up to 100% because of missing data

Follow up

A total of 941/1012 (93%) participants completed 3.5 years of follow up after baseline. The mean duration of follow-up was 51.3 months (SD 15.3), but longer for urban than rural participants (64.5 vs 36.4 months). After enrollment, 38 (3.8%) participants died 21 (5.2%) urban and 17 (2.9%) rural participants. At 3.5 years of follow up, few (3.3%) patients were lost to follow up or transferred out (16 urban and 17 rural participants), and only 15 (1.5%, all urban) participants withdrew study consent.

Risky sexual behavior at baseline (≥ 4 years visit on ART)

Overall, 241 (24.0%) cohort participants reported having engaged in risky sexual behavior at baseline. The type of risky sexual behavior was predominantly inconsistent or no condom use while engaged in a sexual relationship with a single partner (87.1%, 210/241). Engagement in sexual relationships with ≥ 2 partners was less prevalent (12.9%, 32/241). Participants reporting risky sexual behavior at baseline were more likely to be aged 18–34 and 35–44 years, female, married, and rural residency ($p<0.01$ for all) (Table 2).

In univariate logistic regression analysis, rural residence (OR 4.61, 95% CI 3.18–6.68), being male (OR 2.16, 95% CI 1.58–2.94), formal employment (OR 1.54, 95% CI 1.09–2.17), viral load > 1000 copies/ml (OR 1.22, 95% CI 0.80–1.87), and being younger [18–34 years (OR 1.11, 95% CI 0.72–1.72) and 35–44 years (OR 1.43, 95% CI 1.04–1.97) compared with age > 45 years] were associated with an increased odds of risky sexual behavior. Not being married was associated with lower odds of risky sexual behavior (OR 0.11, 95% CI 0.07–0.55).

In multivariable logistic analysis, rural residence (adjusted odds ratio [aOR] 9.54, 95% CI 5.83–15.61) being male (aOR 1.51, 95% CI 1.02–2.31) and younger age, (aOR 3.41, 95% CI 1.87–6.21 for 18–34 years and aOR 2.12, 95% CI 1.40–3.21 for 35–44 years) remained strongly associated with increased odds of risky sexual behavior. Not being married remained associated with lower odds of risky sexual behavior (aOR 0.10; 95% CI 0.06–0.14) (Table 3).

Table 2 Baseline participants risky sexual behavior comparison

Variable	N	Non risky (N = 769) N (%)	Risky sex (N = 241) N (%)
Site	1010		
Urban		363 (47.2)	39 (16.2)
Rural		406 (52.8)	202 (83.8)
Age in years	1010		
18–34		131 (17.1)	38 (15.8)
35–44		331 (43.0)	127 (51.0)
≥ 45		307 (39.9)	80 (33.2)
Gender	1010		
Female		593 (77.0)	147 (61.0)
Male		176 (23.0)	94 (39.0)
Marital status	1010		
Married/cohabiting		265 (34.5)	200 (90.0)
Not married		504 (65.5)	41 (17.0)
Educational level	1010		
No formal education		97 (12.6)	27 (11.2)
Primary Level		343 (44.6)	114 (47.3)
≥ Secondary level		326 (42.8)	100 (41.5)
Employment	996		
Formal employment		231 (30.1)	57 (22.0)
No formal employment		529 (69.9)	184 (80.0)
Baseline viral load	1009		
< 1000 cells/ml		678 (88.3)	207 (85.9)
≥ 1000 cells/ml		90 (11.7)	34 (14.1)
Baseline CD4	1010		
< 200 cells/mm^3		71 (9.2)	29 (12.0)
200–499 cells/mm^3		355 (46.0)	95 (39.4)
> 499 cells/mm^3		345 (44.8)	117 (48.6)

Risky sexual behavior over time

The proportion of rural patients self-reporting risky sexual behavior declined from 33.1% at enrollment to 9.6% at 3.5 additional years of follow up (p-value for trend < 0.01). In contrast, the proportion of urban patients self-reporting risky sexual behavior remained stable: 9.7% at enrollment, 11.2% at 1 year later, 12.6% at 2.5 years later and 9.9% at 3.5 years later of follow up (p value for trend 0.71) (Fig. 1).

In the multivariable (GEE) logistic regression model, taking repeated measures over time into account, rural residence (aOR 4.99, 95% CI 3.64–6.83); male gender (aOR 1.66, 95% CI 1.26–2.19) and younger age; (aOR 5.60 95% CI 3.80–8.25 for 18–34 years and aOR 2.34 95% CI 1.74–3.14 for 35–44 years) were associated with increased odds of risky sexual behavior. Not being married (aOR 0.25, 95% CI 0.19–0.34) and time on ART (aOR 0.71 per year, 95% CI 0.67–0.66), baseline CD4 cell/mm^3 (aOR 0.59, 95% CI 0.38–0.90 for 200–499 cells/mm^3 and aOR 0.52 95% CI 0.33–0.84 for > 499 cells/mm^3) were associated with reduced odds of risky sexual behavior (Table 3).

Educational level, type of employment, the age of first sexual intercourse (aOR 112; 95% CI 0.80–1.78) and number of lifetime sexual partners (aOR 0.95; 95% CI 0.90–1.01) were not associated with risky sexual behavior.

Discussion

Among people on ART for ≥ 4 years we observed that rural residence was associated with increased odds of self-reported risky sexual behavior. Risky sexual behavior was predominately due to poor condom use and much

Table 3 Risky sexual behavior and associations with ART among cohort participants

Variable	Baseline (≥ 4 years risky sexual behavior)		GEE logistic analysis	
	Univariate logistic	Multivariate logistic	Un adjusted GEE	Adjusted GEE
	OR (95% CI)	OR (95% CI)	OR (95% CI)	OR (95% CI
Site				
Urban	Ref	Ref	Ref	Ref
Rural	4.61 (3.18–6.68)	9.54 (5.83–15.61)	2.06 (1.58–2.70)	4.99 (3.64–6.83)
Baseline age in years				
18–34	1.11 (0.72–1.72)	3.41 (1.87–6.21)	2.58 (1.83–3.65)	5.60 (3.80–8.25)
35–44	1.43 (1.04–1.97)	2.12 (1.40–3.21)	1.86 (1.39–2.49)	2.34 (1.74–3.14)
> 45	Ref	Ref	Ref	Ref
Gender				
Female	Ref	Ref	Ref	Ref
Male	2.16 (1.58–2.94)	1.51 (1.0–2.31)	1.82 (1.41–2.35)	1.66 (1.26–2.19)
Marital status				
Married/cohabiting	Ref	Ref	Ref	Ref
Not married	0.11(0.07–0.55)	0.09 (0.06–0.14)	0.26 (0.20–0.34)	0.25 (0.19–0.34)
Educational level				
No formal education	Ref		Ref	
Primary level	1.20 (0.74–1.94)		1.30 (0.85–1.99)	
≥ Secondary level	1.10 (0.68–1.79)		1.45 (0.95–2.22)	
Employment				
No formal employment	Ref	Ref	Ref	
Formal employment	1.54 (1.09–2.17)	0.93 (0.60–1.44)	1.18 (0.89–1.55)	
Viral load				
< 1000 cells/ml	Ref	Ref	Ref	Ref
≥ 1000 cells/ml	1.22 (0.80–1.87)	0.52 (0.23–0.96)	1.26 (0.88–1.79)	0.57 (0.37–0.87)
Baseline CD4				
<200 cells/mm^3	Ref	Ref	Ref	Ref
200–499 cells/mm^3	0.66 (0.49–1.07	0.57 (0.30–1.10	0.67 (0.45–0.99)	0.59 (0.38–0.90)
>499 cells/mm^3	0.51 (0.51–1.34)	0.63 (0.32–1.23)	0.62 (0.42–0.92)	0.52 (0.33–0.84)
Time on ART			0.76 (0.72–0.80)	0.71 (0.67–0.76)
TASO cohort sub-analysis				
No. of life time partners	1.00 (1.10–1.02)		1.01 (1.00–1.02)	
Age of first sex	0.98 (0.92–1.06)		1.02 (0.97–1.07)	

less due to multiple sexual partners. Risky sexual behavior increased with younger age, with a 2.12-fold increased odds among 35–44 years and 3.41-fold higher odds among 18–34 years compared to individuals age 45 years or older. The odds of risky sexual behavior decreased with time of follow up on ART (aOR 0.71), but this decrease over time was only present in the rural cohort. When taking the sexual behavior over the entire period of long-term ART into account, the odds of risky sexual behavior was higher among male compared to female participants (aOR 1.66), while a higher CD4 count (aOR 0.52–0.59) and those who failed to achieve viral load suppression (aOR 0.52) at baseline was associated with a lower odds of risky sexual behavior.

Comparison with other studies in sub-Saharan Africa is difficult as longitudinal data on risky sexual behaviors among people on long-term ART is limited. Our findings do suggest that the reduction in risky sexual behavior observed in the first year(s) of ART in several studies in sub-Saharan Africa [9, 12, 14, 20, 21, 25–31] does not revert into increased risky sexual behavior over time, but instead either stabilizes at a relatively low rate (as observed in the urban cohort) or further decreases over time (as observed in the rural cohort). Even though the risk reduced or stabilized over time, the continued risk-taking emphasizes that it remains important to focus on individual risk reduction practices such as consistent condom use even among patients who are already several years on ART.

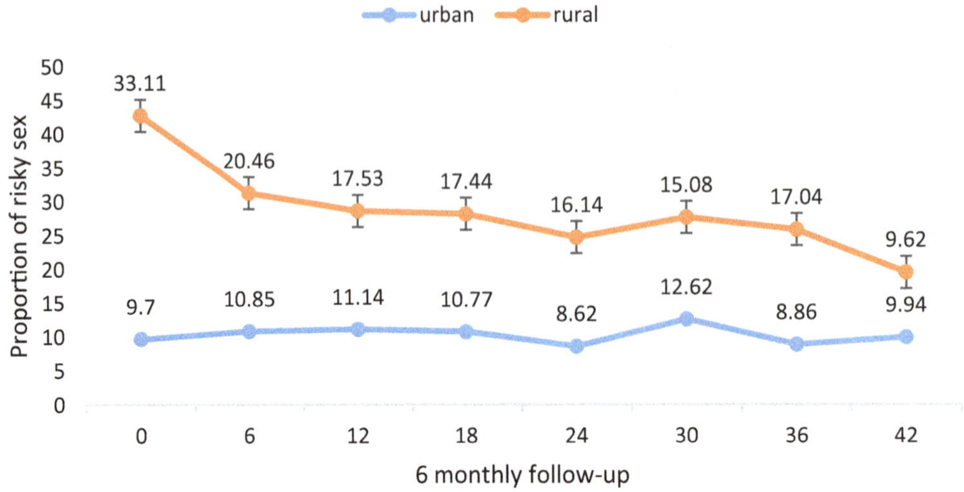

Fig. 1 Trends in risky sexual behavior among urban and rural cohort participants after additional 3.5 years of follow up

We found that rural residence, male gender, and younger age were associated with increased odds of risky sexual behavior, similar to what was observed in sub-Saharan Africa studies of individuals during the first one to 4 years of ART [11–14, 21, 27–29]. For example, in a South African cohort study, people receiving ART at urban and rural health care facilities found younger age, being married and male gender was associated with risky sexual behavior [12]. Our finding of increased risky sexual behavior among males and married is also similar to Ugandan studies that found, among those on ART for one to 4 years, higher or even increased risky sexual behavior among men and those that are married were observed [11, 13, 14, 27, 30]. The increased risky sexual behavior observed among men could be because of the gender and power dynamics, where men are the major decision-makers in sexual issues in Africa. Among the married, the increased risk of sexual behavior is attributed to the desire to have children, fear of HIV status disclosure to the sexual partner(s), and the beliefs that condom use is not necessary for HIV positive couples and reduces sexual satisfaction. The difference in risky sexual behavior among people receiving care at urban and rural facilities could be due to differences in rural vs urban environment with urban participants having greater exposure to HIV prevention messaging and more likely to be of a higher socioeconomic status. Furthermore, condom promotion was mainly done to urban cohort participants.

The reduced odds of risky sexual behavior among participants with higher CD4 cell/mm^3 and suppressed VL at baseline is similar to the findings of other studies in Uganda [11, 13, 14, 27, 30].

Our study had several strengths, including its prospective design, the inclusion of a cohort in both a rural and urban setting, and the large sample size which allowed us to assess and identify factors that are independently associated with risky sexual behavior. Several limitations need to be taken into account when interpreting the results. First, the two cohorts had a 2-year difference in ART initiation timelines and baseline visit included participants who have been on ART for 4 years in the urban cohort or $\geq$ 4 years in the rural cohort, complicating straightforward comparison between these two cohorts. Second, only patients from HIV centers of excellence were included, which may not be representative for smaller centers or primary care settings. Furthermore, at the IDI (urban cohort), patients were asked about sexual behavior from ART initiation by the counsellors which were providing risk-reduction counselling, which may lead to patients being less likely to report risky sexual behavior due to social desirability bias. However, the study team was trained to ask questions in a professional and non-judgmental approach to minimize any social desirability. Third, patients included in the study initiated ART based on CD4 eligibility criteria hence our results may not be generalizable to people receiving long term–term ART under the current WHO 'treat all' strategy. Future studies should monitor trends of risky sexual behavior in high-risk populations on long-term ART and whether low-risk sexual behavior also occurs among patients on long-term ART in the 'treat all' era.

Conclusions

We observed a decline in risky sexual behavior in rural people on long-term ($\geq$ 4 years) ART. Rural, male and young individuals had higher odds of self-reported risky sexual behavior. ART programs should continue

to emphasize risk reduction practices, especially among people receiving care in rural health facilities, males, younger individuals and those who are married.

Abbreviations

ART: antiretroviral therapy; WHO: World Health Organization; TASO: The AIDS Support Organization; IDI: Infectious Diseases Institute; MRC: Medical Research Council.

Authors' contributions

DM, MK, PK, BJ, SO, BC and AK, designed the study. SO, MJ, BT and BC, supervised data collection of the study. SO, MJ and BT abstracted the data. SO, AVR and MJ conducted or contributed to the data analysis. SO, BC, MJ and AVR interpreted the data. SO prepared the original manuscripts, all authors contributed to subsequent revisions. All authors read and approved the final manuscript.

Author details

[1] Infectious Diseases Institute, College of Health Sciences, Makerere University, P.O BOX 22418, Kampala, Uganda. [2] Global Health Institute, University of Antwerp, Antwerp, Belgium. [3] Faculty of Medicine and Health Sciences, University of Antwerp, Antwerp, Belgium. [4] British Columbia Centre for Excellence in HIV/AIDS, Vancouver, Canada. [5] University of British Columbia, Vancouver, Canada. [6] The AIDS Support Organization, Kampala, Uganda. [7] Medical Research Council/Uganda Virus Research Institute, Kampala, Uganda. [8] School of Medicine, College of Health Sciences, Makerere University, Kampala, Uganda.

Acknowledgements

We would like to acknowledge The AIDS Support Organization (TASO) and Infectious Diseases Institute for allowing us to access study data as per their respective data access policy and Dr. Andrew Mujugira, Head of IDI Kasangati HIV prevention research centre of excellence for his on spot mentorship. DMM is supported by a Scholar Award from the Michael Smith Foundation for Health Research.

Competing interests

The authors declare that they have no competing interests.

Funding

This sub study was funded by the Canadian African Preventive Trial network (CAPT-N) as part of my PhD program at the University of Antwerp, Belgium through Institute of Infectious Diseases and Molecular Medicine, University of Cape Town, South Africa. The Long-Term Outcomes Study was funded by the Canadian Institutes for Health Research (Grant Number MOP-119369).

References

1. UNAIDS. Fact sheet: global HIV/AIDS statistics. 2015, 2017.
2. UNAIDS. Fact sheet. UNAIDS report. 2015. p. 1–8. http://www.unaids.org/sites/default/files/media_asset/20150901_FactSheet_2015_en.pdf. Accessed 16 Dec 2017.
3. World Health Organization, March 2014 supplement to the 2013 consolidated guideline on the use ofantiretroviral drugs for treating and prevention HIV infection.
4. Bärnighausen T, Chaiyachati K, Chimbindi N, Peoples A, Haberer J, Newell ML. Interventions to increase antiretroviral adherence in sub-Saharan Africa: a systematic review of evaluation studies. Lancet Infect Dis. 2011;11:70181–5. https://doi.org/10.1016/S1473-3099.
5. UNAIDS. Gap report. 2016.
6. Cohen MS, Dye C, Fraser C, Miller WC, Powers KA, Williams BG. HIV treatment as prevention: debate and commentary-will early infection compromise treatment-as-prevention strategies? PLoS Med. 2012;9(7):e1001232. https://doi.org/10.1371/journal.pmed.1001232.
7. Kirby D. Changes in sexual behavior leading to the decline in the prevalence of HIV in Uganda: confirmation from multiple sources of evidence. Sex Transm Infect. 2008;84(Suppl_2):35–41. https://doi.org/10.1136/sti.2008.029892.
8. Kennedy C, O'Reilly K, Medley A, Sweat M. The impact of HIV treatment on risk behavior in developing countries: a systematic review. AIDS Care. 2007;19(6):707–20. https://doi.org/10.1080/09540120701203261.
9. Sarna A, Luchters SMF, Geibel S, Kaai S, Munyao P, Shikely K, et al. Sexual risk behavior and HAART: a comparative study of HIV-infected persons on HAART and on preventive therapy in Kenya. Int J STD AIDS. 2008;19(2):85–9. https://doi.org/10.1258/ijsa.2007.007097.
10. Ezekiel MJ, Talle A, Juma JM, Mnyika KS, Klepp KI. Attitudes and perceived impact of antiretroviral therapy on sexual risk behavior among young people in Kahe, Moshi Rural District, Tanzania. Tanzania J Health Res. 2008;10(4):203–12.
11. Kembabazi A, Bajunirwe F, Hunt PW, Martin JN, Muzoora C, Haberer JE, et al. Disinhibition in risky sexual behavior in men, but not women, during four years of antiretroviral therapy in rural, southwestern Uganda. PLoS ONE. 2013;8:3–7. https://doi.org/10.1371/journal.pone.0069634.
12. Venkatesh KK, de Bruyn G, Lurie MN, Mohapi L, Pronyk P, Moshabela M. Decreased sexual risk behaviour in the era of HAART among HIV-infected urban and rural South Africans attending primary care clinics. AIDS. 2010;24(17):2687–96. https://doi.org/10.1097/QAD.0b013e32833e78d4.
13. Apondi R, Bunnell R, Ekwaru JP, Moore D, Bechange S, Khana K, et al. Sexual behaviour and HIV transmission risk of Ugandan adults taking antiretroviral therapy: 3-year follow-up. AIDS. 2011;25(10):1317–27. https://doi.org/10.1097/QAD.0b013e328347f775.
14. Bunnell R, Ekwaru JP, Solberg P, Wamai N, Bikaako-Kajura W, Were W, et al. Changes in sexual behaviour and risk of HIV transmission after antiretroviral therapy and prevention interventions in rural Uganda. AIDS. 2005;2006(20):85–92.
15. Eisele T, Mathews C, Chopra M, Lurie MN, Brown L, Dewing S, Kendall C, et al. Changes in risk behaviour among HIV-positive patients during their first year of antiretroviral therapy in Cape Town South Africa. AIDS Behav. 2008;13:1097–105 **(PubMed: 18846418)**.
16. Diabaté S, Alary M, Koffi CK. Short-term increase in unsafe sexual behaviour after initiation of HAART in Côte d'Ivoire. AIDS. 2008;22:154–6 **(PubMed: 18090406)**.
17. Yaya I, Saka B, Landoh DE, Patchali PM, Makawa M-S, Senanou S. Sexual risk behaviour among people living with HIV and AIDS on antiretroviral therapy at the regional hospital of Sokodé, Togo. BMC Public Health. 2014;14(1):636. https://doi.org/10.1186/1471-2458-14-636.
18. Luchters S, Sarna A, Geibel S, Chersich MF, Munyao P, Kaai S, et al. Safer sexual behaviours after 12 months of antiretroviral treatment in Mombasa, Kenya: a prospective cohort. AIDS Patient Care STDs. 2008;22:587–94 **(PubMed: 18601582)**.
19. Wanyama J, Kasibante D, Kayiira P, Wandera B, Kambugu A. Sexual behaviour of HIV+ persons before and after 1 year of ART at the infectious diseases clinic, Kampala, Uganda. In: 17th conference on retroviruses and opportunistic infections; San Francisco. 2010.
20. Berhan A, Berhan Y. Is the sexual behavior of HIV patients on antiretroviral therapy safe or risky in sub-saharan Africa? Meta-analysis and meta-regression. AIDS Res Ther. 2012;9:14. https://doi.org/10.1186/1742-6405-9-14.
21. Doyle JS, Degenhardt L, Pedrana AE, McBryde ES, Guy RJ, Stoové MA, et al. Effects of HIV antiretroviral therapy on sexual and injecting risk-taking behavior: a systematic review and meta-analysis. Clin Infect Dis. 2014;59(10):1483–94. https://doi.org/10.1093/cid/ciu602.
22. Castelnuovo B, Kiragga A, Mubiru F, Kambugu A, Kamya M, Reynolds SJ. First-line antiretroviral therapy durability in a 10-year cohort of naïve adults started on treatment in Uganda. J Int AIDS Soc. 2016;19(1):20773.
23. Okoboi S, Ding E, Persaud S, Wangisi J, Birungi J, Shurgold S, et al. Community-based ART distribution system can effectively facilitate long-term program retention and low-rates of death and virologic failure in rural Uganda. AIDS Res Ther. 2015;12(1):37.
24. Birungi J, Min JE, Muldoon KA, Kaleebu P, King R, Khanakwa S, et al. Lack of effectiveness of antiretroviral therapy in preventing HIV infection in serodiscordant couples in Uganda: an observational study. PLoS ONE. 2015;10(7):e0132182.
25. Allison P. Fixed effects regression methods for longitudinal data using SAS. Cary: SAS Institute Inc; 2005.
26. Shafer LA, Nsubuga RN, White R. Antiretroviral therapy and sexual behaviour in Uganda: a cohort study. AIDS. 2011;25:671–8.
27. Wandera B, Kamya MR, Castelnuovo B, Kiragga A, Kambugu A, Wanyama JN, et al. Sexual behaviors over a 3-year period among individuals with

advanced HIV/AIDS receiving antiretroviral therapy in an urban HIV clinic in Kampala, Uganda. JAIDS J Acquir Immune Defic Syndr. 2011;57(1):62–8.

28. Sarna A, Luchters SM, Geibel S, Kaai S, Munyao P, Shikely KS, et al. Sexual risk behaviour and HAART: a comparative study of HIV-infected persons on HAART and on preventive therapy in Kenya. Int J STD AIDS. 2008;19:85–9 **(PubMed: 18334059)**.
29. Moatti J, Prudhomme J, Traore DC, Juillet-Amari A, Akribi HA, Msellati P, Côte d'Ivoire HIV Drug Access Initiative Socio-Behavioural Evaluation Group. Access to antiretroviral treatment and sexual behaviours of HIV-infected patients aware of their serostatus in Côte d'Ivoire. AIDS. 2003;17:S69–77 **(PubMed: 14565612)**.
30. Bateganya M, Colfax G, Shafer LA, Kityo C, Mugyenyi P, Serwadda D, et al. Antiretroviral therapy and sexual behaviour: a comparative study between antiretroviral-naive and -experienced patients at an urban HIV/AIDS care and research centre in Kampala, Uganda. AIDS Patient Care STDs. 2005;19:760–8 **(PubMed: 16283836)**.
31. Kaida A, Gray G, Bastos FI, Andia I, Maier M, McIntyre J, et al. The relationship between HAART use and sexual activity among HIV-positive women of reproductive age in Brazil, South Africa, and Uganda. AIDS Care. 2008;20:21–5 **(PubMed: 18278611)**.

19

Non-AIDS complexity amongst patients living with HIV in Sydney: risk factors and health outcomes

Derek J. Chan[1,2], Virginia Furner[1], Don E. Smith[1,2*], Mithilesh Dronavalli[1], Rohan I. Bopage[1,2], Jeffrey J. Post[1,3,4] and Anjali K. Bhardwaj[5]

Abstract

Objective: To assess the prevalence of non-AIDS co-morbidities (NACs) and predictors of adverse health outcomes amongst people living with HIV in order to identify health needs and potential gaps in patient management.

Design: Retrospective, non-consecutive medical record audit of patients attending a publicly funded HIV clinic in metropolitan Sydney analysed for predictors of adverse health outcomes. We developed a scoring system based on the validated Charlson score method for NACs, mental health and social issues and confounders were selected using directed acyclic graph theory under the principles of causal inference.

Results: 211 patient files were audited non-consecutively over 6 weeks. 89.5% were male; 41.8% culturally and linguistically diverse and 4.1% were of Aboriginal/Torres Strait Islander origin. Half of patients had no general practitioner and 25% were ineligible for Medicare subsidised care. The most common NACs were: cardiovascular disease (25%), hepatic disease (21%), and endocrinopathies (20%). One-third of patients had clinical anxiety, one-third major depression and almost half of patients had a lifetime history of tobacco smoking. Five predictors of poor health outcomes were identified: (1) *co-morbidity score* was associated with hospitalisation (odds ratio, OR 1.58; 95% CI 1.01–2.46; $p = 0.044$); (2) *mental health score* was associated with hospitalisation (OR 1.79; 95% CI 1.22–2.62; $p = 0.003$) and poor adherence to ART (OR 2.34; 95% CI 1.52–3.59; $p = 0.001$); (3) *social issues score* was associated with genotypic resistance (OR 2.61; 95% CI 1.48–4.59; $p = 0.001$), co-morbidity score (OR 1.69; 95% CI 1.24–2.3; $p = 0.001$) and hospitalisation (OR 1.72; 95% CI 1.1–2.7; $p = 0.018$); (4) *body mass index* < 20 was associated with genotypic resistance (OR 6.25; 95% CI 1.49–26.24; $p = 0.012$); and (5) *Medicare eligibility* was associated with co-morbidity score (OR 2.21; 95% CI 1.24–3.95; $p = 0.007$).

Conclusion: Most HIV patients are healthy due to effective antiretroviral therapy; however, NACs and social/mental health issues are adding to patient complexity. The current findings underpin the need for multidisciplinary management beyond routine viral load and CD4 count monitoring.

Background

The quality of life and life expectancy of people living with HIV infection (PLHIV) are now similar to that of the general population due to effective antiretroviral therapy (ART) [1]. Whilst ART-related co-morbidities such as lipodystrophy syndrome associated with first-generation nucleosides and protease inhibitors do not occur with the newer agents such as integrase inhibitors, non-AIDS co-morbidities (NACs) such as cardiovascular disease, liver disease and malignancy are increasing among PLHIV [1]. Possible reasons include ageing, ongoing low-level immune activation and inflammation despite virological suppression [2] higher rates of modifiable risk factors (such as smoking) and effects of ART itself [3]. Consequently, HIV management now requires holistic management of NACs, poly-pharmacy and identification of

*Correspondence: don.smith@health.nsw.gov.au
[1] Albion Centre, South Eastern Sydney Local Health District, Sydney, NSW 2010, Australia

drug–drug interactions, as well as attention to psychosocial issues that may affect ART compliance.

Australian PLHIV are managed by accredited general practitioners (S100 GPs) and hospital/clinic doctors; however, in our experience marginalised, complex patients (e.g. culturally and linguistically diverse (CALD), aboriginal/torres strait islander (ATSI) patients, those with complex mental health, substance use, socioeconomic problems, or those without federally-funded healthcare (Medicare) may not see GPs due to cost, confidentiality concerns, and lack of appointments or multidisciplinary/multicultural support. The public health system provides care for individuals who, if unlinked to private health care, may potentially become immune-compromised, require hospitalisation, or transmit HIV. Data on the health complexity of this important group is scarce. We assess the prevalence of NACs and predictors of adverse health outcomes for HIV patients attending a publicly funded ambulatory care clinic.

Methods

Setting and participants

The Albion Centre is a publicly funded, ambulatory care clinic in metropolitan Sydney with in-house medical specialists, nurses, psychologists, social workers, dieticians and pharmacists providing same-visit HIV care and treatment. The patients are mostly homosexually-active men, the group most affected by Australia's HIV epidemic.

Design

A checklist was developed to enable a retrospective, non-consecutive audit of medical records for HIV patients presenting for medical care between 1 May–15 June 2014. The project was approved by South Eastern Sydney Human Research Ethics Committee (study number 16/215) adjust.

Data collected included; (1) patients' demographic information, including gender, age, CALD or ATSI background, GP or specialist involvement in care; (2) clinical history; duration of HIV infection, recent HIV RNA viral load, current and nadir CD4 count, HIV genotypic resistance, ART adherence, past AIDS defining conditions, hospital admissions in past year, NACs (cardiac, hepatic, endocrine, renal, neurological, respiratory, neoplastic, musculoskeletal conditions), body mass index (BMI); and (3) psychosocial factors; such as mental health diagnoses, smoking, alcohol and (intravenous) drug use, employment status, housing, financial support and federally-funded Medicare eligibility (only Australian permanent residents and citizens are eligible for Medicare). Regarding categorisation where a particular condition could be reported under more than one NAC domain (e.g. haemochromatosis could be classified as liver, endocrine or cardiac disease) only one NAC was assigned. We did not adjust for frequency of attendance as this was a cross-sectional, non-consecutive analysis of patient records. The mental health diagnoses were made by the attending doctor with or without input from staff clinical psychologists. ATSI and CALD status were defined according to patient registration data including self-declaration of aboriginality, first language spoken at home and year of arrival in Australia if born overseas. The designation of 'social isolation' was derived from the patient's psychosocial history and self-report of same as documented in the records. Refugees were patients who were referred by the Australian Immigration authorities for treatment and care.

Data analysis

Data were analysed using Stata software (StataCorp. 2011, v12: College Station, TX: StataCorp LP). DAG theory was used to determine confounders for each predictor-outcome association (Fig. 1). DAG theory minimises bias and identifies only necessary confounders to increase the power of the analysis (statistical efficiency) [4]. The adverse health outcomes identified in our study were: CD4 count, genotypic resistance, hospital admission, ART adherence and co-morbidity score (health scores are discussed below).

Figure 1 shows the pre-analysis DAG for HIV patients. Arrows in the DAGs in this paper (Figs. 1 and 2) represent a causal association as per syntax of causal inference used by Pearl [5]. This model is not strictly acyclic, as mental health diagnoses may cause social issues and vice versa. For these 'bi-directional' variables, the social issue score was considered a confounder for the mental health score and vice versa in the analysis. This produces conservative effect sizes when assessing causality but the probability rules of the model are maintained.

Associations between predictors with binary outcomes were calculated using logistic regression. The exception is ordinal regression, which is used to calculate the associations between the co-morbidity score and CD4 nadir, social issue score, Medicare eligibility, virological failure, BMI > 30 and CALD. Missing values were ignored (case-wise deletion) and multiple imputation was not performed because some variables in the dataset had more missing observations than others and were likely missing not at random (MNAR) making them unsuitable for multiple imputation.

We developed 'health scores' to facilitate quantitative analysis. These scores, although not validated for PLHIV, follow the principles of the validated Charlson score [6] and are simply a method for counting the total number

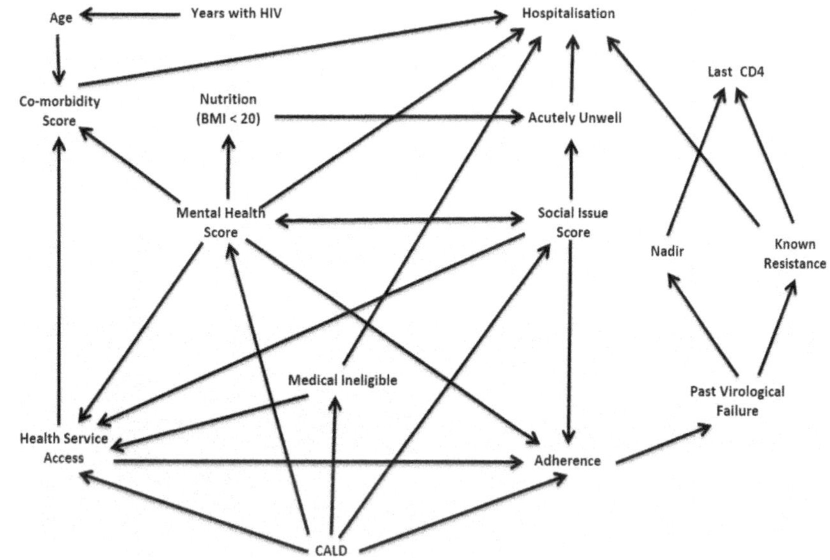

Fig. 1 Pre-analysis direct acyclic graph for HIV patient complexity

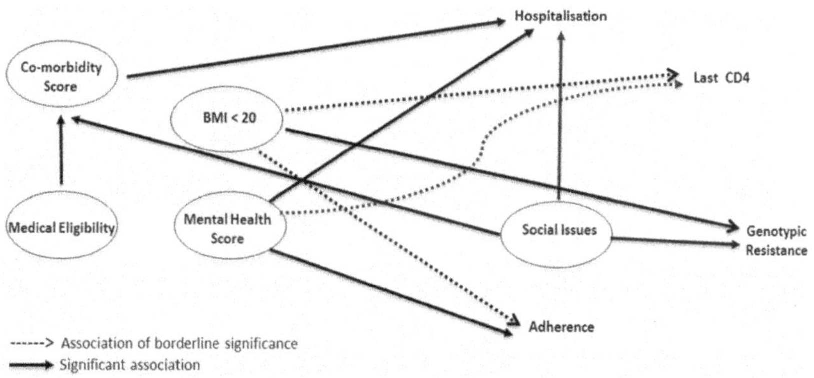

Fig. 2 Post-analysis direct acyclic graph: predictors of adverse health outcomes for HIV patients

or NACs, mental health diagnoses and social issues for each patient. The Comorbidity score was the number of NACs (zero to a maximum seven defined co-morbidities including Cardiac, Renal, Neurological, Liver, Endocrine, Respiratory, Metabolic Bone Disease, Malignancy). The mental health score was the sum of mental health diagnoses (zero to a maximum three diagnoses including anxiety, major depression, drug-dependency, alcohol dependency, personality disorder, schizophrenia and other psychoses). Lastly, the social issues score was the sum of social issues (zero to a maximum of three issues including: unemployment, disability support pension, socially isolated, refugee, retired, homeless, domestic violence).

Results

Demographics

211 files of 264 attendees had audit forms completed in the study period. 89.5% were male, 10% female and 0.5% transgender. Median age was 47.2 years (range 21–73). Many patients were CALD (41.8%) and 4.1% ATSI 95% were taking ART and one-third had HIV infection for 20 years or more. All patients are requested to have a GP as part of our shared-care model, yet only half did. The reasons patients reported for not having a GP included: fear of disclosure, limited GP appointments, cost or lack of multidisciplinary services, or perceived lack of HIV expertise. Half had a specialist managing their NACs. Variables from the DAG model and health scores are given in Table 1.

Table 1 Variables from direct acyclic graph and health scores

	1	0	Yes	Proportion	
				Yes	Total
Predictor/confounder					
CD4 nadir < 200 cells/μL	Yes	No	67	0.4	169
Medicare eligible	Yes	No	157	0.75	210
Virological failure	Yes	No	27	0.14	193
BMI < 20	Yes	No	26	0.23	112
BMI > 30	Yes	No	28	0.25	112
CALD	Yes	No	87	0.42	208
Outcomes					
Last CD4 (cells/μL)	< 200	> 200	74	0.36	206
Genotypic resistance	Yes	No	18	0.1	186
Hospitalisation past 12 months	Yes	No	36	0.17	209
Adherence issue	Yes	No	38	0.18	211
Comorbidity score:	**From 0 to 7**				
	0		90	0.43	211
	1		60	0.28	211
	2		34	0.16	211
	3		16	0.08	211
	4		5	0.02	211
	5		3	0.01	211
	6		2	0.01	211
	7		1	0.005	211
Mental health score:	**From 0 to 3**				**211**
	0		97	0.47	
	1		66	0.32	
	2		34	0.16	
	3		13	0.06	
Social issue score:	**From 0 to 3**				**211**
	0		57	0.27	
	1		103	0.49	
	2		35	0.17	
	3		16	0.08	

Clinical parameters

The patients were generally healthy: 94% were taking ART and 82.3% had undetectable viral load. 18% had poor ART adherence (as determined by doctor), 8.1% past genotypic resistance and 12.8% past virological failure. 12.4% were underweight (BMI < 20) and 12.9% were obese (BMI > 30). 17% had been hospitalised in the past 12 months (most not HIV-related) and 13% had a past AIDS-defining condition. Polypharmacy was common with 20% prescribed five or more non-ART medications. Approximately one-third had been living with HIV for 10–20 years and one-third more than 20 years.

Non-AIDS comorbidities

43% of patients had no NAC. 28.1% had at least one NAC and some had multiple NACs. The prevalence of specific NACs (with predominant condition) was: cardiovascular disease (hypercholesterolaemia, hypertension) 26.8%; liver disease (hepatitis B or C co-infection, alcoholic liver disease) 22.1%; endocrinopathy (e.g.: type 2 diabetes, dyslipidemia) 21.7%; neurological disease (peripheral neuropathy, HIV-associated neurocognitive disorder) 12%; renal impairment (eGFR < 60 mL/min) 7.8%; osteoporosis 6%; respiratory disease (chronic obstructive pulmonary disease) 6.9%; and malignancy 4.6%.

Psychosocial issues

There was a significant burden of mental health and social issues in this sample. 54% had at least one psychiatric diagnosis: predominantly anxiety disorder (one-third) and major depression (one-third), followed by drug dependence (12.9%), alcohol dependence (4.3%), personality disorder (3.7%), schizophrenia (3.1%), other psychosis, e.g. drug-induced (3.1%), post-traumatic stress disorder (2.4%), bipolar affective disorder (1.8%) and adjustment disorder (1.8%). Dual mental health diagnoses occurred in 20% of patients. 49% were past/current smokers, 14.3% were past or current intravenous drug users, and 1.8% were homeless. About one-fifth of patients were unemployed (22.1%), receiving disability support pension (22.6%) or were Medicare ineligible (25%).

Predictors of poor health outcomes

We identified five predictors of poor health outcomes for our HIV patients adjusting for appropriate confounders as per DAG (Table 2).

Firstly, the comorbidity score was causally associated with hospitalisation in the previous year, odds ratio, OR 1.58; 95% CI 1.01–2.46; $p=0.044$ (adjusting for Medicare eligibility, mental health score, social issue score, CALD, ART adherence, BMI > 30 as confounders). Interestingly, CALD status was causally associated with a lower risk of hospitalisation, OR 0.31; 95% CI 0.13–0.74; $p=0.008$.

The mental health score was also causally associated with hospitalisation, OR 1.79; 95% CI 1.22–2.62; $p=0.003$ (adjusting for CALD) and poor ART adherence, OR 2.34; 95% CI 1.52–3.59; $p=0.001$ (adjusting for social issue score, CALD).

Table 2 Logistic regression for associations between predictors and outcomes

	OR (95% CI)	*p* value	L 95% CI	U 95% CI	Confounders
Last CD4					
CD4 nadir	3.13 (1.62–6.05)	0.001	1.62	6.05	Crude
ART adherence	3.3	0.001	1.59	6.87	Crude
Mental health score	1.35	0.081	0.96	1.88	Social issue score, CALD
BMI < 20	2.61	0.062	0.95	7.15	ARV adherence
Genotypic resistance					
Virological failure	421.33	0.001	47.7	3721.87	Crude
Social issue score	2.61	0.001	1.48	4.59	CALD
BMI < 20	6.25	0.012	1.49	26.24	Crude
ART adherence	6.64	0.001	2.38	18.53	Crude
Hospital admission					
Co-morbidity score	1.58	0.044	1.01	2.46	Medicare eligibility, mental health score, CALD, social issue score, ART adherence, BMI > 30
Social issue score	1.72	0.018	1.1	2.7	ART adherence, CALD, mental health score
Age	1.04	0.03	1	1.07	Crude
CALD	0.31	0.008	0.13	0.74	Crude
Mental health score	1.79	0.003	1.22	2.62	CALD
Poor ART adherence					
CD4 nadir	2.15	0.064	0.96	4.82	Crude
Virological failure	12.75	0.001	5.1	31.9	Crude
BMI < 20	2.65	0.077	0.9	7.81	Social
Mental health score	2.34	0.001	1.52	3.59	CALD, social issue score
Comorbidity score[a]					
CD4 nadir	2.28	0.005	1.28	4.05	ART adherence
Social issue score	1.69	0.001	1.24	2.3	CALD, mental health score
Medicare eligibility	2.21	0.007	1.24	3.95	CALD
Virological failure	3.15	0.006	1.39	7.13	ART adherence
BMI > 30	3.59	0.002	1.59	8.11	Social issue score, mental health score
CALD	0.62	0.064	0.37	1.03	Crude

OR odds ratio; *L95% CI* lower limit, 95% confidence interval; *U95% CI* upper limit, 95% confidence interval; *BMI* body mass index; Crude adjustment for confounding not required; *CALD* culturally and linguistically diverse background

[a] Calculated by ordinal regression

The social issue score was causally associated with: (1) hospitalisation, OR 1.72; 95% CI 1.1–2.7; $p=0.018$ (adjusting for ART adherence, CALD, mental health score); (2) genotypic resistance, OR 2.61; 95% CI 1.48–4.59; $p=0.001$ (adjusting for CALD); and (3) the co-morbidity score, OR 1.69; 95% CI 1.24–2.3; $p=0.001$ (adjusting for CALD, mental health score).

A low BMI was causally associated with genotypic resistance, OR 6.25; 95% CI 1.49–26.24; $p=0.012$ (adjusting for CALD).

Finally, Medicare eligibility was causally associated with the co-morbidity score, even when adjusting for CALD as a confounder, OR 2.21; 95% CI 1.24–3.95; $p=0.007$.

The final DAG model shows the significant predictors of adverse health outcomes supported by our data (Fig. 2). Notably, it identifies potential specific roles for multidisciplinary management of health predictors in virologically stable patients, underpinning our current model of HIV care.

Discussion

An audit of PLHIV attending our service revealed a significant number of NACs within this population. A mixture of medical conditions, mental health and social issues reflect the complexity of current management for this population. Within the Australian HIV Observational Database cohort, a recent review of people seen predominantly in general practice showed similar levels of NACs, with rates of depression and anxiety of 35 and 18%, respectively—which is consistent with our findings [7]. As expected in a publicly funded service such as ours, there is an over-representation of Medicare ineligible PLHIV and those with social disadvantage.

Similar scoring methods to assess patient complexity are used elsewhere in medicine. The Comprehensive Geriatric Assessment, for example, is 'a multidimensional, interdisciplinary diagnostic process to determine the medical, psychological, and functional capabilities of a frail elderly person in order to develop a coordinated and integrated plan for treatment and long-term follow-up' [8] and a global frailty scoring system for use in the elderly is well recognised [9]. In relation to PLHIV, our development of co-morbidity, mental health and social scores to quantify HIV patient complexity is similar to work conducted by Guaraldi et al. [10] who have developed scoring indices that specifically assess frailty amongst PLHIV.

DAGs can provide an understanding of the complex interrelationships between clinical, psychological and social factors with specific health outcomes and their use is well recognised in modern epidemiology [4]. DAGs have been used widely throughout clinical medicine to identify the minimum set of confounders in order to reduce bias in studies of assessing causation. Examples include nephrology [11], cardiology [12], feto-maternal medicine [13] and orthopaedics [14]. To our knowledge we are the first group to use DAG theory in a study of PLHIV. Our DAG analysis selected confounders and identified five predictors of poor health outcomes within our cohort: i.e., higher comorbidity score, higher mental health score, low social issue score, low BMI and eligibility for Medicare. The association between having a comorbidity and poor health outcomes seems logical, as does mental health issues and poor health outcomes where ARV compliance and health seeking behaviour may be compromised. The association between social deprivation and poor health is also well known across a range of chronic diseases. However, low BMI is difficult to explain when increasing BMI within the general population is associated with a number of chronic diseases such as diabetes, hypertension and cardiovascular disease. This finding may be related to past HIV wasting syndrome or current food insecurity and malnourishment amongst our patients.

The protective effect of being ineligible for Medicare and of CALD status against hospitalisation may seem paradoxical. It is likely that cost of diagnostic tests and hospitalisation are a barrier for our non-Medicare, CALD patients to attending hospital for all except life threatening events, or a reflection of these patients being generally younger within our cohort.

Limitations of this study include that it was conducted at a single site, possible sampling bias due to more unwell patients with NACs perhaps presenting more frequently to our service and not a GP and relatively small sample size and lack of an intervention to test the hypotheses generated. However, by using DAGs only the minimum set of confounders required were used in the analysis making out analyses sample size efficient. The method by which patient records were audited cannot eliminate selection bias but we believe our non-consecutive approach makes this less plausible. Also the complexity score has not been previously validated for use in HIV patients but follows the general principles of the Charlson score in that it accumulates points by body system. The complexity score also summates points without weightings for particular body systems in order to be transparent, easily interpretable and not data driven [6]. Our results cannot, however, be generalised to the entire Australian HIV cohort due to the limitations of the study and the particular patient demographics seen in our clinic.

The study demonstrated associations between mental health and social issues with medical outcomes, suggesting an ongoing need for a biopsychosocial model of multidisciplinary care to overcome the potential disadvantage of PLHIV.

Conclusion

Although ART has been simplified so that most patients need only take a single, effective and well-tolerated tablet per day, contemporary HIV management by clinicians is not simply a matter of prescribing ARVs and obtaining periodic blood tests for essentially healthy patients. PLHIV are living much longer and, on a background on chronic immune activation, are at increased risk for developing NACs from the interplay of medical, psychological and social factors that may influence long term health [15]. Mental health and social issues may adversely affect adherence to ARVs and clinic attendance, and lifestyle factors such as smoking, alcohol and recreational drug use can further affect the development and progression of some NACs such as cardiovascular disease. Publicly-funded HIV services play a pivotal role in providing a 'safety net' for disadvantaged and vulnerable PLHIV who cannot access private health care and require ARV and management of NACs. Engaging individuals with HIV in complex care management may reduce hospitalisation from HIV-related complications and prevent ongoing transmission.

Authors' contributions

DC: writing of manuscript, introduction, analysis and discussion of results. DS: designed the project concept, developed data collection tool, analysis and interpretation of results, writing manuscript. MD developed the database, analysed the data, undertook the regression models, constructed the DAG model, summarized the results, and helped edit the paper. VF contributed to the concept design including data collection form, data collection on designated patients, contribution to draft paper. RB contributed to the study design and interpretation of the data. JP edited the manuscript and assisted in the development of the data collection tool. AB developed the audit questionnaire after consultation with the core working group for this project. She also developed the database, conducted data analysis and contributed to the writing of the manuscript. All authors read and approved the final manuscript.

Author details

[1] Albion Centre, South Eastern Sydney Local Health District, Sydney, NSW 2010, Australia. [2] School of Public Health and Community Medicine, Faculty of Medicine, University of New South Wales, Sydney, NSW 2052, Australia. [3] Department of Infectious Diseases, Prince of Wales Hospital, South Eastern Sydney Local Health District, Sydney, NSW 2010, Australia. [4] Prince of Wales Clinical School, UNSW, Sydney, NSW 2051, Australia. [5] University of Sydney, Sydney, Australia.

Acknowledgements

Albion Centre is a facility of South Eastern Sydney Local Hospital Network.

Competing interests

The authors declare that they have no competing interests.

Funding

No additional funding was required for this work.

References

1. Weber R, Ruppik M, Rickenbach M, Spoerri A, Furrer H, Battegay M, et al. Decreasing mortality and changing patterns of causes of death in the Swiss HIV Cohort Study. HIV Med. 2013;14:195–207.
2. Phillips AN, Neaton J, Lundgren JD. The role of HIV in serious diseases other than AIDS. AIDS. 2008;22:2409–18.
3. Friis-Moller N, Weber R, Reiss P, Thiébaut R, Kirk O, d'Arminio Monforte A, et al. Cardiovascular disease risk factors in HIV patients—association with antiretroviral therapy. Results from the DAD study. AIDS. 2003;17:1179–93.
4. Shrier I, Platt RW. Reducing bias through directed acyclic graphs. BMC Med Res Methodol. 2008;8:70.
5. Pearl J. Causal inference from indirect experiments. Artif Intell Med. 1995;7:561–82.
6. Austin SR, Wong YN, Uzzo RG, Beck JR, Egleston BL. Why summary comorbidity measures such as the Charlson comorbidity index and Elixhauser score work. Med Care. 2015;53(9):e65–72.
7. Petoumenos K, Huang R, Hoy J, Bloch M, Templeton D, Baker D et al. APPLES—the australian positive & peers longevity evaluation study. In: Conference on retroviruses and opportunistic infections. 2017, Seattle.
8. Wieland D, Hirth V. Comprehensive geriatric assessment. Cancer Control. 2003;10(6):454–62.
9. Guaraldi G, Brothers TD, Zona S, Stentarelli C, Carli F, Malagoli A, et al. A frailty index predicts survival and incident multimorbidity independent of markers of HIV disease severity. AIDS. 2015;29(13):1633–41. https://doi.org/10.1097/qad.0000000000000753.
10. Rockwood K, Song X, MacKnight C, Bergman H, Hogan DB, McDowell I, Mitnitski A. A global clinical measure of fitness and frailty in elderly people. CMAJ. 2005;173(5):489–95.
11. Suttorp MM, Siegerink B, Jager KJ, Zoccali C, Friedo W, Dekker FW. Graphical presentation of confounding in directed acyclic graphs. Nephrol Dial Transplant. 2015;30(9):1418–23. https://doi.org/10.1093/ndt/gfu325.
12. Thornley S, Marshall RJ, Wells S, Jackson R. Using directed acyclic graphs for investigating causal paths for cardiovascular disease. J Biomet Biostat. 2013;4:182. https://doi.org/10.4172/2155-6180.1000182.
13. Pizzi C, De Stavola BL, Pearce N, Lazzarato F, Ghiotti P, Merletti F, et al. Selection bias and patterns of confounding in cohort studies: the case of the NINFEA web-based birth cohort. J Epidemiol Community Health. 2012;66(11):976–81. https://doi.org/10.1136/jech-2011-200065.
14. Thelaus A, Pettersson T, Gordon M, Krupic F, Sköldenberg O. A prospective observational cohort study on orthopaedic and anaesthetic registrars performing femoral nerve block on patients with an acute hip fracture. Surg Res Pract. 2016. https://doi.org/10.1155/2016/7512360.
15. Lau B, Gange, Stephen J, Moore R. Risk of non-AIDS-related mortality may exceed risk of AIDS-related mortality among individuals enrolling into care with CD4 + counts greater than 200 cells/mm3. J Acquir Immune Defic Syndr. 2007;44(2):179–87.

20

Multivariate analysis of covariates of adherence among HIV-positive mothers with low viral suppression

Tamara Nsubuga-Nyombi[1], Simon Sensalire[1*], Esther Karamagi[1], Judith Aloyo[1], John Byabagambi[1], Mirwais Rahimzai[1], Linda Kisaakye Nabitaka[2] and Jacqueline Calnan[3]

Abstract

Background: As part of efforts to improve the prevention of mother-to-child transmission in Northern Uganda, we explored reasons for poor viral suppression among 122 pregnant and lactating women who were in care, received viral load tests, but had not achieved viral suppression and had more than 1000 copies/mL. Understanding the patient factors associated with low viral suppression was of interest to the Ministry of Health to guide the development of tools and interventions to achieve viral suppression for pregnant and lactating women newly initiating on ART as well as those on ART with unsuppressed viral load.

Methods: A facility-based cross-sectional and mixed methods study design was used, with retrospective medical record review. We assessed 122 HIV-positive mothers with known low viral suppression across 31 health facilities in Northern Uganda. Adjusted odds ratios were used to determine the covariates of adherence among HIV positive mothers using logistic regression. A study among health care providers shed further light on predictors of low viral suppression and a history of low early retention. This study was part of a larger national evaluation of the performance of integrated care services for mothers.

Results: Adherence defined as taking antiretroviral medications correctly everyday was low at 67.2%. The covariates of low adherence are: taking other medications in addition to ART, missed appointments in the past 6 months, experienced violence in the past 6 months, and faces obstacles to treatment. Mothers who were experiencing each of these covariates were less likely to adhere to treatment. These covariates were triangulated with perspectives of health providers as covariates of low adherence and included: long distances to health facility, missed appointments, running out of pills, sharing antiretroviral drugs, violence, and social lifestyles such as multiple sexual partners coupled with non-disclosure to partners. Inadequate counseling, stigma, and lack of client identity are the frontline factors accounting for the early loss of mothers from care.

Conclusions: Adherence of 67% was low for reliable viral suppression and accounts for the low viral suppression among HIV-positive mothers studied, in absence of any other factors. This study provided insights into the covariates for low adherence to ART and low viral load suppression; these covariates included taking other medications in addition to ART, missed appointments in the past 6 months, feels like giving up, doesn't have someone with whom to share private concerns, experienced violence in the past 6 months, and faces obstacles to treatment and confirmed by health providers. To improve adherence, we recommend use of a screening tool to identify mothers with any of these covariates so that more intensive adherence support can be provided to these mothers.

Keywords: Low viral suppression, Retention, Mothers, ART

*Correspondence: ssensalire@urc-chs.com

[1] USAID Applying Science To Strengthen and Improve Systems (ASSIST) Project, USAID, University Research Co., LLC, Plot 40, Ntinda II Road, P.O. Box 28745, Kampala, Uganda

Background

Human immunodeficiency virus (HIV) causes a chronic infection that leads to a progressive disease. Without treatment, most persons with HIV develop acquired immunodeficiency syndrome (AIDS) within 10 years of infection, which results in HIV transmission to sex partners, substantial morbidity, and eventually death [1]. Testing identifies infected persons and is the entry point to a continuum of HIV health care and social services that improve health outcomes, including survival. This continuum includes diagnosis (HIV testing), linkage to and retention in continuous medical care for HIV, prevention counseling and other services that reduce transmission, and consistent antiretroviral therapy (ART) for viral suppression [1].

While the ultimate goal of ART is to reduce HIV-related morbidity and mortality, the initial goal is full and durable viral suppression. Full viral suppression allows for utmost reconstitution or maintenance of immune function and minimizes the emergence of drug-resistant viruses caused by ongoing replication in the presence of antiretroviral drugs. The current guidelines in Uganda define viral suppression as reducing the function and replication of the HIV virus to fewer than 1000 copies/mL [2]. In addition to reducing HIV-associated morbidity and mortality for the individual patient, viral suppression is an important goal for epidemic control at the population level, since when viral suppression is achieved and maintained, HIV transmission is substantially decreased [2].

In general, people with HIV need to use a combined antiretroviral therapy also known as highly active antiretroviral therapy (HAART) to achieve long-term viral suppression. Combination ART is necessary because HIV can mutate when a single drug (also referred to as monotherapy) is used. Sometimes, a particular ART regimen cannot help an HIV-positive patient achieve an undetectable viral load. In such cases, new combinations of drugs need to be tried until full viral suppression is achieved [3].

The World Health Organization recommends viral load testing as the preferred method for monitoring the clinical response to ART of people living with HIV infection (PLHIV). Viral load monitoring of patients on ART helps ensure early identification and confirmation of ART failure and enables clinicians to take an appropriate course of action for patient management.

While the ultimate goal of ART is to reduce HIV-related morbidity and mortality, the initial goal is full and durable viral suppression. Long-term viral suppression requires near-perfect adherence to antiretroviral medications [3]. Other factors include genetic differences in drug metabolism, severe baseline immune suppression, prior drug resistance, and concurrent opportunistic infections. In practice, highly consistent adherence requires a patient on a twice-daily regimen not to miss or substantially delay more than three doses of antiretroviral medications per month [4] and as few as one dose per month if the regimen consists of a once-daily backbone drug. This degree of adherence is far greater than that commonly associated with other chronic diseases and is quite difficult for most patients to maintain over the course of a lifelong illness [4].

In Uganda, despite being an early success story in the reduction of HIV infection rates, there are myriad challenges in the recent era of accelerated ART scale-up, including low viral suppression among PLHIV on antiretroviral drugs, with adherence being a major predictor. Ongoing vulnerabilities of poverty, famine, inadequate monitoring of clients on ART, stigma, and violence compound treatment-related costs and concerns [5].

With funding support from the U.S. President's Emergency Plan for AIDS Relief (PEPFAR), the United States Agency for International Development (USAID) Applying Science to Strengthen and Improve Systems (ASSIST) Project supported interventions for the elimination and prevention of mother-to-child transmission of HIV (PMTCT) through quality improvement activities in PMTCT implementing sites in Northern Uganda. Under this initiative, Ministry of Health (MoH) PMTCT sites were supported to monitor viral load in HIV-positive mothers on ART, retain these mothers in care, and maintain adherence to treatment in order to reduce the risk of transmission to their HIV-exposed babies. Facility teams identified mothers who were eligible for viral load testing and to ensure follow-up for those with low viral suppression. Health workers were trained to interpret viral load results and provide intensive adherence counselling for mothers that were not suppressing. Community-based linkage facilitators were also trained to provide health education for adherence and follow up mothers in the community so as to keep them in care. Linkage facilitators also identified mothers who give birth in the community and referred them for HIV testing so as to initiate those positive on ART.

In December 2016, results generated from the MoH central public health laboratory showed that 217 pregnant and lactating women receiving care in health facilities in 15 districts of Northern Uganda had not achieved viral suppression and had viral load values of more than 1000 copies/mL. The present study was carried out to gain further insight into the reasons for non-viral load suppression amongst HIV-positive pregnant and lactating women in Northern Uganda in order to inform improvement interventions to increase viral load suppression in this particularly vulnerable population.

Adherence in this study was operationally defined to mean taking antiretroviral medication correctly every day.

Methods

Study subjects

The study was conducted among 122 HIV-positive pregnant and lactating mothers known to have low or no viral suppression based on the results of their most recent viral load test results. The current guidelines in Uganda define viral suppression as reducing the function and replication of the HIV virus to fewer than 1000 copies/mL. Mothers who had not attained viral suppression as per these guidelines were therefore considered to have low or no viral suppression for purposes of this study. Study participants were identified from 13 health facilities in 15 districts of Northern Uganda where the USAID ASSIST Project was supporting PMTCT services. All HIV-positive pregnant women known in these 13 facilities to have low viral suppression and were present at the study sites at the time of the study were included. Additional information was collected through focus group discussions with health care providers and linkage facilitators connected to these 13 facilities, to understand their perceptions of the underlying causes of low viral load suppression, non-adherence, and low early retention among their clients.

Study design

The evaluation was a facility-based, cross-sectional study with retrospective medical record review for the study subjects for whom medical records could be located. The study utilized a mixed methods approach to enrich information to inform improvement strategies and the development of tools to address the covariates of low adherence responsible for low viral suppression. Cross-sectional data was collected through interviews with the identified HIV-positive mothers with low viral suppression on factors identified from the literature underlying low early retention in care. Focus group discussions were conducted with service providers to obtain their perspectives on predictors of low viral suppression. Retrospective data was collected for 68 of the 122 subjects on recorded adherence at the time of taking the viral load sample, clinical failure in the past 12 months, and immunological failure in the past 12 months. This constituted the sample whose records could be located at the facility at the time of the study.

Data collection

The structured interview questionnaire asked about mothers' socio-economic and demographic characteristics, HIV disclosure, social support and isolation, stigma and discrimination, treatment with ARVs and other drugs including traditional medicine, adherence to treatment, length of treatment, exposure to violence, and satisfaction with the adequacy of ART preparation counseling.

Focus group discussions (FGDs) with health care providers and linkage facilitators in the care of PLHIV obtained information on the category of mothers who have low viral suppression, the underlying causes of low viral suppression and low early retention, adherence to treatment, reasons for non-adherence, and suggestions on addressing low viral suppression, non-adherence, and low early retention within the facility context. A total of eight FGDs were conducted and comprised of both male and female health care providers and community linkage facilitators from different level facilities. Retrospective data was extracted from patient files and covered clinical assessments for clinical failure, immunological failure, treatment regimen, and adherence at the time of taking last viral load test.

Analysis

Quantitative data was analyzed using SPSS 16 and comprised of participant interviews and clinical records data. Univariate analysis was conducted to describe clinical records data related with adherence. Multivariate analysis was carried out to estimate covariates of adherence among HIV-positive mothers with low viral suppression. To assess the effect sizes of covariates of adherence, we analyzed data from the participant interviews using logistic regression model. The effect size of the covariates and strength of association was depicted using the adjusted odds ratios (AOR). Necessary model diagnostics and exploratory data analysis were checked at the respective stages of the analysis.

Focus group discussions with health care providers were transcribed verbatim into full text and coded using a thematic analysis. The quotations included in the text best represented the range of ideas voiced around key themes. The quotations were carefully edited without altering the meaning. To maintain anonymity, these quotes are identified by place of discussion only.

Ethical considerations

This study was reviewed and approved in accordance with the guidelines for conducting research and was part of a wider study of mothers under integrated care. It was reviewed by an approved local Institutional Review Board, and the Uganda National Council of Science and Technology. Administrative clearances were obtained from district health management teams and from the community leaders within the intervention areas. Participation was entirely voluntary, and consent was based on full information about the study and intervention.

Table 1 Characteristics of HIV-positive mothers

Socio-demographic information	Number (n = 22)	Percentage
Age		
15–24	26	21.3
25–29	28	23.0
30–34	67	54.9
45+	1	0.8
Level of education		
None	31	25.4
Primary	81	66.4
O level	10	8.2
Marital status		
Married	78	63.9
Single	10	8.2
Divorced/separated	22	18.0
Widowed	12	9.8
Has non-regular partner	28	23
Distance from home to the health facility		
Less than a km	10	8.2
2–3 km	19	15.6
4–5 km	27	22.1
6–10 km	19	15.6
More than 10 km	47	38.5
Cost of each visit to the facility		
Less than $0.2	2	1.6
Between $0.2 and $0.6	19	15.6
$0.8–$1.4	23	18.9
$1.6–$2.7	34	27.9
More than $2.7	30	24.6
Walks to the facility	14	11.5
Lives with other people in household		
Lives alone	3	2.5
Lives with other people above 5 years	199	97.5
Victim of violence in last 6 months		
Yes	63	51.6
No	59	48.4
Takes alcohol		
Yes	20	16.4
No	102	83.6

Results

Profile of HIV-positive mothers

The majority (78%) of the HIV-positive mothers interviewed were aged 25–34. They were largely illiterate with primary education (66.4%). More than half of them (54.1%) traveled 6 km or more to the health facility for treatment. Of these, 38.5% travelled as far as between 10 and 20 km to the health facility and spent at least 1.6 US dollars on transport alone for each visit to the facility. Almost all of these women lived with someone aged above 5 years (98%). They were predominantly married (63.9%). However, 23% of all mothers had non-regular partner in the past 12 months preceding the study. This was corroborated by health providers and linkage facilitators, who indicated that the majority of these mothers were in unstable relationships and/or multiple sexual relationships. More than half (51.6%) of mothers had experienced some form of violence in the last 6 months and 16% take alcohol. These results are contained in Table 1.

Table 2 provides information on use of ART and traditional medicine among mothers with low viral suppression. Results in Table 2 show that only 67% of the mothers were taking ARVs daily and about 19% were taking ARVs along with other medicines, including traditional medicine/local herbs (8.2%). Close to a quarter of the mothers with low viral suppression had changed ARVs since starting on treatment and 18% of all mothers had been admitted in the hospital in the past 1 year preceding the study.

The study investigated early retention of mothers in care so as to determine its effect on low viral suppression. Early retention was operationally defined to mean retention in care for the first 3 months after enrollment for ART. We found out that only 22.1% (n = 27) of the mothers studied had dropped out of treatment with 3 months after initiation on ART.

Table 2 Consistence in the use of ARVs and traditional medicine

Medication	Number (n = 122)	Percentage
Frequency with which ARVs are taken		
Everyday	82	67.2
Not every day	40	32.8
Taking other medication with ARVs		
Yes	23	18.9
No	99	81.1
Takes traditional medicine and ARVs		
Yes	10	8.2
No	112	91.8
Changed ARVs since starting ART		
Yes	29	23.8
No	93	76.2
Fall out of treatment 3 months after initiation on ART		
Yes	27	22.1
No	95	77.9
Admitted in hospital in the past 1 year		
Yes	22	18.0
No	100	82.0

Clinical characteristics of the study participants

During the assessment, we extracted clinical data from patient records for only 68 of the 122 mothers due to documentation gaps. The findings are contained in Table 3. We found that 41% of the mothers out of the 68 whose clinical data was extracted, were on tenofovir, lamivudine, and efavirenz (TDF–3TC–EFV) at the time of taking the last viral load measurement.

Eighty-three percent (83%) of the mothers (n = 122) received adherence counselling before initiation on ART including the common side effects of ARV drugs while they received the drugs. Close to 54% of mothers had missed appointments in the last 6 months. Only 78% of the 55 mothers whose adherence charts were accessed at the time of the interview recorded good adherence. Close to 43% had immunological failure. Nearly three quarters of mothers had taken ARVs for more than 3 years.

Covariates of low viral suppression

Multivariate analysis examined the association between the different characteristics of mothers and adherence. We used adherence to treatment as the common predictor to low viral suppression, as in the case of studies in other jurisdictions [3]. In this study adherence was operationally defined to mean taking drugs every day as prescribed by the health worker. Results in Table 4 indicate that the covariates of low adherence are: taking other medications in addition to ART, missed appointments in the past 6 months, feels like giving up, and experienced violence in the past 6 months ($p \leq 0.05$).

Specifically, HIV-positive mothers who were not taking other medications were six times more likely to adhere to treatment than those who were taking other medication alongside ARVs ($p < 0.001$). We further found out that HIV-positive mothers who had missed their appointments in the past 6 months were two times more likely not to adhere to treatment than those who had not missed their appointment ($p = 0.001$). Mothers who felt like giving up on taking ARVs were almost five times more likely not to adhere to treatment than those who stated expressed no desire to stop medication. Similarly, mothers who experienced some form of violence in the last 6 months were three times more likely not to adhere to treatment than those who never experienced violence.

Table 3 Clinical characteristics of study participants

Clinical information	Frequency	Percent
Patient regimen at the time of taking last viral load	n = 68	
AZT/3TC/NVP	15	12.3
TDF/3TC/EFV	50	41.0
TDF/3TC/NVP	2	1.6
AZT/3TC/EFV	1	0.8
Received adherence counseling before ART	n = 122	
Yes	101	82.8
No	21	17.2
Recorded adherence on the chart at the time of taking the viral load	n = 55	
Good	43	78.2
Poor	12	21.8
Missed appointments in the last 1 year	n = 122	
Yes	65	53.7
No	57	46.3
Clinical failure in the last 12 months	n = 54	
Yes	5	9.3
No	49	90.7
Immunological failure	n = 54	
Yes	23	42.6
No	31	57.4
Duration on ART	n = 122	
Less than 3 years	40	32.8
3–5 years	39	32.0
More than 5 years	43	35.2

Provider perspectives

The results of the focus group discussions with health care providers and linkage facilitators complemented the quantitative survey of HIV-positive mothers and shed further light on its findings. The thematic analysis suggested a range of factors which negatively influenced adherence to ART and put low viral suppression into perspective.

Health care provider description of mothers with low viral suppression

The characteristics of mothers with low viral suppression was one of the most discussed themes under the study. FGD participants mainly described them as; illiterate, with poor economic backgrounds and who survive on selling food stuffs, lacking support of their husbands, in unstable relationships and having multiple sexual partners and/or marriages and therefore hardly reside in one place, having many children, inconsistently taking their medication because of lack of food or drug stock-out, sharing antiretroviral drugs with husbands or peers, having not disclosed their HIV status to their partners and therefore discreetly taking drugs or not at all, never coming to the facility for scheduled appointments, experiencing different forms of torture and violence, living far away from the health facilities, and mainly in late adolescence.

These comments resonate with the social demographic characteristics described in Table 1 and can be validated by one or more of the following quotations of the FGD participants:

Table 4 Covariates of low viral suppression among HIV-positive mothers

Background information	Adherent *n* (%)	Non-adherent *n* (%)	Sig	Adjusted (odds ratios)
Mother is taking other medication alongside ARVs				
Yes[a]	12 (52.2)	11 (47.8)	0.000	1.000
No	70 (70.7)	29 (29.3)		6.044
Received adherence counseling before ART				
Yes[a]	71 (70.3)	30 (29.7)	0.527	1.000
No	11 (52.4)	10 (47.6)		0.790
Mothers feels was adequately prepared to start ART				
Yes[a]	63 (71.6)	25 (28.4)	0.178	1.000
No	19 (55.9)	15 (44.1)		0.572
Missed appointments in the last 6 months				
Yes[a]	35 (53.8)	30 (46.2)	0.001	1.000
No	47 (82.5)	10 (17.5)		2.707
Treated differently since disclosing HIV status				
Yes[a]	25 (58.1)	18 (41.9)	0.201	1.000
No	57 (73.1)	21 (26.9)		1.287
There are instances when mother feels like giving up with ARVs				
Yes[a]	12 (50)	12 (50)	0.030	1.000
No	70 (71.4)	28 (28.6)		4.867
Has someone to share with private concerns				
Yes[a]	65 (71.4)	26 (28.6)	0.90	1.000
No	16 (53.3)	14 (46.7)		0.627
Experience violence in the last 6 months				
Yes[a]	34 (54.0)	29 (46.0)	0.053	1.000
No	48 (81.4)	11 (18.6)		2.931
Mother has obstacles to treatment				
Yes[a]	48 (59.3)	33 (40.7)	0.11	1.000
No	34 (82.9)	7 (17.1)		0.299

[a] Reference category

"Some [of the mothers] don't have real husbands. They are up and down. That's why you will not get them easily because they are not in one place," FGD participant, Nwoya.

"Most of them [mothers] lack support of their partners, most of them are not educated and earn a living by selling food stuff that they grow," FGD participant, Nwoya.

"Many of the newly initiated mothers [on ART] have disclosure problems and sometimes don't disclose their [HIV] status to their spouses," FGD participant, Kitgum.

"These are mothers who have not disclosed their [HIV positive] status to their husbands. They are mothers whose husbands are not aware that their wives are taking drugs…," FGD participant, Lira

"Mothers come from poor families. They lack transport and move on foot. They take drugs on empty stomach. There is gender based violence, [and when] husband chases the woman away, [and] they never come back for refill. Some would [could] stay 2 months without refill," FGD participant, Gulu.

Health care provider adherence assessment

The practice of assessing adherence had mixed responses. Some providers reported making use of appointment dates or pill count if the mother comes with a bottle, while others depended on self-recall by the mother on the number pills left. In some cases, providers reported to use both methods concurrently. However, it was also common for health providers to qualify their statements by adding that the heavy workload and long queues made it difficult for them to count pills as a way of assessing adherence.

At a FGD in Awach, all providers agreed that the adherence rating on record in the registers was not accurate because it was not based on real adherence analysis but rather on the provider's quick guess for purposes of recording. This was not so different with other providers elsewhere who mostly attributed this to the workload on any particular clinic day. There was mention that adherence cards which were used to assess adherence in the past are now stocked out. The following quotations support these findings.

> *"We ask mothers to come with the remaining pills, but majority do not come with their pills and in this case, we use appointment dates,"* FGD participant, Lira.

> *"The good or fair assessment of adherence in registers is not real because we don't delve into pill count because of the large numbers [of clients]...,"* FGD participant, Gulu.

> *"From the ART card there is that column for adherence where if a mother comes for refill we normally ask them looking at the appointment. Then we ask them of the number of the pills they have swallowed,"* FGD participant, Apac.

Health care provider experiences with adherence

Health care providers commonly shared, on the basis of their own experience, that mothers miss their appointments and therefore run out of medicine, they share drugs between themselves and/or with their husbands when either party is unable to come to the facility, and that they stop taking drugs whenever they get new unsuspecting partners. Participants often cited various forms of distress including violence from husbands as prohibitive to mothers taking drugs. It was common for health care providers to state that mothers miss taking drugs especially when they have travelled away, while others think they have recovered from ill health and need not take drugs anymore. The following quotations represent the most common sentiments of providers with regard to mothers' adherence.

> *"I have one mother who told me that her husband does not allow her to take her medicine. So she hides and whenever the man discovers that she has the drugs he throws it in the pit latrine. And right now she has shifted to her mother's place,"* FGD participant, Apac.

> *"Some mothers think they are healthy. So [they see] no need to take ARVs. When they get psychological reconstruction, they feel they are healthy,"* FGD participant, Gulu.

> *"Poor adherence [is a result of] some of the women combine [combining] drugs for morning and evening and take [taking] them once in the evening,"* FGD participant, Kitgum.

Health care provider perspectives on non-viral suppression

A key area of exploration in the qualitative component of the study was to obtain providers' perspectives about why mothers were not suppressing. Common reasons why the respondents believed mothers don't suppress included: missing appointments and dropping out of care for some time without close monitoring, taking drugs erratically on the account of recovery and good health, torture and violence from their partners, or over time, failing to respond well to the medication. Long distances to the health facility and lack of transport also keep mothers away from care. The shortage of food affects drug use, as mothers will not take drugs on an empty stomach. Similarly, negative perceptions about ARVs, mothers experiencing side effects and stopping taking the drugs, or using them occasionally as and when they feel unwell, and stigma and discrimination keep clients in self-denial and affect adherence and appointments. Representative comments from providers in this regard:

> *"...there's one who stays in [the] village, [and doesn't follow appointment. She feels cured when she feels her body is fine. That's what she always says,"* FGD participant, Apac.

> *"Most of them don't have supportive husbands. They [husbands] want to take their drugs [away from them claiming that]. .....That this transport you are wasting you can use for paying [school fees for] children in school after all you will still die even if you swallow the medicine,"* FGD participant, Apac.

> *"I have a client who kept piling her drugs because [she] believed that the drug will [would] kill her,"* FGD participant, Lira.

> *"Other mothers mistake Septrin for ARVs such that they are confidently swallowing cotrimoxazole in place of ARVs e.g. [we see this] when they run out of stock,"* FGD participant, Lira.

> *"...Pill burden, especially for those with other OIs [opportunistic infections] like TB,"* FGD participant, Kitgum.

Provider's perspectives on early retention

We inquired from health care providers why mothers drop out of care just 3 months after initiation on ART. They identified as contributing factors, that mothers lack proper identifying information for follow-up and non-disclosure to their partners for fear of reprimand, violence or separation. The following quotes provide an account of this phenomenon:

> *"They use common names in villages like maama John, and follow-up is not easy [with such names],"* FGD participant, Gulu.

> *"Disclosure to husband will cause divorce and cause mother [to] move back [be chased away] to her parents. So she keeps quiet and disappears [from routine care],"* FGD participant, Apac.

Results of the study among HIV-positive mothers revealed that 17% of the 122 mothers never received adherence counseling before initiation on ART. This was confirmed by providers as follows:

> *"Sometimes midwives counsel them, but not to [their] expectation, especially that the [HIV] positive person needs a lot of time,"* FGD participant, Gulu.

> *"It's the pregnancy that will lead them [to] know their status and once they know, it's shocking and [they end up] leave [leaving] the facility. HIV status is detected only during ANC so it's a shocking moment,"* FGD participant, Gulu.

> *"Some mothers will enter denial stage and go to another health facility. So one client can be registered twice, [and this is] common in town,"* FGD participant, Kitgum.

> *"[They have for the] Disbelief of the results and [they] will deny the results and they will go away....,"* FGD participant, Gulu.

Discussion of results

This study collected data on different variables from HIV-positive mothers with known low viral suppression only, since looking at these characteristics in all HIV-positive women would bias results; given that their characteristics may not be similar or have the same distribution in the women with good viral suppression.

Unfortunately, the rate of adherence in our sample was significantly lower (67.2%) than has been observed in many other studies in Africa, even when it was self-reported adherence. For example, a study on adherence and low viral response in Kisumu, Kenya found adherence at 87.1% among women on Option B+ [6]. Many factors identified in this study would explain this problem. While socio-economic factors in this study are consistent with other literature in influencing adherence, the majority of our sample comprised a relatively young population with unique characteristics.

Up to 23% of women in this study had multiple sexual partners. This was corroborated by health care providers that most women who have not achieved the required suppression have unstable relationships and were less likely to disclose their HIV status to their non-regular partners for fear of breakdown of their relationship. They were more prone to violence and vulnerable to discrimination by others even before the effect of other socio-economic conditions that generally affect women on ARVs. These could be termed as frontline factors, both of which could be used to explain this finding and were corroborated by the health care providers.

The cultural context in Northern Uganda, a post-conflict region, is such that women are sexual subordinates and most often responsible for care of the household and children, and as a consequence, these practical barriers may adversely affect adherence among women. Perhaps, these among other factors, make the sample not comparable with women in other studies whose socio-economic variables could have different levels of influence on treatment adherence.

Another key adherence barrier raised during the interviews included violence from their partners. Our findings reinforce the importance of partner counseling, including obtaining remedies for victims of violence whenever they exceed the confines of counseling.

Adherence counseling prior to initiation of ART was associated with consistency in taking drugs. It was further discovered that mothers who had missed appointments in the last 6 months were more than two times less likely to adhere to their treatment than HIV-positive mothers who never missed their appointments at all. Adherence counseling before ART is one way to determine readiness to start treatment, diagnosing and addressing stigma, depression, and initiating a patient-provider relationship to even understand the patient better [7]. Such a missed opportunity has long-term effects that would not be reversed when clients slowly become complacent to treatment.

Even HIV-positive mothers who were treated discriminately since disclosure of their HIV status were only slightly less likely to take their drugs consistently as compared to those who were not discriminated/stigmatized. It is possible that patients with limited literacy might be reluctant to ask others for the kind of help they need to take their medicines correctly. Better-educated patients who are convinced of ART efficacy, perhaps as a result of educational programs, show a propensity towards better adherence [8]. Therefore, adherence interventions among our sample which was predominantly illiterate need to consider these factors when reinforcing continuing adherence practices. It may be necessary to schedule follow-ups that are more frequent, monitor adherence more closely, and ensure that education and discussions take place in a safe environment.

Patients' beliefs, knowledge, and expectations regarding treatment strongly influence medical decision making [9]. Our findings from both mothers and health care providers showed that a few mothers believed that ARVs kill, are like any other medication such as Panadol, or have the same effect as cotrimoxazole prophylaxis or even think that one can take substitute ARVs with Septrin. Therefore, misconceptions towards the disease and treatment regimens could explain the poor therapeutic outcomes that in turn may impede achievement of optimal levels of adherence. However, this argument is limited by the fact that this study did not ascertain whether the mothers had received health education on PMTCT, an important aspect that could have influenced mother's beliefs, knowledge and expectations regarding treatment as well as adherence to ART.

Although ART is free of charge throughout Uganda's public health system, there are ART-associated costs such as expenses in transport and food. These obstacles were cited by mothers and corroborated by health care providers. Mothers cited skipping medication because of lack of food or went without medication because they could not reach the health facility. This is consistent with other studies which have linked costs with poor adherence to treatment [6].

A study in Botswana showed that adherence was higher when cost was not an obstacle and that poor patients were able to achieve excellent rates of adherence when they had access to free laboratory monitoring and subsidized ART [10]. This is a useful finding, and it is important that policy makers use this information to introduce outreach programs for ART to cut key costs associated with transport.

In the FGDs, participants raised the issue that mothers were worried of disclosing their status to partners for fear of losing them. As such they either take drugs in hiding or cease taking them completely. Like many other studies, non-disclosure of HIV status was associated with poorer adherence. Our findings suggest unless mothers disclose, they cannot effectively take their drugs. This could perhaps explain the high rates of missed appointments (53.7%). This is a fundamental issue that disclosure health education and individual counselling sessions should embrace with utmost importance.

Distance to health facilities was a common cause of missed appointments, as was drug stock-out as reported by mothers and validated by health care providers in the FGDs. Over half of the mothers come as far as 10 or more kilometers to the health facilities and find the transport cost prohibitive. This coupled with the seasonal deterioration of poorer roads during the rainy season makes it even harder to access facilities. Deliberate outreaches in hard-to-reach areas would offset this limitation as much as possible.

ART regimens have toxicities and adverse side effects that vary from mild to severe and acute to chronic, which can prevent adherence [11]. Our study revealed that both mothers and health care providers cited side effects as one of the key barriers to taking medication promptly. This is worsened by the scarcity of food to support treatment. Adherence counseling together with follow-up and clinical support for mothers, especially at early initiation onto ART, would help guide mothers on how to cope with side effects. These may be tackled by informing patients in advance what side effects to expect and how they might be managed, as well as prescribing antiemetic or anti-diarrheal agents to alleviate these side effects.

Food was an important barrier to medication in this study. Previous research has shown a relationship between food insecurity (uncertain access to safe and nutritious food) and lower rates of viral suppression among ART-treated patients in the US and Uganda. Pregnant and breastfeeding women may be especially vulnerable to food insecurity and insufficiency [12].

Conclusions

Adherence of 67.2% among mothers with low viral suppression in this study is very low. The main covariates were distance to travel to health facility leading to missed appointments and running out of drugs, sharing antiretroviral drugs, drug side effects, lack of pre-ART counseling, gender-based violence, social lifestyles such as multiple sexual partners, non-disclosure to partners, and stigma and discrimination. Qualitative findings from providers corroborated these findings. To improve the quality of care provided to mothers, the information from this study can be used to screen pregnant women and lactating mothers on ART for any of the factors strongly associated with low adherence to ART (and thus low viral load suppression) and then provide support through intensive adherence counselling and self-management or peer-to-peer support.

Abbreviations

ART: antiretroviral therapy; ARVs: antiretroviral drugs; AIDS: acquired immune deficiency syndrome; ASSIST: Applying Science to Strengthen and Improve Systems; AZT: zidovudine; CDC: Centers of Disease Control and Prevention;

CD4: cluster of differentiation 4-positive cell; CI: confidence interval; EFV: efavirenz; EPIDATA: epidemiological data version 3; EMTCT: elimination of mother-to-child transmission; EID: early infant diagnosis; FGD: focus group discussion; HAART: highly active antiretroviral therapy; HIV: human immunodeficiency virus; HC: Health Center; HCT: HIV counseling and testing; 3TC: lamivudine; MTCT: mother-to-child transmission; MOH: Ministry of Health; NVP: nevirapine; OR: odds ratio; PEPFAR: U.S. President's Emergency Plan for AIDS Relief; PLHIV: people living with HIV/AIDS; PMTCT: prevention of mother-to-child transmission; TDF: tenofovir; UNAIDS: Joint United Nations Programme on HIV/AIDS; USAID: United States Agency for International Development.

Authors' contributions

LNK gave strategic direction to have this study conducted. SS perceived the study, conducted the study, performed the statistical analysis and drafted the manuscript. TNN participated in the design of the study and reviewed the manuscript. JA, EK, MR, JB, JC reviewed the manuscript. All authors critically appraised and reviewed the manuscript submitted for publication. All authors read and approved the final manuscript.

Author details

[1] USAID Applying Science To Strengthen and Improve Systems (ASSIST) Project, USAID, University Research Co., LLC, Plot 40, Ntinda II Road, P.O. Box 28745, Kampala, Uganda. [2] Ministry of Health, Kampala, Uganda. [3] United States Agency for International Development (USAID), Kampala, Uganda.

Acknowledgements

We sincerely thank all the participants in the study and the district and health facility for the administrative clearance to conduct the study for their support. Support for this work was provided by PEPFAR through USAID. The authors acknowledge the HIV positive mothers who participated in the study.

Competing interests

The authors declare that they have no competing interests.

Funding

This study and the intervention described were made possible by the support of the American people through PEPFAR and USAID, through the USAID Applying Science to Strengthen and Improve Systems (ASSIST) Project, implemented by University Research Co., LLC under Cooperative Agreement Number AID-OAA-A-12-00101.

References

1. Centers for Disease Control and Prevention. Vital signs: HIV prevention through care and treatment—United States. MMWR Morb Mortal Wkly Rep. 2011;60(47):1618–23.
2. Ng'ambi WF, Tweya H, Speight C, Man-Bourdon C, Hosseinpour M, Phiri S. Determinants of antiretroviral treatment adherence among women accessing PMTCT "Option B+": a retrospective study at Bwaila Hospital, Malawi. In: IAS conference on HIV pathogenesis, treatment and prevention, 30 June–03 July 2013-Kuala Lumpur, Malaysia.
3. Engell CA, Pham VP, Holzman RS, Aberg JA. Virologic outcome of using tenofovir/emtricitabine to treat hepatitis B in HIV-coinfected patients. ISRN Gastroenterol. 2011; 2011:405390.
4. Mannheimer S, Friedland G, Matts J, Child C, Chesney M. The consistency of adherence to antiretroviral therapy predicts biologic outcomes for human immunodeficiency virus-infected persons in clinical trials. Clin Infect Dis. 2002;34(8):1115–21.
5. Winchester MS. Synergistic vulnerabilities: antiretroviral treatment among women in Uganda. Glob Public Health. 2015;10(7):881–94. https://doi.org/10.1080/17441692.2015.1007468.
6. Okonji JA. CD4, viral load response, and adherence among antiretroviral-naive breast-feeding women receiving triple antiretroviral prophylaxis for prevention of mother-to-child transmission. JAIDS J Acquir Immune Defic Syndr. 2012;61(2):249–57.
7. Simoni JM, Amico KR, Pearson CR, Malow R. Strategies for promoting adherence to antiretroviral therapy: a review of the literature. Curr Infect Dis Rep. 2008;10(6):515–21.
8. Johnson VR, Jacobson KL, Gazmararian JA, Blake SC. Does social support help limited-literacy patients with medication adherence?: a mixed methods study of patients in the Pharmacy Intervention for Limited Literacy (PILL) study 2010. Patient Educ Couns. 2010;79(1):14–24. https://doi.org/10.1016/j.pec.2009.07.002 **(Epub 2009 Aug 3)**.
9. Adam BD, Maticka-Tyndale E, Cohen JJ. Adherence practices among people living with HIV. AIDS Care. 2003;15:263–74.
10. Weiser S, Wolfe W, Bangsberg D, Thior I, Gilbert P, et al. Barriers to antiretroviral adherence for patients living with HIV infection and AIDS in Botswana. J Acquir Immune Defic Syndr. 2003;34:281–8.
11. Catz SL, Kelly JA, Bogart LM, Benotsch EG, McAuliffe TL. Patterns, correlates, and barriers to medication adherence among persons prescribed new treatments for HIV disease. Health Psychol. 2000;19(2):124–33.
12. Kobin AB, Sheth NU. Levels of adherence required for virologic suppression among newer antiretroviral medications. Ann Pharmacother. 2011;45(3):372–9 **(Epub 2011/03/10)**.

21

CD4/CD8 ratio normalization rates and low ratio as prognostic marker for non-AIDS defining events among long-term virologically suppressed people living with HIV

Win Min Han[1*], Tanakorn Apornpong[1], Stephen J. Kerr[1,2], Akarin Hiransuthikul[1], Sivaporn Gatechompol[1], Tanya Do[1], Kiat Ruxrungtham[1,2] and Anchalee Avihingsanon[1,2]

Abstract

Background: Immune restoration is often incomplete after ART in HIV patients, both quantitatively and qualitatively. We studied the incidence and probability of CD4/CD8 normalization in an adult Thai HIV cohort and explored the predictive value of the ratio for developing of non-AIDS defining events (NAEs).

Methods: We analyzed data from HIV-infected Thai adults between 1996 and 2017 in the HIV-NAT 006 prospective long-term cohort in Bangkok, Thailand. Normalization was defined as CD4/CD8 ratio ≥ 1 on two consecutive visits, and normalization probability was calculated using the Kaplan–Meier method. NAEs were a composite endpoint including cardiovascular or cerebrovascular diseases, chronic kidney diseases, non-AIDS defining malignancies and death. Multivariate Cox regression was used to evaluate demographic, disease and treatment characteristics associated with CD4/CD8 ratio normalization and NAEs.

Results: A total of 800 ART-naïve patients with baseline CD4/CD8 ratio of < 0.8 who started combination ART, and had sustained virological suppression were enrolled. Participants were on ART for a median of 8.9 years and virologically suppressed for 6.1 years. The probabilities of CD4/CD8 normalization at 2, 5 and 10 years after virological suppression were 5.1%, 18.6% and 39.1%, respectively. Factors associated with normalization in multivariate analysis were female sex (hazard ratio [HR]: 2.47, 95% CI 1.71–3.56, $p < 0.001$) and baseline CD4 counts ≥ 350 cells/mm^3 (HR: 3.62, 95% CI 2.36–5.55), $p < 0.001$) vs. < 200 cells/mm^3 as reference. The second analysis explored the predictive value of CD4/CD8 ratio for NAEs. Older age (HR: 1.09, 95% CI 1.05–1.13, $p < 0.01$) and current CD4/CD8 ratio < 0.3 (HR: 3.02, 95% CI 1.27–7.21, $p = 0.01$) or between 0.3 and 0.45 (HR: 2.03, 95% CI 1.03–3.98, $p = 0.04$) vs. > 0.45 were independently associated with higher risk of progression to NAEs in the multivariate analysis.

Conclusions: Our findings showed that complete immune recovery is uncommon in an Asian setting and earlier ART initiation at higher CD4 counts may have increased the ratio sooner. The findings demonstrate the use of CD4/CD8 ratio as a prognostic marker for clinical progression of NAEs.

Keywords: CD4/CD8 ratio, Immune restoration, Non-AIDS events, Long-term virological suppression, Asia

*Correspondence: win.m@hivnat.org
[1] HIV-NAT, The Thai Red Cross AIDS Research Center, 104 Ratchadamri Rd., Pathumwan, Bangkok 10330, Thailand
Full list of author information is available at the end of the article
All authors belongs to HIV-NAT 006 team.

Background

Survival of HIV-infected individuals has significantly improved with the introduction of combination antiretroviral therapy (cART). Nowadays, since antiretrovirals (ARVs) are initiated in earlier stages of infection, HIV-associated illnesses or complications of acquired immunodeficiency syndrome (AIDS) are less frequently observed in most HIV-infected individuals [1]. Despite low risks of AIDS in many patients who are treated with cART, immune recovery or restoration is rarely achieved [2, 3]. The incidence of several serious non-AIDS defining events (NAEs) including cardiovascular disease, cerebrovascular disease, renal disease and non-ADIS-related cancers have risen as longevity has increased among PLHIV [4]. Lifestyle factors and ageing play a role, but the impact of HIV infection and associated chronic inflammatory states on the incidence of these NAEs is still not fully understood.

Chronic inflammation includes persistent ongoing immune activation, bacterial translocation caused by injured mucosa-associated lymphoid tissue, asymptomatic replication of HIV itself and co-pathogens such as cytomegalovirus infection. These conditions lead to immune activation, and hence potentially increase the risk for all-cause mortality in HIV patients [5–8]. The ratio of $CD4^+$ T cells to $CD8^+$ T cells (CD4/CD8 ratio) has been used as a surrogate marker of immunosenescence in both the general population [9, 10] and PLHIV [11]. Additionally, the CD4/CD8 ratio has shown an independent association with NAEs and mortality in people living with HIV (PLHIV) whereas CD4 counts alone do not predict the risk of NAEs [12, 13]. Studies have reported the ratio remains low, with a slow rate of recovery in a substantial proportion of patients, including those with adequate $CD4^+$ T cell count recovery, over years of cART [12, 14]. The clinical significance of this ongoing immune dysfunction needs further exploration.

The majority of previous published studies exploring associations with CD4/CD8 ratios and their prognostic value for predicting NAE have been from Western countries, and evidence to inform an association in HIV-infected Asians is still limited. A study comparing Asian and Caucasian cohorts has shown that the baseline CD4/CD8 ratio before cART initiation was significantly lower in Asians but there were no differences in the odds of achieving the ratio value of > 1 between two cohorts [15].

In this study, we aimed to firstly evaluate the incidence and probability of CD4/CD8 normalization and to explore factors associated with normalization among patients from a Thai HIV cohort with sustained virologic suppression and long-term follow-up. Secondly, we explored the value of CD4/CD8 ratio in predicting NAEs including cardiovascular or cerebrovascular diseases, kidney diseases, non-AIDS malignancies and deaths.

Methods

Study design and population

This is a prospective study in an ongoing HIV Thai adult cohort (HIV-NAT 006 cohort, clinical trial number: NCT00411983). The details of this cohort have previously been described [16–18]. Participants were eligible for inclusion in this analysis if they achieved and maintained suppressed viremia at HIV-RNA < 50 copies/mL after starting cART. Once a participant had detectable viral load after achieving suppression, follow-up for that participant was censored. All patients had regular clinic visits where medical history, including the occurrence of NAEs was documented.

Definition of endpoints

The normalization of CD4/CD8 ratio, defined as two consecutive values ratios ≥ 1 [19], was the primary endpoint of the initial analysis. For the second analysis, we defined NAEs as cardiovascular or cerebrovascular diseases (including coronary artery diseases, myocardial ischemia, cerebral artery occlusion and stroke), chronic kidney diseases (defined as confirmed estimated glomerular filtrate rate < 60 mL/min with Modification of Diet in Renal Disease MDRD formula), non-AIDS defining malignancies and deaths (excluding 1 death from heroin overdose, 1 unknown cause of death, 3 suicide cases).

Statistical analysis

Firstly, the probabilities of CD4/CD8 ratio normalization and associated factors were identified. Baseline for CD4/CD8 normalization analysis was the first of two consecutive virological suppressions after initiating cART. The normalization incidence rate was calculated by dividing the number of normalization events by total person-years of follow-up (PYFU) after achieving viral suppression. The Kaplan–Meier method was used to assess independent predictors associated with a normalized CD4/CD8 ratio. Baseline covariates modelled were age, sex, mode of HIV transmission, HIV-RNA levels, CD4 and CD8 cell counts, Centers for Disease Control and Prevention (CDC) staging, hepatitis B surface antigen (HBsAg), anti-hepatitis-C antibody (anti-HCV ab).

Secondly, the incidence rate of NAEs was analyzed as a composite endpoint by combining deaths and other NAE in time to event models. CD4/CD8 ratio was fitted as categories with cutoff values of < 0.30, 0.30–0.45 and > 0.45 [11, 12], for the interests of applicability in clinical practice. A value of CD4/CD8 ratio < 0.4 showed the best cutoff to predict NAEs [11] and to link the association with different T-cell activation markers [2]. In these models,

NAEs or deaths were modelled as a first event; patients not reaching the endpoint were censored at their most recent clinic visit. Time-updated covariates modelled included were age, body mass index (BMI) and tuberculosis infection. Diabetes mellitus was defined by two consecutive values of fasting blood glucose ≥ 126 mg/dL or initiation of anti-diabetic medications. Covariates in univariate analysis with p value <0.15 were included in the multivariate model.

Results

CD4/CD8 ratio normalization

After excluding participants treated with cART before the enrollment into the 006 cohort and who did not have baseline CD4/CD8 ratio measurements, 1236 participants were evaluated. We then excluded the patients who had baseline CD4/CD8 ratio ≥ 0.8 and those who commenced on mono or dual ART regimens which may have biased ratio recovery times (Fig. 1). Finally, a total of 800 HIV-infected adults, with 67% male, median age of 32.3 (interquartile range, IQR, 27.4–37.5) years and median baseline HIV-RNA level of 4.8 (IQR, 4.39–5.24) $\log_{10}$ copies/mL, achieved viral suppression and were included in the analysis. Of 800 participants, most were heterosexual (54%) and the rest were homosexual or bisexual (35%) injecting drug users (0.8%) and others (11%), with a median duration of 7 (IQR, 4–35) months to achieve the first virological suppression. Median duration of cART over follow-up was 8.9 (IQR, 5.2–13.7) years. Most participants (47%) achieved virological suppression within 6 months and their median duration of suppression was 6.08 (IQR, 2.97–10.75) years (Table 1). Participants who achieved virological suppression within 6 months had higher pre-cART CD4/CD8 ratio (0.23 vs. 0.21, $p=0.04$) and lower pre-cART HIV RNA level (4.72 $\log_{10}$ vs. 4.85 $\log_{10}$ copies/mL, $p<0.005$), compared to those achieving virological suppression later. There were no differences in pre-cART CD4, CD8 counts or CDC staging between the two groups. Overall baseline CD4/CD8 ratio before cART initiation was 0.22 (IQR, 0.12–0.32) and median CD4/CD8 ratio at confirmed first time of virological suppression was 0.42 (IRQ: 0.27–0.56).

The overall incidence rate of CD4/CD8 ratio normalization was 4.38 per 100 PYFU (95% confidence interval [CI] 3.81–5.04) with 4289 PYFU. With Kaplan–Meier estimation methods, we found that the probabilities of normalization at 2, 5 and 10 years after virological suppression were 5.1%, 18.6% and 39.1%, respectively (Figs. 2 and 3). Thirty-six percent of those who achieved normalization had pre-cART CD4 counts ≤ 200 cell counts, compared to 52% of patients who failed to achieve normalization ($p<0.001$). Median pre-cART CD4/CD8 ratios for participants achieving

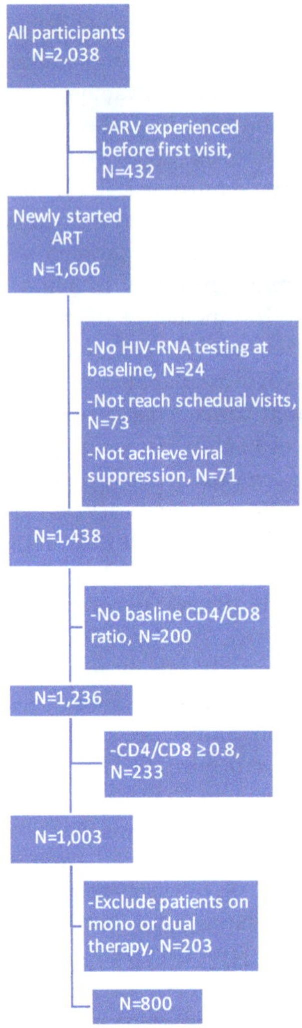

Fig. 1 Flow diagram for patients for inclusion to study analysis

normalization and the non-achiever group were 0.20 (IQR, 0.10–0.30) and 0.28 (IQR, 0.18–0.39), respectively. Of note, the duration of virological suppression was longer among the patients who achieved the normalization target than the non-normalization group (10.8 years [IQR: 7.5–12.7] vs. 4.9 years, [IQR: 2.3–9.1], $p<0.001$). However, there was no significant difference in the time to first virological suppression between patients who achieved normalization and who did not have normal ratios ($p=0.243$). Additionally, there was significant difference in CD4/CD8 ratio at first virological suppression between two groups, with median value of 0.38 (IQR: 0.24–0.5) in patients without CD4/CD8 normalization and 0.54 (0.42–0.69) in the group achieving normalization ($p<0.001$).

In multivariate analysis (Table 2), after adjusting for CDC category, months since starting cART to first viological suppression, HBsAg status and baseline cART

Table 1 Patient characteristics

	N	Descriptive, median (IQR) or n (%)	Not achieved CD4/CD8 ratio < 1 (N = 606)	Achieved CD4/CD8 ratio ≥ 1 (N = 194)	p-value
Gender, n (%)	800				< 0.001
Male		533 (66.63)	439 (72.44)	94 (48.45)	
Female		267 (33.38)	167 (27.56)	100 (51.55)	
Age at start ARV	800	32.3 (27.4–37.5)	31.8 (26.7–37.1)	33.7 (28.6–38.5)	0.006
Pre-cART HIV-RNA level (log_{10} copies/mL)	800	4.8 (4.39–5.24)	4.83 (4.44–5.25)	4.67 (4.18–5.2)	0.003
Pre-cART CD4 count (cells/mm^3)	799	206 (102–291)	193 (80–282)	229 (170–316)	0.0001
Pre-cART CD8 count (cells/mm^3)	769	853 (611–1190)	890 (616–1219)	818 (596–1109)	0.16
Pre-ART CD4/CD8 ratio	769	0.22 (0.12–0.32)	0.20 (0.10–0.30)	0.28 (0.18–0.39)	< 0.001
CDC grading, n (%)	790				0.045
A		466 (58.99)	338 (56.71)	128 (65.98)	
B		223 (28.23)	174 (29.19)	49 (25.26)	
C		101 (12.78)	84 (14.09)	17 (8.76)	
Route of transmission, n (%)	800				0.002
Heterosexual		433 (54.13)	305 (50.33)	128 (65.98)	
MSM/bisexual		280 (35)	233 (38.45)	47 (24.23)	
IDU		6 (0.75)	5 (0.83)	1 (0.52)	
Others		4 (0.5)	4 (0.66)	0 (0)	
Unknown		77 (9.63)	59 (9.74)	18 (9.28)	
Months since cART start to first virological suppression		7 (4–35)	7 (3–34)	9 (4–38)	0.51
Duration of cART (years)	800	8.9 (5.2–13.7)	7.0 (4.2–12.1)	13.5 (9.3–16.7)	< 0.001
Duration of viral suppression (years)	800	6.08 (2.97–10.75)	4.91 (2.26–9.12)	10.77 (7.49–12.74)	< 0.001
CD4/CD8 ratio at first viral suppression, median (IQR)	800	0.42 (0.27–0.56)	0.38 (0.24–0.5)	0.54 (0.42–0.69)	< 0.001
CD4/CD8 ratio at first viral suppression, n (%)	800				< 0.001
< 0.3		224 (28.00)	209 (34.49)	15 (7.73)	
0.30–0.45		228 (28.50)	182 (30.03)	46 (23.71)	
> 0.45		348 (43.50)	215 (35.48)	133 (68.56)	
Positive HBsAg, n (%)	784	130/784 (16.58)	108/592 (18.24)	22/192 (11.46)	0.028
Positive anti-HCV Ab, n (%)	796	66/796 (8.29)	50/602 (8.31)	16/194 (8.25)	0.980
Baseline ARV regimen, n (%)	800				< 0.001
PI-based regimen		272 (34)	178 (29.37)	94 (48.45)	
NNRTI-based regimen		509 (63.63)	411 (67.82)	98 (50.52)	
INSTI-based regimen		19 (2.38)	17 (2.81)	2 (1.03)	

Descriptive data are n (%) or median (*IQR* interquartile range), *ART* antiretroviral therapy, *MSM* men who have sex with men, *IDU* injecting drug users, *ARV* antiretroviral drugs, *NNRTI* non-nucleoside reverse transcriptase inhibitor, *PI* protease inhibitor, *INSTI* integrase strand transfer inhibitors

regimen, factors independently associated with CD4/CD8 ratio normalization were female sex (hazard ratio [HR]: 2.47, 95% CI 1.71–3.56, p < 0.001) and baseline CD4 counts ≥350 cells/mm^3 (HR: 3.62, 95% CI 2.36–5.55, p < 0.001) or between 200 and 350 cells/mm^3 (HR: 1.95, 95% CI 1.40–2.72, p < 0.001) vs. < 200 cells/mm^3 as reference. The interaction between age and CD4/CD8 ratio was tested in the model by using the ratio as continuous, and grouped in categories that matched the analysis. However, no interactions were found.

Non-AIDS defining events

We next explored the associations of CD4/CD8 ratio and NAEs in the second part of our analysis. A total of 123 NAEs occurred in a total of 4071 person-years of follow up. Among them, 108 participants developed chronic kidney disease, 5 developed cardiovascular or cerebrovascular events, 12 developed non-AIDS malignancies and 15 participants died. Among them, 16 patients had more than one of the events mentioned. Overall incidence of NAEs as first events was 3.02 (2.53–3.61) per 100 person-years of follow-up (100 PYS). The incidence

Table 2 Factors associated with normalisation of CD4/CD8 (ratio ≥ 1)

Variables	Univariate			Multivariate		
	HR	95% CI	p-value	HR	95% CI	p-value
Gender						
Male	Ref					
Female	1.99	(1.5–2.64)	*< 0.001*	2.47	(1.71–3.56)	*< 0.001*
Age, (per year older)	1.001	(0.98–1.02)	0.906			
Body mass index (BMI, kg/m^2)						
< 25	1.11	(0.75–1.64)	0.606			
≥ 25	Ref					
Pre-cART HIV-RNA level (log_{10} copies/mL)	0.79	(0.65–0.96)	0.017			
Pre-cART CD4 count (per 100 cell/mm^3 increased)	1.40	(1.28–1.54)	*< 0.001*			
Pre-cART CD4 count (cells/mm^3)			*< 0.001*			*< 0.001*
0–200	Ref			Ref		
201–350	2.05	(1.5–2.81)	*< 0.001*	1.95	(1.4–2.72)	*< 0.001*
≥ 351	3.47	(2.31–5.2)	*< 0.001*	3.62	(2.36–5.55)	*< 0.001*
Pre-cART CD8 count (per 50 cell/mm^3 increase)	0.99	(0.97–1.004)	0.139			
CDC grading						
A, or B	1.81	(1.1–2.99)	0.019	1.2	(0.71–2.02)	0.503
C	Ref			Ref		
Months since ART start to first virological suppression			0.057			0.25
< 6 months	Ref			Ref		
6–12 months	0.48	(0.22–1.06)	0.07	1.30	(0.84–2.02)	0.24
≥ 12 months	1.14	(0.79–1.64)	0.49	1.49	(0.89–2.51)	0.13
HBsAg status						
Negative	1.62	(1.04–2.52)	0.04	1.26	(0.79–2.01)	0.33
Positive	Ref			Ref		
Anti-HCV Ab status						
Negative	1.08	(0.65–1.81)	0.76			
Positive	Ref					
Baseline ARV regimen			*0.017*			0.14
NNRTI based	Ref					
PI based	1.50	(1.13–1.99)	0.01	1.35	(0.99–1.82)	0.051
INSTI based	2.01	(0.49–8.27)	0.33	1.60	(0.38–6.70)	0.52
cART by calendar year						
< 2007	Ref					
≥ 2007	0.85	(0.61–1.2)	0.37			

IQR interquartile range, *ART* antiretroviral therapy, *MSM* men who have sex with men, *IDU* injecting drug users, *ARV* antiretroviral drugs, *NNRTI* non-nucleoside reverse transcriptase inhibitor, *PI* protease inhibitor, *INSTI* integrase strand transfer inhibitors

Significant *p*-values are in italics ($p < 0.001$)

rates of non-AIDS composite events were significantly different between the cutoffs for CD4/CD8 ratio, with 11.42 per 100 PYS (95% CI 7.45–17.52) for current CD4/CD8 ratio < 0.3 and 2.23 per 100 PYS (1.77–2.81) for ratio > 0.45 (Table 3).

Univariate and multivariate analyses of the risk factors associated with composite endpoint of NAEs are summarized in Table 4. Older age, MSM or bisexual (vs. heterosexual), time updated CD4/CD8 ratio (< 0.3 and 0.3–0.45 vs. > 0.45), diabetes mellitus (DM), baseline protease inhibitors-based regimen and cART initiation after calendar year 2007 (vs. before 2007) were associated with higher chances of non-AIDS composite end point in univariate analysis. However, after adjusting the potential cofounders from the univariate analysis, older age (HR: 1.09, 95% CI 1.05–1.13, p < 0.01) and CD4/CD8 ratio (HR: 3.02, 95% CI 1.27–7.21, p = 0.01) for ratio < 0.3 and between 0.3 and 0.45 (HR: 2.03, 95% CI 1.03–3.98, p = 0.04) vs. > 0.45 were independently associated with higher risks of progression to NAEs in the multivariate

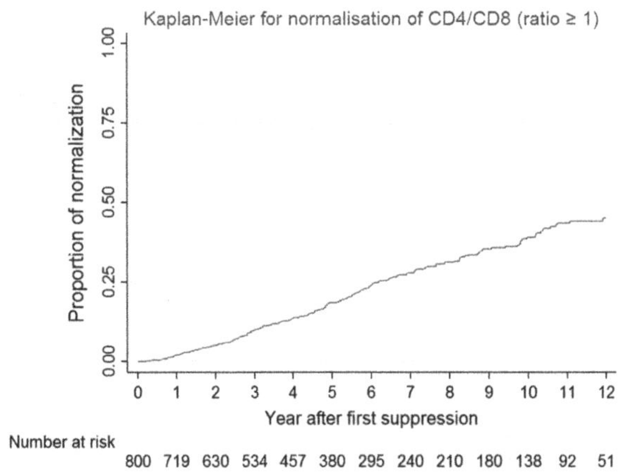

Fig. 2 Kaplan–Meier curve showing probabilities of CD4/CD8 ratio normalization

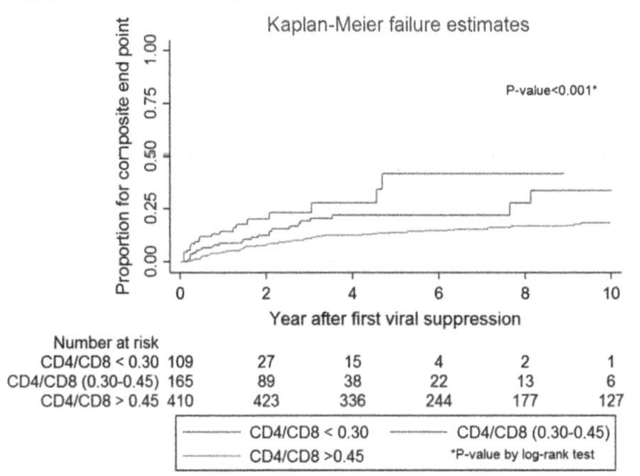

Fig. 3 Kaplan–Meier curves showing probabilities of composite end point with CD4/CD8 ratio

Table 3 Number of composite endpoint events with CD4/CD8 ratio

	No. of event	Person-year of follow-up	Rate per 100 person-year, 95% CI
Composite end-point (n=692)	123	4071	3.02 (2.53–3.61)
Current CD4/CD8 ratio*			
<0.3	21	184	11.42 (7.45–17.52)
0.30–0.45	28	496	5.64 (3.90–8.17)
>0.45	72	3227	2.23 (1.77–2.81)

* $P<0.001$ for long rank test

analysis. Since the majority of NAE in our cohort were from CKD, the diagnosis of which is derived from an equation, we conducted a sensitivity analysis where CKD was confirmed at 2 consecutive visits. Using this method, 48 patients met criteria for CKD, and we found significantly elevated risks of NAE in multivariate models: HR 3.29 (95% CI 1.66–6.50; p = 0.001) for current CD4/CD8 ratio < 0.3) and HR 2.46 (95% CI 1.44–4.20; p = 0.001) for those with ratios between 0.3 and 0.45, vs. > 0.45 as the reference group.

Discussion

In our cohort with median duration cART of 8.9 years and median duration of virological suppression of 6.1 years, the probability of achieving CD4/CD8 normalization at 5 and 10 years was 19% and 39% respectively. These Kaplan–Meier probabilities are consistent with our incidence rate of approximately 4% per year. Our data confirmed the previous few available data demonstrating the prolonged duration of recovery to normal CD4/CD8 ratio among PLHIV with suppressive cART, with a median of 10 years to reach normalization target [12]. This study also demonstrated that low ratio was a higher risk for clinical progression of NAEs. This can be translated into that persistent disparity between CD4 and CD8 cell counts, even with CD4 recovery after cART, could be a critical marker for evaluating the prognosis of long-term virologically suppressed PLHIV. Our patients had a relatively lower incidence of CD4/CD8 ratio normalization compared to an Italian cohort. The Italian cohort that included only patients with undetectable HIV viral load (HIV-RNA level < 80 copies/mL) after cART initiation, showed 29% achieved ratio normalization by 5 years whereas it was 19% by 5 years from our study [12]. However, the baseline median CD4/CD8 ratio and median nadir CD4 count in the Italian cohort were higher than those of our Thai cohort (0.39 vs. 0.22, and 378 vs. 206 cells/mm3, respectively). Our study showed that higher chances of normalization were associated with higher baseline CD4 counts (> 350 cells/mm^3). This is consistent with previous studies suggesting baseline CD4 counts < 200 cells/mm^3 was an unfavorable predictor towards CD4/CD8 ratio normalization [3, 12], and that low CD4 T-cell counts at baseline before cART are associated with incomplete immune response even after years of viral suppression [20]. Moreover, improvement of CD4/CD8 ratio was seen in both normalization and non-normalization groups after having suppressed viremia, compared to baseline values before cART initiation. This suggests that current ART guidelines recommending initiation of cART treatment with higher CD4 cell counts will have benefits in increasing the number of participants achieved higher CD4/CD8 ratios earlier.

The literature is conflicting regarding the use of CD4/CD8 ratio as a surrogate marker to describe immune dysfunction and to predict the progression towards NAEs

Table 4 Factors associated with composite end point

Variables	Univariate model			Multivariate model		
	HR	95% CI	p-value	HR	95% CI	p-value
Gender						
Male	Ref					
Female	1.09	(0.75–1.58)	0.65			
Age[a], year	1.07	(1.04–1.09)	< 0.001	1.09	(1.05–1.13)	*< 0.001*
BMI[a], kg/m^2						
< 25	Ref			Ref		
≥ 25	1.68	(0.89–3.16)	0.11	1.42	(0.73–2.76)	0.30
Route of transmission			0.008			0.19
Heterosexual	Ref			Ref		
MSM/bisexual	0.54	(0.35–0.82)	0.004	1.74	(0.95–3.21)	0.07
IDU/others/unknown	0.66	(0.33–1.30)	0.23	1.06	(0.32–3.53)	0.93
Ever smoking	0.82	(0.56–1.20)	0.31			
Ever alcohol drinking	0.82	(0.38–1.77)	0.62			
Baseline HIV-RNA level (log_{10} copies/mL)	1.19	(0.92–1.54)	0.19			
Baseline CDC grading						
Stage A or B	Ref					
Stage C	1.03	(0.61–1.74)	0.92			
Tuberculosis infection[a]						
No	Ref					
Yes	1.24	(0.17–8.93)	0.83			
Time since ART initiation to first viral suppression			0.057			
< 6 months	Ref					
6–12 months	0.48	(0.22–1.06)	0.07			
≥ 12 months	1.14	(0.79–1.64)	0.49			
Current CD4 counts per 100 increased	0.93	(0.85–1.02)	0.12			
Current CD4/CD8						
< 0.3	3.10	(1.87–5.14)	< 0.001	3.02	(1.27–7.21)	*0.001*
0.30–0.45	1.76	(1.13–2.75)	0.01	2.03	(1.03–3.98)	*0.04*
> 0.45	Ref			Ref		
Diabetes mellitus	2.27	(1.52–3.39)	< 0.001	3.02	(0.06–163.26)	0.59
HBs Ag status						
Negative	Ref					
Positive	0.69	(0.40–1.18)	0.17			
Anti-HCV Ab status						
Negative	Ref					
Positive	1.04	(0.54–1.98)	0.92			
Baseline ARV regimen						
NNRTI-based	Ref			Ref		
PI-based	1.55	(1.09–2.22)	0.015	1.09	(0.6–1.99)	0.77
cART by calendar year						
< 2007	Ref			Ref		
≥ 2007	0.40	(0.27–0.61)	< 0.001	1.29	(0.7–2.36)	0.42

Significant *p*-values are in italics

IQR interquartile range, *BMI* body mass index, *MSM* men who have sex with men, *IDU* injecting drug users, *ARV* antiretroviral drugs, *ART* antiretroviral therapy, *NNRTI* non-nucleoside reverse transcriptase inhibitor, *PI* protease inhibitor, *INSTI* integrase strand transfer inhibitors

[a] Time-updated variables include age, BMI and tuberculosis infections

and mortality [12, 13, 21]. A report from Mussini et al. [12] suggested the predictive value of CD4/CD8 ratio for clinical progression of severe NAEs and deaths among patients with prolonged cART treatment in a large Italian cohort, with the same cutoff values of the ratio used in our study. In contrast, in a large collaborative study of European and North American cohorts failed to show a link between low CD4/CD8 ratio and non-AIDS related mortality among virologically suppressed patients on cART [21]. Of note, the study showed low ratio and high CD8 counts were associated with AIDS-related mortalities. We sought to carry out an additional analysis to explore whether CD4/CD8 ratio has an association with development of NAEs. Our case definition of NAEs was similar to the ones used in previous studies, which included cardiovascular and cerebrovascular diseases, non-AIDS defining cancers, kidney diseases and deaths [12, 13]. The incidence rates of composite non-AIDS endpoints were significantly different among categories with different CD4/CD8 ratio cutoff values in our study. Patients with low CD4/CD8 ratio had higher incidence rates of NAEs than those with higher ratios. In multivariate analysis, we also found the independent associations of low CD4/CD8 ratio with composite end point or deaths after adjusting for potential confounders that were significant in the univariate analysis.

Previous reports have also suggested the association of CD4/CD8 ratio in T-cell activation or senescence [22, 23]. A plausible explanation associations with NAEs is that low CD4/CD8 ratio could be a marker of ongoing immune dysfunction among prolonged virologically suppressed HIV patients on stable cART since immune activation is been associated with clinical events and mortality in PLHIV [24].

One of the strengths of our study is the prolonged follow-up time with a median of 8.9 (IQR, 5.2–13.7) years of cART treatment. Our participants were taking cART with prolonged duration of virological suppression of 6.1 (IQR, 3–10.8) years. Another strength of our study is that we evaluated the probabilities of normalization among virologically suppressed participants up to 10 years. This is relatively longer than other studies which showed the normalization probabilities just up to 2 years [3] and 5 years [12], respectively.

Several important limitations in this study should be acknowledged. First, we could not provide the association of low CD4/CD8 ratio with each particular non-AIDS incident due to low numbers of events in each category. Second, we could not include some potential factors that have previously suggested may have influences on immune activation or persistent inflammation such as cytomegalovirus (CMV) co-infection [25, 26] in our study analysis. Third, our study population could be considered low risk, since they started cART, and maintained good adherence and virological suppression. Nevertheless, this also allowed us to assess CD4/CD8 ratio recovery without the confounding effect of viremia. Fourth, the study was a retrospective analysis from a prospective cohort. The conclusion for causal inference between low CD4/CD8 ratio and NAEs is therefore low due to the observational nature of the cohort. Lastly, although CD4/CD8 ratios may be a useful marker, there is no known strategy apart from taking cART to improve ratios that are low. Further analyses should explore whether newer therapies for HIV treatment such integrase strand inhibitors or monoclonal antibodies have additional impact on CD4/CD8 ratio recovery.

Conclusions

Probabilities of immune recovery among patients on cART is relatively low in our cohort, suggesting the ongoing immune dysfunctions even after years of treatment. Patients with low baseline CD4 counts were less likely to achieve ratio normalization. Earlier ART initiation may result in increased normalization rates. We also sought to use multiple NAEs as a composite endpoint to determine its association with the ratio. The finding of low ratio with the linkage to NAEs highlights the potential use of CD4/CD8 ratios as a marker for the clinical progression of non-communicable diseases and mortality among PLHIV with prolonged suppression of viremia.

Authors' contributions

WMH drafted the manuscript. AA, SK reviewed and edited the manuscript. WMH, SK, TA interpreted the data and TA performed statistical analysis. AA, SG, AH, WMH oversaw the participants. KR, AA lead the study. All authors read and approved the final manuscript.

Author details

[1] HIV-NAT, The Thai Red Cross AIDS Research Center, 104 Ratchadamri Rd., Pathumwan, Bangkok 10330, Thailand. [2] Faculty of Medicine, Chulalongkorn University, Bangkok, Thailand.

Acknowledgements

We thank to the study participants and all team members from the HIV-NAT 006 cohort.

Competing interests

KR has received the Senior Research Scholar from Thailand Research Fund (TRF), and has received honoraria or consultation fees from Merck, Roche, Jensen-Cilag, Tibotec, Mylan and GPO (Governmental pharmaceutical organization, Thailand). He also has participated in company sponsored speaker's bureaus for Abbott, Gilead, Bristol-Myers Squibb, Merck, Roche, Jensen-Cilag, GlaxoSmithKline, and GPO (Governmental pharmaceutical organization). AA participated in a company sponsored speaker's bureau from Jensen-Cilag, Gilead and Bristol-Meyer Squibb. The rest of the authors declare that they have no competing interests.

Funding
Not applicable.

References

1. Low A, Gavriilidis G, Larke N, B-Lajoie MR, Drouin O, Stover J, et al. Incidence of opportunistic infections and the impact of antiretroviral therapy among HIV-infected adults in low- and middle-income countries: a systematic review and meta-analysis. Clin Infect Dis. 2016;62(12):1595–603.
2. Serrano-Villar S, Sainz T, Lee SA, Hunt PW, Sinclair E, Shacklett BL, et al. HIV-infected individuals with low CD4/CD8 ratio despite effective antiretroviral therapy exhibit altered T cell subsets, heightened $CD8^+$ T cell activation, and increased risk of non-AIDS morbidity and mortality. PLoS Pathog. 2014;10(5):e1004078.
3. Leung V, Gillis J, Raboud J, Cooper C, Hogg RS, Loutfy MR, et al. Predictors of CD4:CD8 ratio normalization and its effect on health outcomes in the era of combination antiretroviral therapy. PLoS ONE. 2013;8(10):e77665.
4. Mocroft A, Reiss P, Gasiorowski J, Ledergerber B, Kowalska J, Chiesi A, et al. Serious fatal and nonfatal non-AIDS-defining illnesses in Europe. J Acquir Immune Defic Syndr. 2010;55(2):262–70.
5. Brenchley JM, Price DA, Schacker TW, Asher TE, Silvestri G, Rao S, et al. Microbial translocation is a cause of systemic immune activation in chronic HIV infection. Nat Med. 2006;12(12):1365–71.
6. Appay V, Sauce D. Immune activation and inflammation in HIV-1 infection: causes and consequences. J Pathol. 2008;214(2):231–41.
7. Dock JN, Effros RB. Role of CD8 T cell replicative senescence in human aging and in HIV-mediated immunosenescence. Aging Dis. 2011;2(5):382–97.
8. Hunt PW, Martin JN, Sinclair E, Epling L, Teague J, Jacobson MA, et al. Valganciclovir reduces T cell activation in HIV-infected individuals with incomplete $CD4^+$ T cell recovery on antiretroviral therapy. J Infect Dis. 2011;203(10):1474–83.
9. Hadrup SR, Strindhall J, Kollgaard T, Seremet T, Johansson B, Pawelec G, et al. Longitudinal studies of clonally expanded CD8 T cells reveal a repertoire shrinkage predicting mortality and an increased number of dysfunctional cytomegalovirus-specific T cells in the very elderly. J Immunol. 2006;176(4):2645–53.
10. Wikby A, Maxson P, Olsson J, Johansson B, Ferguson FG. Changes in CD8 and CD4 lymphocyte subsets, T cell proliferation responses and non-survival in the very old: the Swedish longitudinal OCTO-immune study. Mech Ageing Dev. 1998;102(2–3):187–98.
11. Guiguet M, Kendjo E, Carcelain G, Abgrall S, Mary-Krause M, Tattevin P, et al. $CD4^+$ T-cell percentage is an independent predictor of clinical progression in AIDS-free antiretroviral-naive patients with $CD4^+$ T-cell counts > 200 cells/mm^3. Antivir Ther. 2009;14(3):451–7.
12. Mussini C, Lorenzini P, Cozzi-Lepri A, Lapadula G, Marchetti G, Nicastri E, et al. CD4/CD8 ratio normalisation and non-AIDS-related events in individuals with HIV who achieve viral load suppression with antiretroviral therapy: an observational cohort study. Lancet HIV. 2015;2(3):e98–106.
13. Serrano-Villar S, Perez-Elias MJ, Dronda F, Casado JL, Moreno A, Royuela A, et al. Increased risk of serious non-AIDS-related events in HIV-infected subjects on antiretroviral therapy associated with a low CD4/CD8 ratio. PLoS ONE. 2014;9(1):e85798.
14. Caby F, Guihot A, Lambert-Niclot S, Guiguet M, Boutolleau D, Agher R, et al. Determinants of a low CD4/CD8 ratio in HIV-1-infected individuals despite long-term viral suppression. Clin Infect Dis. 2016;62(10):1297–303.
15. Petoumenos K, Choi JY, Hoy J, Kiertiburanakul S, Ng OT, Boyd M, et al. CD4:CD8 ratio comparison between cohorts of HIV-positive Asians and Caucasians upon commencement of antiretroviral therapy. Antivir Ther. 2017;22(8):659–68.
16. Putcharoen O, Wattanachanya L, Sophonphan J, Siwamogsatham S, Sapsirisavat V, Gatechompol S, et al. New-onset diabetes in HIV-treated adults: predictors, long-term renal and cardiovascular outcomes. AIDS. 2017;31(11):1535–43.
17. Durier N, Ananworanich J, Apornpong T, Ubolyam S, Kerr SJ, Mahanontharit A, et al. Cytomegalovirus viremia in Thai HIV-infected patients on antiretroviral therapy: prevalence and associated mortality. Clin Infect Dis. 2013;57(1):147–55.
18. Edwards-Jackson N, Kerr S, Tieu H, Ananworanich J, Hammer S, Ruxrungtham K, et al. Cardiovascular risk assessment in persons with HIV infection in the developing world: comparing three risk equations in a cohort of HIV-infected Thais. HIV Med. 2011;12(8):510–5.
19. Tinago W, Coghlan E, Macken A, McAndrews J, Doak B, Prior-Fuller C, et al. Clinical, immunological and treatment-related factors associated with normalised $CD4^+/CD8^+$ T-cell ratio: effect of naive and memory T-cell subsets. PLoS ONE. 2014;9(5):e97011.
20. Falster K, Petoumenos K, Chuah J, Mijch A, Mulhall B, Kelly M, et al. Poor baseline immune function predicts an incomplete immune response to combination antiretroviral treatment despite sustained viral suppression. J Acquir Immune Defic Syndr. 2009;50(3):307–13.
21. Trickey A, May MT, Schommers P, Tate J, Ingle SM, Guest JL, et al. CD4:CD8 ratio and CD8 count as prognostic markers for mortality in human immunodeficiency virus-infected patients on antiretroviral therapy: the antiretroviral therapy cohort collaboration (ART-CC). Clin Infect Dis. 2017;65(6):959–66.
22. Serrano-Villar S, Gutierrez C, Vallejo A, Hernandez-Novoa B, Diaz L, Abad Fernandez M, et al. The CD4/CD8 ratio in HIV-infected subjects is independently associated with T-cell activation despite long-term viral suppression. J Infect. 2013;66(1):57–66.
23. Sainz T, Serrano-Villar S, Diaz L, Gonzalez Tome MI, Gurbindo MD, de Jose MI, et al. The CD4/CD8 ratio as a marker T-cell activation, senescence and activation/exhaustion in treated HIV-infected children and young adults. AIDS. 2013;27(9):1513–6.
24. Sandler NG, Wand H, Roque A, Law M, Nason MC, Nixon DE, et al. Plasma levels of soluble CD14 independently predict mortality in HIV infection. J Infect Dis. 2011;203(6):780–90.
25. Barrett L, Stapleton SN, Fudge NJ, Grant MD. Immune resilience in HIV-infected individuals seronegative for cytomegalovirus. AIDS. 2014;28(14):2045–9.
26. Freeman ML, Mudd JC, Shive CL, Younes SA, Panigrahi S, Sieg SF, et al. CD8 T-cell expansion and inflammation linked to CMV coinfection in ART-treated HIV infection. Clin Infect Dis. 2016;62(3):392–6.

22

Mental health service utilization is associated with retention in care among persons living with HIV at a university-affiliated HIV clinic

Lauren A. Saag[1], Ashutosh R. Tamhane[2], D. Scott Batey[3], Michael J. Mugavero[2] and Ellen F. Eaton[2*]

Abstract

Background: Mental health (MH) comorbidities reduce retention in care for persons living with HIV (PLWH) and are associated with poor health outcomes. Optimizing retention in primary care is vital, as poor retention is associated with delayed receipt of antiretroviral (ARV) therapy, ARV non-adherence, and poor health outcomes, including failure to suppress viral load, decreased CD4 counts, and clinically significant ARV drug resistance. We hypothesized that MH service utilization would be associated with improved retention in care for patients with HIV and MH comorbidities.

Methods: This is a retrospective analysis of PLWH initiating outpatient HIV health care at a university-affiliated HIV clinic between January 2007 and December 2013. We examined the association between MH service utilization and retention in care, the outcome of interest, using univariate and multivariable logistic regression.

Results: Overall, 627 (84.4%) out of 743 patients were retained in care using the Health Resources & Services Administration HIV/AIDS Bureau (HRSA/HAB) metric. A multivariable model adjusted for several sociodemographic factors, MH comorbidities, and MH service utilization. The results suggest that lack of health insurance (public ORadj = 0.3, $p < 0.01$; no insurance ORadj = 0.4, $p < 0.01$) and ≥ 3 MH comorbidities (ORadj = 0.3, P = 0.01) were associated with decreased retention in care. Conversely, older age (> 45 years, ORadj. = 1.6, p = 0.14) and ≥ 3 MH service utilization visits (ORadj. = 6.8, $p < 0.01$) were associated with increased retention in care.

Conclusions: Even in the absence of documented MH comorbidities, improved retention in care was observed with increasing MH service utilization. In order to achieve the US-based National HIV/AIDS Strategy goal of 90% retention in care for PLWH, MH service utilization should be considered along with other evidence-based interventions to improve retention for PLWH newly engaged in care.

Keywords: HIV, Mental illness, Substance use, Mental health services, Retention in care

Background

The goals of the US-based National HIV/AIDS Strategy (NHAS) include increasing the percentage of persons living with HIV (PLWH) who are retained in HIV primary medical care to at least 90% [1]. Currently, 56.9% of all persons ≥ 13 years with diagnosed HIV are retained in care [2]. Optimizing retention in care is vital as poor retention is associated with delayed receipt of antiretroviral (ARV) therapy, ARV non-adherence, HIV viremia, decreased CD4 counts, and drug resistance [3–7].

The "triple diagnosis" of HIV, psychiatric conditions, and substance use disorders (encompassing drug and alcohol use) complicates the management of HIV infection [8]. Mental health comorbidities (MHC), which include depression, drug use, and high-risk alcohol use [9], are common in PLWH. Major depression is over three times more prevalent in PLWH [10]. Half of PLWH

*Correspondence: eeaton@uabmc.edu
[2] Division of Infectious Diseases, Department of Medicine, University of Alabama at Birmingham, 845 19th St. South, Birmingham, AL 35294, USA

report drug use [11], and rates of heavy drinking among PLWH are almost twice that of the general population [12]. Ten to 28% of PLWH have co-occurring substance use disorders and psychiatric disorders [13]. MHCs predispose PLWH to poor retention in HIV primary care (i.e. more missed visits) [14, 15] and contribute to negative health outcomes (i.e. HIV viremia, lower CD4 cell counts) [13, 16, 17]. This is not surprising given mental health disorders limit one's ability to access health care leading to partial or no medical treatment and progressive disease.

Due to the prevalence and co-existence of MHCs in PLWH and their deleterious effects on retention in care, optimizing MHCs has the potential to foster retention in care and improve HIV-related outcomes [16, 18]. In select populations, integrating needs-based case management has been shown to increase retention in care and improve depression and drug and alcohol use [19–22] Additionally, strengths-based case management and stigma-reducing interventions [19] may ameliorate the effects of MHC on health outcomes in PLWH [23, 24]. Due to the stigma surrounding HIV, a diagnosis can be a very stressful, life-altering event [25–27] Even those without a MHC may be best managed with mental health care, such as counseling to cope with this diagnosis [25].

We hypothesized that PLWH, with and without the three examined MHCs, would experience greater retention in care if they utilized mental health services. The objective of this study is to elucidate the association between mental health (MH) service utilization (e.g. psychiatry, psychology, and substance use counseling appointments) and retention in HIV medical care. We analyzed PLWH with and without MHCs initiating HIV medical care at a US-based comprehensive clinic, which relies on federally appropriated Ryan White-safety net funds for uninsured and underinsured patients (see "Methods").

Methods

Study setting and population

This retrospective study was conducted at a university-affiliated HIV Clinic. This is the largest HIV outpatient center in Alabama, and it provides comprehensive medical and mental health care and case management with assistance from the Ryan White HIV/AIDS program (RWHAP). The RWHAP is federal funding that supports primary medical care and ancillary services for uninsured or underinsured PLWH [28]. The clinic maintains an electronic database including over 3200 active patients with details of clinical, socio-demographic, and psychosocial patient data. The institutional review board of the university approved this study, study forms, and protocols.

Eligibility criteria

Treatment naïve patients newly initiating HIV care and completing a Project CONNECT (see below) visit between January 1, 2007 and December 31, 2013 were included. Treatment naïve persons are more likely to be newly diagnosed and experiencing similar life stressors associated with HIV diagnosis and treatment. Participants were included regardless of the presence or absence of MHC. We excluded treatment-experienced persons because they have received HIV treatment and care, often including mental health services, at other clinics making them a more complex population.

Data collection

Data was collected through two existing research protocols at the clinic. Participant data was obtained through the CFAR Network of Integrated Clinical Systems (CNICS) database, which integrates clinical data from outpatient and inpatient encounters. Clinic visit data, including the number of mental health service utilizations and primary care appointments, were obtained from CNICS to calculate exposure and outcome measures as defined below. Project CONNECT (Client-Oriented New Patient Navigation to Encourage Connection to Treatment) was initiated at the clinic in 2007 to improve linkage to medical care and has been recognized by the Centers for Disease Control and Prevention (CDC) among its compendium of best practices, and was founded on CNICS methodology, [29]. All new patients (newly-diagnosed, transferring care, or re-engaging in care after > 12 months out of care) receive Project CONNECT services including a semi-structured interview to assess a variety of sociodemographic domains (e.g., housing, HIV disclosure, transportation) and a behavioral patient-reported outcomes (PRO) questionnaire using standardized, validated instruments such as the Patient Health Questionnaire-9 (PHQ-9) [30] for depression, the Alcohol Use Disorder Identification Test-Consumption (AUDIT-C) [31] for alcohol use, and the Alcohol, Smoking and Substance Involvement Screening Test (ASSIST) [32] for substance use (alcohol use questions are excluded in ASSIST questionnaire). Project CONNECT was used as the single source for PROS. PROS are collected with touch-screen tablets or PC computers and web-based survey software developed specifically for PROs and prompt additional referrals, including mental health services from co-located psychiatry, psychology/counselor, and substance use counselors, if necessary. Data collected at the Project CONNECT visit are considered baseline and will hereafter be referred as such.

Outcome of interest

The outcome of interest was retention in HIV primary medical care 12 months following the Project CONNECT orientation visit. Using the Health Resources & Services Administration–HIV/AIDS Bureau (HRSA/HAB) metric [33–35] retention in care was defined as those having attended at least two primary HIV care appointments within a period of 12 months separated by at least 90 days. The number of HIV primary medical care appoints was obtained from the CNICS database.

Independent variables

Mental health comorbidities: Patients were categorized by the presence or absence of MHCs, obtained by PROs at the Project CONNECT visit. Depressive symptoms were defined by the PHQ-9 [30] and categorized into "major" (score $\geq$ 10) versus "mild/no" depressive symptoms (score $\leq$ 9) [36, 37]. The ASSIST assessed drug use and was categorized into "current" and "past/never" use [32]. We are not aware of any literature suggesting a relationship with tobacco and retention in HIV care; therefore data on tobacco usage was excluded. Because there is some evidence that marijuana may improve rather than reduce HIV treatment adherence [38], we did not include marijuana alongside other drugs which are known to negatively impact HIV outcomes. The AUDIT-C, an instrument for screening alcohol use disorders, was used to measure alcohol use in terms of "no/low risk" and "at risk" [31]. For women, a score of $\geq$ 3 was considered "at risk," and < 3 was considered "no/low" risk. For men, a score of $\geq$ 4 was considered "at risk," and < 4 was considered "no/low" risk. Missing data was included in the referent category, as follows: 36 (4.9%) missing depression score were categorized as "mild/no" depression, 11 (1.5%) missing drug use score were categorized as "past/never" drug use, and 13 (1.8%) missing alcohol use were categorized as "no/low risk" alcohol.

Mental health service utilization: MH service utilization, obtained from the CNICS database, was defined as the number of individual psychiatry, psychology, and substance use counseling visits attended in the 12 months following the Project CONNECT visit. Group therapy sessions were not included as utilization data was not available. Due to a small number of participants utilizing 4 or more MH services, MH service utilization was categorized as 0, 1, 2 or $\geq$ 3.

Other variables: Age, sex (male or female), race (white, black, other), transmission risk [heterosexual sex, intravenous drug use (IVDU), men who have sex with men (MSM), and unknown], and insurance status (public, private, uninsured) were collected from the semi-structured interview at the initial visit. The only public insurers of study participants were Medicare and Medicaid. For this analysis, insurance status is as a proxy for socioeconomic status, a common practice in health services research [39–41]. Baseline CD4 cell count and HIV RNA viral load were obtained at the initial visit.

Statistical analysis

Descriptive evaluation was performed for the total study population and by grouping participants as "retained" or "not retained" in primary care based on the HRSA-HAB definition. Continuous variables were reported as means (with standard deviations, SDs) when the distribution was normal and as medians (with quartiles, Q1 = first quartile, Q3 = third quartile) for non-normal distribution. Categorical variables were reported as frequencies (with percentages).

Associations of factors with retention in primary HIV medical care (outcome of interest) were evaluated by univariate and multivariable logistic regression. Variables were considered for inclusion into the multivariable model based on clinical relevance and statistical consideration of collinearity with other variables in the model [34]. Results are reported with unadjusted and adjusted odds ratios (OR and ORadj., respectively) and 95% confidence intervals (CIs). Age, race, sex, transmission risk factor, insurance status, number of MHCs, and number of MH service utilization visits in 12 months study period were included in the multivariable model. Model performance was examined using c-statistics, max-rescaled r-square and Hosmer–Lemeshow test for model fit. Multicollinearity of the independent factors was examined with variance inflation factor (VIF) by adjusting the linear combinations by the weight matrix used in the maximum likelihood algorithm [42]. Because the number of MHCs and each individual MHC (depression, drug use, at-risk alcohol use) were collinear, separate multivariable models were built. The first model used the 'number of MHC' (presented model) and the second, using each individual MH condition separately (not presented). Both models produced similar results. The VIF for all other factors was < 1.6, indicating no additional multicollinearity. While examining the effect of MHCs on the association of retention in care and MH service utilization, we encountered quasi-complete separation due to zero cell frequency. Therefore, Firth's penalized likelihood method [43] was used to produce ORs and corresponding profile-likelihood CIs.

Statistical significance was set at 0.05 (two-tailed). All analyses were performed using SAS statistical software, version 9.3 (SAS Institute, Cary, NC).

Table 1 Demographic and clinical characteristics of HIV-positive patients[a] receiving care at UAB, 2007–2013 (N = 743)

Characteristic	Total N = 743 N (col%)	Retained[b] N = 627 (84.4) n (row%)	Not retained[b] N = 116 (15.6) n (row%)
Age (years), mean (SD)	34.8 ± 11.3	34.9 ± 11.4	34.2 ± 10.3
Age (years)[c]			
< 30	312 (42.0)	264 (84.6)	48 (15.4)
30–45	288 (38.8)	238 (82.6)	50 (17.4)
> 45	143 (19.2)	125 (87.4)	18 (12.6)
Race			
White	259 (34.9)	222 (85.7)	37 (14.3)
Black	458 (61.6)	385 (84.1)	73 (15.9)
Other	26 (3.5)	20 (76.9)	6 (23.1)
Sex			
Female	133 (17.9)	113 (85.0)	20 (15.0)
Male	610 (82.1)	514 (84.3)	96 (15.7)
Transmission risk			
Heterosexual	234 (31.5)	193 (82.5)	41 (17.5)
IVDU	45 (6.0)	38 (84.4)	7 (15.6)
MSM	407 (54.8)	351 (86.2)	56 (13.8)
Unknown	57 (7.7)	45 (79.0)	12 (21.0)
Insurance[c]			
Private	282 (38.0)	255 (90.4)	27 (9.6)
Public	84 (11.3)	64 (76.2)	20 (23.8)
Uninsured/unknown	377 (50.7)	308 (81.7)	69 (18.3)
CD4 count, cells/uL[c]			
< 200	244 (33.7)	211 (86.5)	33 (13.5)
≥ 200	481 (66.3)	404 (84.0)	77 (16.0)
Viral load[c]			
< 200	18 (2.5)	15 (83.3)	3 (16.7)
≥ 200	709 (97.5)	603 (85.0)	106 (15.0)
Depression[c,d]			
Yes	251 (33.7)	211 (84.1)	40 (16.0)
Mild/No	462 (61.5)	387 (83.8)	75 (16.2)
Unknown	36 (4.8)	31 (86.1)	5 (13.9)
Drug use[c,e]			
Current	129 (17.1)	103 (79.8)	26 (20.2)
Past/never	609 (81.4)	515 (81.9)	94 (15.4)
Unknown	11 (1.5)	11 (100.0)	0 (0)
At risk alcohol use[c,f,g]			
Yes	253 (34.0)	209 (82.6)	44 (17.4)
No/Low	477 (64.2)	408 (85.5)	44 (14.5)
Unknown	13 (1.7)	10 (76.9)	3 (23.1)
Number of MHCs[c,h]			
0	307 (41.3)	259 (84.4)	48 (15.6)
1	270 (36.3)	235 (87.0)	35 (13.0)
2	138 (18.6)	113 (81.9)	25 (18.1)
3	28 (3.8)	20 (71.4)	8 (28.6)
Mental healthcare utilization[i]			
0	559 (75.2)	461 (82.5)	98 (17.5)
1–2	98 (13.2)	84 (85.7)	14 (14.3)
3+	86 (11.6)	82 (95.4)	4 (4.6)

IVDU intravenous drug use, *MHC* mental health co-morbidities, *MSM* men who have sex with men, *SD* standard deviation, *UAB* University of Alabama at Birmingham (Birmingham, AL, USA)

[a] Treatment naïve and newly engaged in care

[b] Definition: at least two primary care appointments being attended within a period of 12 months but separated by at least 90 days

[c] Measured at baseline (time of clinic enrollment interview)

[d] Patient Health Questionnaire-9

[e] Alcohol, smoking and substance involvement screening test

[f] Alcohol use disorder identification test-consumption

[g] Drug use excludes marijuana

[h] Measured as total count of depression, drug use, and alcohol use

[i] Measured within 12 months

Results

Overall, 2797 PLWH had an initial visit between January 1, 2007 and December 31, 2013. Of these, 743 patients met inclusion criteria: treatment naïve and initiating outpatient HIV medical care. Notably, 627 (84.4%) were retained in care at 12 months. The mean age was 34.8 years (SD ± 11.3). A majority were male (82.1%), African American (61.6%), and MSM (54.8%) (Table 1). Additional patient characteristics are summarized in Table 1.

Over half of patients reported ≥ one MHC based upon PRO self-assessment: 41.3% reported one MH condition, 18.6% reported two MHCs (53.6% of those with depression and alcohol use, 18.1% with depression and drug abuse, and 28.2% with alcohol use and drug abuse), and 3.8% reported all three MHCs. At-risk alcohol use was the most commonly reported MHC (34.0%), followed by "major" depressive symptoms (33.7%) and current drug use (17.1%). Despite the high burden of MHCs, three quarters (75.2%) of the sample did not have any MH service utilization: 13.2% had between one and two MH service utilizations, and 11.6% had three or more MH service utilizations during their 12-month observation period.

In Table 2, univariate and multivariable analyses examining association of retention in care with MH service utilization, MHCs, and socio-demographic variables are presented. Although none of the mental health conditions

Table 2 Unadjusted and adjusted odds ratios examining association of retention[a] in care with demographic and clinical characteristics in HIV-positive patients[b] receiving care at UAB, 2007–2013 (N = 743)

Characteristic	Univariate analysis[c]		Multivariable analysis[c,d]	
	Unadjusted OR (95% CI)	*p*	Adjusted OR (95% CI)	*p*
Age (years)[e]				
< 30[l]	1.0	–	1.0	–
30–45	0.9 (0.6, 1.3)	0.51	0.9 (0.6, 1.4)	0.69
> 45	1.3 (0.7, 2.3)	0.43	1.6 (0.8, 3.2)	0.14
Race				
White[l]	1.0	–	1.0	–
Black	0.9 (0.6, 1.3)	0.55	1.3 (0.8, 2.2)	0.27
Other/unk	0.6 (0.2, 1.5)	0.24	0.9 (0.3, 2.5)	0.83
Sex				
Female[l]	1.0	–	1.0	–
Male	0.9 (0.6, 1.6)	0.84	0.7 (0.4, 1.4)	0.32
Transmission risk				
Heterosexual[l]	1.0	–	1.0	–
IVDU	1.2 (0.5, 2.8)	0.75	1.6 (0.6, 4.5)	0.31
MSM	1.3 (0.9, 2.1)	0.20	1.5 (0.9, 2.7)	0.13
Unknown	0.8 (0.4, 1.6)	0.54	1.1 (0.5, 2.4)	0.78
Insurance[e]				
Private[l]	1.0	–	1.0	–
Public	*0.3 (0.2, 0.6)*	*< 0.001*	*0.3 (0.1, 0.6)*	*< 0.001*
Uninsured/unknown	*0.5 (0.3, 0.8)*	*0.002*	*0.4 (0.3, 0.7)*	*0.001*
CD4 count, cells/uL[e]				
< 200	1.2 (0.8, 1.9)	0.38	–	–
≥ 200[l]	1.0	–		
Viral Load[e]				
< 200	0.9 (0.2, 3.1)	0.84	–	–
≥ 200[l]	1.0	–		
Depression[e,f]				
Yes	1.0 (0.6, 1.5)	0.83	–	–
No[l]	1.0	–		
Drug use[e,g]				
Current	0.7 (0.4, 1.2)	0.17	–	–
Past/never[l]	1.0	–		
At risk alcohol use[e,h,i]				
Yes	0.8 (0.5, 1.2)	0.34	–	–
No/low[l]	1.0	–		
Number of MHCs[e,j]				
0[l]	1.0	–	1.0	–
1	1.2 (0.9, 1.9)	0.36	1.2 (0.7, 1.9)	0.50
2	0.8 (0.5, 1.4)	0.51	0.7 (0.4, 1.1)	0.13
3	0.5 (0.2, 1.1)	0.09	*0.3 (0.1, 0.7)*	*0.01*

were significantly associated with retention in care in univariate analysis, an inverse dose–response relationship was observed for the number of MHCs (Table 2). In other words, as the number of MHCs increased, the odds of retention decreased. Although not statistically significant, the odds of retention for those with 3 MHC was approximately 50% lower than those without any MHC (3 MHCs = 0.5, 95% CI 0.2–1.1). Higher MH service utilization was associated with increased odds of retention in care; the association was strongest for the group utilizing ≥ 3 MH services ($OR_{unadj} = 4.4$; 95% CI 1.6–12.2; $p = 0.01$).

Table 2 continued

Characteristic	Univariate analysis[c]		Multivariable analysis[c,d]	
	Unadjusted OR (95% CI)	*p*	Adjusted OR (95% CI)	*p*
Mental healthcare utilization[k]				
0[l]	1.00		1.0	–
1–2	1.3 (0.7, 2.3)	0.43	1.6 (0.8, 3.0)	0.15
≥ 3	*4.4 (1.6, 12.2)*	*0.01*	*6.8 (2.3, 20.4)*	*<0.001*

CI confidence Interval, *IDU* intravenous drug use, *MHC* mental health co-morbidities, *MSM* men who have sex with men, *OR* odds Ratio, *SD* standard deviation, *UAB* University of Alabama at Birmingham (Birmingham, AL, USA)

Italic type face are statistically significant at 0.05 level

[a] Definition: at least two primary care appointments being attended within a period of 12 months but separated by at least 90 days

[b] Treatment naïve and newly engaged in care

[c] Logistic regression method

[d] Model performance: C-statistics = 0.677; Max-rescaled r-square = 9.1%; Hosmer–Lemeshow test *p* value = 0.62

[e] Measured at baseline (time of clinic enrollment interview)

[f] Patient Health Questionnaire-9

[g] Alcohol, Smoking and Substance Involvement Screening Test

[h] Alcohol Use Disorder Identification Test-Consumption Test

[i] Drug use excludes marijuana

[j] Measured as total count of depression, drug use, and alcohol use

[k] Measured within 12 months

[l] Reference category

In multivariable analyses (Table 2), persons with public insurance (OR_{adj} = 0.3; 95% CI 0.1–0.6; p < 0.001) and no insurance (OR_{adj} = 0.4; 95% CI 0.3–0.7; p = 0.001) were significantly less likely to be retained in care than privately insured PLWH. The dose response relationships for both MHCs and MH service utilization in multivariable analysis was similar to univariate analysis. There was an inverse association between 3 MHCs (OR_{adj} = 0.3; 95% CI0.1–0.7; p = 0.01) and retention in care and a positive association between ≥ 3 MH service utilization (OR_{adj} = 6.8, 95% CI 2.3, 20.4; p < 0.001) with retention in care. Both were statistically significant.

An additional multivariable model (not shown) with the individual MH conditions instead of number of MHCs was examined due to collinearity between these two variables. The strength of association and statistical significance for the individual MH conditions remained the same as in univariate analyses. The results for the other predictors were similar to the model presented in Table 2. Additional analyses were completed to examine whether presence of any MH comorbidity(s) had an effect on the association between MH service utilization and retention in HIV primary care (Table 3, Fig. 1). Due to large variability and wide confidence intervals produced by Firth's correction method, only point estimates are graphed with 95% CI labelled in Fig. 1. Among those without MH service utilization, those with ≥ 1 MHCs had reduced odds of retention (OR = 0.9; 95% CI 0.6–1.4; p = 0.74), which did not meet statistical significance. Of those with zero MHCs, odds of retention in care increased as MH service utilization increased from 0 to 1–2 and ≥ 3 service utilization visits. These associations were stronger in those without MHCs as compared to those with MHCs (1–2 MH utilization, OR = 1.8, 95% CI 0.5–9.0 vs OR = 1.0, 95% CI 0.5–2.2 and ≥ 3 MH service utilization, OR = 5.6, 95% CI 0.7–720 vs. OR = 3.2, 95% CI 1.3–10.0). In the absence of MHCs, the effect of MH service utilization on retention was increased. These relationships remained the same even when adjusted for age, race, sex, and transmission risk (data not shown on Figure).

Discussion

This study evaluated the association between MH service utilization and retention in HIV medical care and found a positive dose–response relationship: as utilization of mental health services increased, retention in care improved. Patients using ≥ 1mental health service were more likely to be retained in primary care at 12 months relative to those who did not. PLWH receive the greatest benefit when utilizing ≥ 3 mental health services during their first year of care regardless of the presence or absence of self-reported MHCs (depressive symptoms, drug use, and/or at-risk alcohol use, see "Methods"), which are often comorbid with HIV.

Table 3 Effect of mental health comorbidities[a] on the association of retention[b] in care and mental health utilization in HIV-positive patients[c] receiving care at UAB, 2007–2013 (N = 743)

Mental health utilization	Univariate analysis[d]		Multivariable analysis[d,e]	
	Mental health comorbidity		Mental health comorbidity	
	0	≥ 1	0	≥ 1
0	N = 271 OR = 1.0 (Reference category)	N = 288 OR = 0.9 (95% CI: 0.6, 1.4) P = 0.74	OR = 1.0 (Reference category)	OR = 1.0 (95% CI: 0.6, 1.5) P = 0.96
1–2	N = 23 OR = 1.8 (95% CI 0.5, 9.0) P = 0.37	N = 75 OR = 1.0 (95% CI 0.5, 2.2) P = 0.89	OR = 2.3 (95% CI 0.7, 11.8) P = 0.19	OR = 1.2 (95% CI 0.6, 2.4) P = 0.69
≥ 3	N = 13 OR = 5.6 (95% CI 0.7, 720.0) P = 0.12	N = 73 OR = 3.2 (95% CI 1.3, 10.0) P = 0.01	OR = 5.7 (95% CI 0.7, 738.8) P = 0.12	OR = 3.8 (95% CI 1.5, 12.2) P = 0.005

CI confidence interval, *OR* odds ratio, *UAB* University of Alabama at Birmingham (Birmingham, AL, USA)

[a] Measured as total count of depression, drug use, and alcohol use

[b] Definition: at least two primary care appointments being attended within a period of 12 months but separated by at least 90 days

[c] Treatment naïve and newly engaged in care

[d] Logistic regression method with Firth's bias correction

[e] Adjusted for age, race, sex, and transmission risk

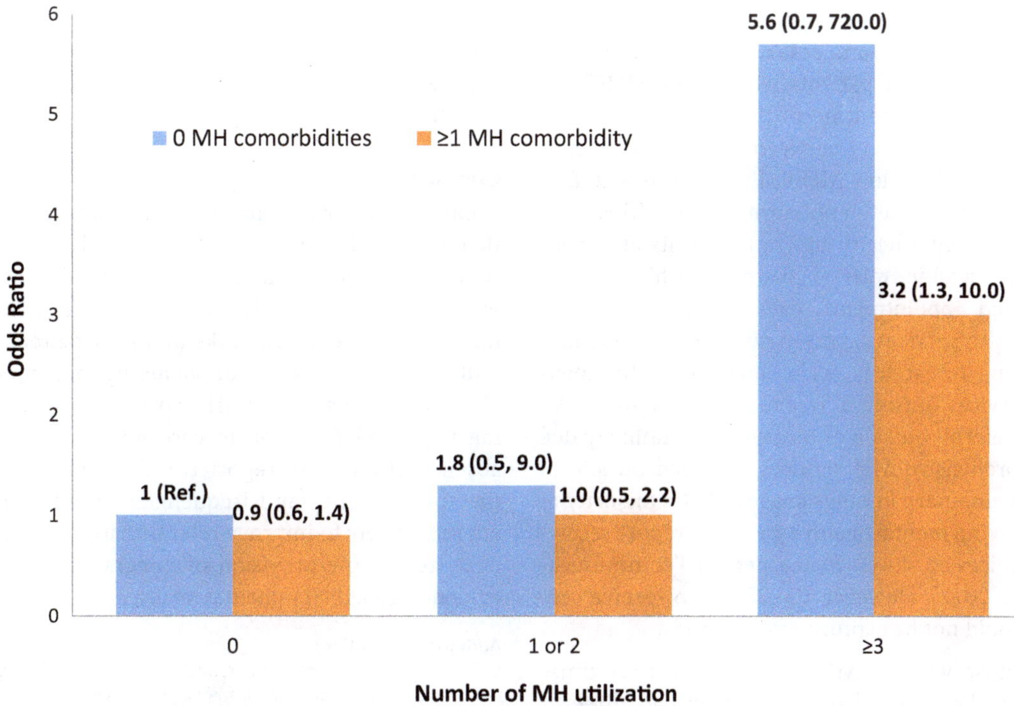

Fig. 1 Univariate analysis of the effect of mental health comorbidities on the association of retention in care and mental health utilization in HIV-positive patients receiving care at UAB, 2007–2013 (N = 743)

There are several explanations for the dose–response relationship between MH service utilization and retention in care. It is known that effective MHC treatment requires attention to the complex relationship between HIV and MHCs [8, 44], and integrated treatment approaches have been proven to improve the care of both HIV and MHCs [45, 46]. Additionally, contact with mental health professionals may reinforce the importance of HIV care [47]. When attending mental health appointments, patients may receive more reminders about HIV clinic appointments. For example, in our clinic, upcoming appointment reminders are printed for patients at each visit. Regardless, it is clear that exposure to more mental health services has a positive effect on clinic retention in our study both for PLWH with and without the three aforementioned MHCs. It is also noteworthy that our study evaluated PLWH newly initiating outpatient HIV medical care, a group that can be overwhelmed with their diagnosis and may benefit from case management and/or counseling [25]. Even in the absence of MHCs, contact with a mental health specialist may prompt referrals for additional support services (e.g., food supplements, travel vouchers) which may have eased the transition and attenuated the challenges often faced among persons establishing HIV medical care [34].

Our population has a high prevalence of MHCs with about one-third reporting depressive symptoms and slightly more than one-third reporting high risk alcohol use. However, a minority of patients (24.8%) received MH services during the first year of care. This is surprising as providers, social workers, and case managers in our clinic have the option to refer patients who report MHCs for mental health care at the time of PRO assessment. It is possible that the disconnect between the high prevalence of MHCs and relatively low MH utilization is due to failure to attend mental health appointments [48]. This analysis evaluated mental health utilization (visits attended) but did not include referral patterns, which would include missed appointments, cancelled appointments, or mental health services accessed outside our clinic network. Ongoing research is evaluating referral for mental health services outside of our healthcare system. We expect MH referral outside of our system is unlikely due to the comprehensive MH services provided on site in our clinic. Preliminary findings suggest that a majority of patients receiving mental health care (75%) report receiving these services on site (B. Pence, personal communication, June 26, 2017). However, the 25% who receive care elsewhere would not be captured in this study.

Notably, those with no MHCs were almost six times more likely to be retained in care if they had three or more MH utilizations in the first year. Perhaps this speaks to the prevalence of other MHCs (anxiety, schizophrenia) or the presence of unmet needs (food and/or housing) which are common in PLWH. Neither additional psychiatric conditions and unmet needs were measured in this analysis but may improve with support and resources provided through increased use of health care services, leading to improved retention in care [47, 49]. Furthermore, additional encounters with the clinic, be it for mental health care or other ancillary services, may lead to subsequent referrals for supportive care and resources. Meeting these additional needs related to food, housing, and/or transportation increases retention in HIV care [34]. By increasing the number of supportive services offered, each mental health encounter may indirectly increase retention in care. Alternatively, as clinicians, we observe the profound effect that an HIV diagnosis has on mental health and, therefore, suspect that counseling may benefit all PLWH [25–27].

This study is a moderate sized, single site assessment of MH utilization and HIV retention in care and is limited by 12-month follow-up time. Only three MHC were included (depressive symptoms, at-risk alcohol use, and drug use) and defined via self-report at the time of entry to care, which may exclude additional psychiatric conditions that may respond to MH services. Our clinic employs additional interventions including cognitive-behavioral therapy (CBT), intensive case management, and support group referrals which we were unable to query and/or measure during the study period. Study participants with MHC may have received these unmeasured services, which would potentially increase important outcomes (e.g., retention in care) due to these services rather than MH service utilization as defined by this study.

Conclusions

Improving retention in HIV care, adherence to ARV therapies, and achieving sustained viral load suppression is critical to halting the HIV epidemic. For many PLWH with MHCs, specifically depression, drug use, and alcohol abuse, these benchmarks may only be reached with a multidisciplinary care team including mental health care. Our results suggest that MH care is important in achieving improved retention in care for PLWH, even in the absence of a patient-reported indication. Understanding the specific types and frequencies of MH services that are most likely to improve retention in care is an essential next step to the provision of integrated, comprehensive evidence-based HIV mental health care.

Authors' contributions

LAS was primarily responsible for study design, acquisition of data, interpretation of data, and drafting manuscript. EFE was responsible for revising manuscript and approving final version and overseeing data interpretation. ART conducted data analysis and assisted in data interpretation, reviewing, and revising the manuscript. DSB and MJM assisted with study conception, data interpretation and revising the original manuscript. All authors read and approved the final manuscript.

Author details
[1] Division of Epidemiology, Department of Epidemiology, Vanderbilt University, 2525 West End Ave, Suite 600, Nashville, TN 37235, USA. [2] Division of Infectious Diseases, Department of Medicine, University of Alabama at Birmingham, 845 19th St. South, Birmingham, AL 35294, USA. [3] Department of Social Work, University of Alabama at Birmingham, 900 13th Street South, Birmingham, AL 35294, USA.

Acknowledgements
Not applicable.

Competing interests
LAS, ART, and DSB have nothing to disclose. EFE is supported by grant K12HS023009 from the Agency for Health Research and Quality and the UAB Center for AIDS Research (CFAR; P30-A1027767) and has received funds (to UAB) from the Bristol Myers Squibb Virology Fellowship and Merck. MJM has received grant support (to UAB) from Bristol Myers Squibb Virology Fellows Research Training Program and consulting fees from Gilead Sciences.

Funding
This study was supported by grant K12HS023009 from the Agency for Health Research and Quality and the UAB Center for AIDS Research (CFAR; P30-A1027767).

References

1. White House. National HIV/AIDS Strategy for the United States: Updated to 2020, 2015. https://www.hiv.gov/federal-resources/national-hiv-aids-strategy/nhas-update.pdf. Accessed 3 Dec 2017.
2. Centers for disease control and prevention. Selected national HIV prevention and care outcomes in the United States. 2017:2014–2016.
3. Horstmann E, Brown J, Islam F, Buck J, Agins BD. Retaining HIV-infected patients in care: where are we? where do we go from here? Clin Infect Dis. 2010;50(5):752–61. https://doi.org/10.1086/649933.
4. Giordano TP, Gifford AL, White ACJ, et al. Retention in care: a challenge to survival with HIV infection. Clin Infect Dis. 2007;44(11):1493–9. https://doi.org/10.1086/516778.
5. Berg MB, Safren SA, Mimiaga MJ, Grasso C, Boswell S, Mayer KH. Nonadherence to medical appointments is associated with increased plasma HIV RNA and decreased CD4 cell counts in a community-based HIV primary care clinic. AIDS Care. 2005;17(7):902–7. https://doi.org/10.1080/09540120500101658.
6. Nemes MIB, Carvalho HB, Souza MFM. Antiretroviral therapy adherence in Brazil. AIDS. 2004;18(Suppl 3):S15–20.
7. Mugavero MJ, Amico KR, Westfall AO, et al. Early retention in HIV care and viral load suppression: implications for a test and treat approach to HIV prevention. J Acquir Immune Defic Syndr. 2012;59(1):86–93. https://doi.org/10.1097/QAI.0b013e318236f7d2.
8. Durvasula R, Miller TR. Substance abuse treatment in persons with HIV/AIDS: challenges in managing triple diagnosis. Behav Med. 2014;40(2):43–52. https://doi.org/10.1080/08964289.2013.866540.
9. Hasin DS, O'Brien CP, Auriacombe M, et al. DSM-5 criteria for substance use disorders: recommendations and rationale. Am J Psychiatry. 2013;170(8):834–51. https://doi.org/10.1176/appi.ajp.2013.12060782.
10. Do AN, Rosenberg ES, Sullivan PS, et al. Excess burden of depression among HIV-infected persons receiving medical care in the united states: data from the medical monitoring project and the behavioral risk factor surveillance system. PLoS ONE. 2014;9(3):e92842. https://doi.org/10.1371/journal.pone.0092842.
11. Justice A, Sullivan L, Fiellin D. HIV/AIDS, comorbidity, and alcohol: can we make a difference? Alcohol Res Health. 2010;33(3):258–66.
12. Galvan FH, Bing EG, Fleishman JA, et al. The prevalence of alcohol consumption and heavy drinking among people with HIV in the United States: results from the HIV cost and services utilization study. J Stud Alcohol. 2002;63(2):179–86.
13. Chander G, Himelhoch S, Moore R. Substance abuse and psychiatric disorders in HIV-positive patients. Drugs. 2006;66(6):769–89. https://doi.org/10.2165/00003495-200666060-00004
14. Howe CJ, Cole SR, Napravnik S, et al. The role of at-risk alcohol/drug use and treatment in appointment attendance and virologic suppression among HIV(+) African Americans. AIDS Res Hum Retroviruses. 2014;30(3):233–40. https://doi.org/10.1089/AID.2013.0163.
15. Mugavero MJ, Westfall AO, Zinski A, et al. Measuring retention in HIV care: the elusive gold standard. J Acquir Immune Defic Syndr. 2012;61(5):574–80. https://doi.org/10.1097/QAI.0b013e318273762f.
16. Azar MM, Springer SA, Meyer JP, Altice FL. A systematic review of the impact of alcohol use disorders on HIV treatment outcomes, adherence to antiretroviral therapy and health care utilization. Drug Alcohol Depend. 2010;112(3):178–93. https://doi.org/10.1016/j.drugalcdep.2010.06.014.
17. De Hert M, Correll CU, Bobes J, et al. Physical illness in patients with severe mental disorders. I. Prevalence, impact of medications and disparities in health care. World Psychiatry. 2011;10(1):52–77. http://www.embase.com/search/results?subaction=viewrecord&from=export&id=L361401218. Accessed 3 Dec 2017.
18. Yehia BR, Stewart L, Momplaisir F, et al. Barriers and facilitators to patient retention in HIV care. BMC Infect Dis. 2015;15(1):1–10. https://doi.org/10.1186/s12879-015-0990-0.
19. Messeri PA, Abramson DM, Aidala AA, Lee F, Lee G. The impact of ancillary HIV services on engagement in medical care in New York City. AIDS Care. 2002;14(Suppl 1):S15–29. https://doi.org/10.1080/09540120220149948.
20. Calsyn RJ, Klinkenberg WD, Morse GA, Miller J, Cruthis R. Recruitment, engagement, and retention of people living with HIV and co-occurring mental health and substance use disorders. AIDS Care. 2004;16(Suppl 1):S56–70.
21. Cunningham WE, Wong M, Hays RD. Case management and health-related quality of life outcomes in a national sample of persons with HIV/AIDS. J Natl Med Assoc. 2008;100(7):840–7.
22. Flores D, Leblanc N, Barroso J. Enroling and retaining human immunodeficiency virus (HIV) patients in their care: a metasynthesis of qualitative studies. Int J Nurs Stud. 2016;62:126–36. https://doi.org/10.1016/j.ijnurstu.2016.07.016.
23. Higa DH, Marks G, Crepaz N, Liau A, Lyles CM. Interventions to improve retention in HIV primary care: a systematic review of U.S. studies. Curr HIV/AIDS Rep. 2012;9(4):313–25. https://doi.org/10.1007/s11904-012-0136-6.
24. Turan B, Hatcher AM, Weiser SD, Johnson MO, Rice WS, Turan JM. Framing mechanisms linking HIV-related stigma, adherence to treatment, and health outcomes. Am J Public Health. 2017;107(6):863–9. https://doi.org/10.2105/AJPH.2017.303744.
25. Honiden S, Sundaram V, Nease RF, et al. The effect of diagnosis with HIV infection on health-related quality of life. Qual Life Res. 2006;15(1):69–82. https://doi.org/10.1007/s11136-005-8485-x.
26. Emlet CA, Brennan DJ, Brennenstuhl S, Rueda S, Hart TA, Rourke SB. The impact of HIV-related stigma on older and younger adults living with HIV disease: does age matter? AIDS Care. 2015;27(4):520–8. https://doi.org/10.1080/09540121.2014.978734.
27. Earnshaw VA, Lang SM, Lippitt M, Jin H, Chaudoir SR. HIV stigma and physical health symptoms: do social support, adaptive coping, and/or identity centrality act as resilience resources? AIDS Behav. 2015;19(1):41–9. https://doi.org/10.1007/s10461-014-0758-3.
28. Policy HB. Clarifications regarding clients eligible for private health insurance and coverage of services by Ryan White HIV/AIDS Program. http://hab.hrsa.gov/manageyourgrant/pinspals/pcn1304privateinsurance.pdf. Accessed 3 Dec 2017.
29. Compendium of evidence-based interventions and best practices for HIV prevention. Centers for disease control. Published 2015. http://www.cdc.gov/hiv/prevention/research/compendium/lrc/index.html. Accessed 5 Jan 2016.
30. Kroenke K, Spitzer RL, Williams JB. The PHQ-9: validity of a brief depression severity measure. J Gen Intern Med. 2001;16(9):606–13.
31. Hodgson RJ, John B, Abbasi T, et al. Fast screening for alcohol misuse. Addict Behav. 2003;28(8):1453–63.
32. Humeniuk R, Ali R, Babor TF, et al. Validation of the alcohol, smoking and substance involvement screening test (ASSIST). Addiction. 2008;103(6):1039–47. https://doi.org/10.1111/j.1360-0443.2007.02114.x.
33. Mugavero MJ, Davila JA, Nevin CR, Giordano TP. From access to engagement: measuring retention in outpatient HIV clinical care. AIDS Patient Care STDS. 2010;24(10):607–13. https://doi.org/10.1089/apc.2010.0086.
34. Thompson MA, Mugavero MJ, Amico KR, et al. Guidelines for improving entry into and retention in care and antiretroviral adher-

ence for persons with HIV: evidence-based recommendations from an International Association of Physicians in AIDS Care panel. Ann Intern Med. 2012;156(11):817–33, W-284–289. https://doi.org/10.7326/0003-4819-156-11-201206050-00419.

35. HRSA HAB. HIV/AIDS Bureau Revised Performance Measure Portfolio. 2015.
36. Manea L, Gilbody S, McMillan D. A diagnostic meta-analysis of the Patient Health Questionnaire-9 (PHQ-9) algorithm scoring method as a screen for depression. Gen Hosp Psychiatry. 2015;37(1):67–75. https://doi.org/10.1016/j.genhosppsych.2014.09.009.
37. Edwards M, Quinlivan EB, Bess K, et al. Implementation of PHQ-9 depression screening for HIV-infected patients in a real-world setting. J Assoc Nurses AIDS Care. 2014;25(3):243–52. https://doi.org/10.1016/j.jana.2013.05.004.
38. de Jong BC, Prentiss D, McFarland W, Machekano R, Israelski DM. Marijuana use and its association with adherence to antiretroviral therapy among HIV-infected persons with moderate to severe nausea. J Acquir Immune Defic Syndr. 2005;38(1):43–6.
39. Eaton EF, Tamhane AR, Burkholder GA, Willig JH, Saag MS, Mugavero MJ. Unanticipated effects of new drug availability on antiretroviral durability: implications for comparative effectiveness research. Open forum Infect Dis. 2016;3(2):ofw109. https://doi.org/10.1093/ofid/ofw109.
40. Marcin JP, Schembri MS, He J, Romano PS. A population-based analysis of socioeconomic status and insurance status and their relationship with pediatric trauma hospitalization and mortality rates. Am J Public Health. 2003;93(3):461–6. https://doi.org/10.2105/AJPH.93.3.461.
41. Smith SA, Hasan AK, Binkley PF, Foraker RE. The impact of insurance and socioeconomic status on outcomes for patients with left ventricular assist devices. J Surg Res. 2014;191(2):302–8. https://doi.org/10.1016/j.jss.2014.05.004.
42. Allison PD. Logistic regression using SAS: theory and application. In: Institute S, editor. NC: Cary; 2003.
43. Firth D. Bias reduction of maximum likelihood estimates. Biometrika. 1993;80(1):27–38. https://doi.org/10.2307/2336755.
44. Halkitis PN, Wolitski RJ, Millett GA. A holistic approach to addressing HIV infection disparities in gay, bisexual, and other men who have sex with men. Am Psychol. 2013;68(4):261–73. https://doi.org/10.1037/a0032746.
45. Zaller N, Gillani FS, Rich JD. A model of integrated primary care for HIV-positive patients with underlying substance use and mental illness. AIDS Care. 2007;19(9):1128–33. https://doi.org/10.1080/09540120701335196.
46. Gardner EM, McLees MP, Steiner JF, Del Rio C, Burman WJ. The spectrum of engagement in HIV care and its relevance to test-and-treat strategies for prevention of HIV infection. Clin Infect Dis. 2011;52(6):793–800. https://doi.org/10.1093/cid/ciq243.
47. Gardner LI, Giordano TP, Marks G, et al. Enhanced personal contact with HIV patients improves retention in primary care: a randomized trial in 6 US HIV clinics. Clin Infect Dis. 2014;59(5):725–34. https://doi.org/10.1093/cid/ciu357.
48. Ho CP, Zinski A, Fogger SA, et al. Factors associated with missed psychiatry visits in an urban HIV clinic. AIDS Behav. 2015;19(8):1423–9. https://doi.org/10.1007/s10461-014-0967-9.
49. Katz MH, Cunningham WE, Fleishman JA, et al. Effect of case management on unmet needs and utilization of medical care and medications among HIV-infected persons. Ann Intern Med. 2001;135(8_Part_1):557–65. https://doi.org/10.7326/0003-4819-135-8_Part_1-200110160-00006.

23

A meta-analysis comparing 48-week treatment outcomes of single and multi-tablet antiretroviral regimens for the treatment of people living with HIV

Patrick G. Clay[1*], Wei C. Yuet[1], Christiane H. Moecklinghoff[2], Inge Duchesne[3], Krzysztof L. Tronczyński[4], Sandip Shah[5] and Dong Shao[5]

Abstract

Objectives: To compare outcomes with single tablet regimens (STR) versus multi-tablet regimens (MTR) for human immunodeficiency virus (HIV) treatment using published data.

Design: Systematic review and random-effects meta-analysis of literature on approved and investigational HIV regimens.

Methods: The research followed the Preferred Reporting Items for Systematic Reviews and Meta-Analyses guidelines. Single or un-blinded studies reporting a direct comparison between STR and MTR were eligible for the meta-analysis. Double-blinded studies were excluded due to lack of difference in pill burden between cohorts. The key outcomes of interest included: adherence rates/proportion meeting target, efficacy, safety/tolerability, non-clinical and economic outcomes.

Results: After screening 63 full-text articles and posters, 14 studies were eligible for the meta-analysis. The analysis showed that patients taking STR had improved outcomes over those taking MTR. Patients were significantly more adherent regardless of daily dosing frequency (odds ratio [OR]: 1.96, $p < 0.001$) and were more likely to achieve virological suppression (relative risk [RR]: 1.05, $p = 0.002$). There was a trend toward a lower discontinuation risk in the STR cohort, together with reported higher therapy satisfaction, better symptom control, improved health status, reduced healthcare resource utilization and demonstrated cost-effectiveness compared to MTR. There were no differences in CD4 cell count increase (at 48 weeks) or safety outcomes.

Conclusions: The findings of this study confirm previously reported preliminary findings of the advantages of STR over MTR for HIV treatment in adherence, therapy continuation, viral suppression, tolerability, quality of life improvement, cost-effectiveness and healthcare resource utilization.

Keywords: Human immunodeficiency virus, Treatment adherence and compliance, Treatment outcome, Quality of life, Economics pharmaceutical

*Correspondence: Patrick.Clay@unthsc.edu
[1] University of North Texas System College of Pharmacy, 3500 Camp Bowie Blvd, Fort Worth, TX 76107, USA

Introduction

Although treatment options have expanded significantly, human immunodeficiency virus (HIV) remains an important global public health issue. In 2017, the number of people living with HIV (PLWH) was approximately 36.9 million [1] and about 1.1 million people died of acquired immune deficiency syndrome (AIDS)-related illnesses [1]. The annual rate of new infections remained relatively constant between 2005 and 2017, however, the number of PLWH receiving antiretroviral therapy (ART) increased dramatically from 2.2 million to 21.7 million [1].

ART has evolved significantly in the past two decades. Beginning with protease inhibitors in 1995, through multiple drug single class combination tablets in 2001 and multiple drug, multiple class combination tablets in 2006, to the most recent and sixth ART class, post-attachment inhibitors (ibalizumab), in 2018. Today, multiple class, multiple drug, fixed-dose, single tablet regimens (STR) dominate use [2]. Collectively, these advances have improved outcomes, have enhanced tolerability and reduced pill burden and enabled more PLWH to reach goal adherence levels [3]. With each newly approved STR, there is potential for treatment guidelines/practice patterns to change in PLWH naïve to therapy, yet the needs of the individual is paramount [4, 5]. Efforts continue to develop long-acting mechanisms to deliver ART that may improve durability [3, 6].

Simplified regimens improve adherence and clinical outcomes and have long been proven in other conditions, such as hypertension, diabetes and asthma [3, 7]. With the advent of STR, HIV has become a treatable, chronic disease [8] with both the Joint United Nations Programme on HIV and AIDS (UNAIDS) and the World Health Organization (WHO) highly recommending once daily fixed-dose combinations (FDC) to improve adherence [6, 9].

FDC can include multiple classes of ART and may represent an entire recommended regimen taken once daily (e.g., one 'tablet' once daily). FDC reduce the number of total daily pills (pill burden) and contain at least two active agents, rather than a single dosing unit with a single active agent with a pharmacokinetic enhancer/booster, such as Kaletra™ (lopinavir/ritonavir), Prezcobix™ (darunavir/cobicistat [DRV/COBI]) and Evotaz™ (atazanavir/cobicistat [ATV/COBI]) [10].

When a FDC constitutes an entire regimen and is provided as one 'tablet' for use once daily, it is known as an STR. However, FDC can be co-administered with another ART agent to create a multiple-tablet regimen (MTR). MTR can be taken once or more times per day, dependent upon the MTR components. Since 2014, a number of STR and MTR have been approved and are now recommended by treatment guidelines as first-line treatment for treatment-naïve patients. The newly included STR regimens include elvitegravir/cobicistat/emtricitabine/tenofovir alafenamide (EVG/COBI/FTC/TAF), darunavir/cobicistat/emtricitabine/tenofovir alafenamide (DRV/COBI/FTC/TAF) and emtricitabine/rilpivirine/tenofovir alafenamide (FTC/RPV/TAF). MTR component agents include ATV/COBI, DRV/COBI and emtricitabine/tenofovir alafenamide (FTC/TAF). As none of these combinations have been compared in a systematic review [11], the objective of this study is to compare the clinical (adherence, virologic and safety/tolerability), economic and non-clinical or humanistic outcomes of all currently available STR and MTR.

Methods

Search strategy and study selection

A literature review and meta-analysis was conducted to include all currently approved FDC, both STR and MTR. The study followed the Preferred Reporting Items for Systematic Reviews and Meta-Analyses (PRISMA) guidelines and the PICOS principles (Patient, Intervention, Comparator, Outcome, and Study Design) based on an internal study protocol (available upon request) [12]. Databases including Embase, PubMed and ClinicalTrials.gov were searched to capture relevant literature published from 2005 to 2017, with filters to include only studies conducted in humans and published in English.

The endpoints of interest included adherence, efficacy, safety and healthcare resource utilization along with an emerging element for decision makers, humanistic outcomes [11]. Data included published, publicly available randomized controlled trials (RCT) and observational studies. Case studies, abstracts without posters or full-text, letters, reviews, editorials and comments were excluded. Two reviewers conducted a two level screening process. A first-pass screening of bibliographic details, titles and abstracts of all citations eliminated duplicates and irrelevant studies. Full-text of studies meeting the eligibility criteria and reported outcomes of interest were included for data extraction and screened for inclusion. For all quantitative outcomes, only studies with outcome measures in evaluable format (n/N, mean, standard deviation, N or median and inter-quartile range) with a clear comparison between STR and MTR arms were included. Double-blind studies were excluded as enrolled subjects would receive the same number of tablets, thus removing direct comparison between MTR and STR. Qualitative evidence data capture reporting in the literature precluded use of this standard, thus data was included when provided and resulted in slight variance in studies used. For all studies however, the methodological quality of RCTs was assessed using the Cochrane handbook, focusing on the risk of bias across five different categories (selection, performance, detection, reporting and attrition) [13]. For observational studies, the Critical Appraisal Skills Programme (CASP) Cohort Study Checklist was used to evaluate the overall study quality [14]. A random-effects meta-analysis was conducted using Comprehensive Meta-Analysis Software (version 2) for data analysis and to create the forest plots.

Endpoints

The 48-week primary endpoints were used in all analyses. Adherence outcomes included achieving a protocol specific threshold measure (yes/no, dichotomous) and as author reported adherence frequency (pill count, percentage adherence or proportion of days covered, etc.). Efficacy outcomes included the percentage of patients achieving viral load suppression (i.e., < 50 copies/ml) and changes in mean CD4 counts from baseline. Safety outcomes included the percentage of patients experiencing any severe adverse event (SAE), mortality or any grade 3 to 4 clinically significant event or laboratory abnormality. Tolerability outcomes included the percentage of patients discontinuing their STR or MTR for any reason. Economic and humanistic outcomes are summarized in the review to provide a single-source review of STR compared with MTR to inform healthcare providers as well as policymakers.

Statistical methods

Inverse variance methods were used in a random-effects model to analyze both dichotomous and continuous data and to assess heterogeneity [15]. Heterogeneity was evaluated using the Chi squared test and quantified using the I^2 statistic [16]. Alpha < 0.05 was used to determine statistical significance. I^2 values of 25, 50 and 75% correspond to low, medium and high levels of heterogeneity, respectively. Summary statistics were calculated for each study to describe observed treatment effects; mean and standard deviation values were calculated where studies reported median and inter-quartile range. When necessary, 95% confidence intervals (CI) were converted to standard deviations via the formula $SD = (\sqrt{N})*((\text{upper limit} - \text{lower limit})/3.96)$. A pooled treatment effect estimate was then calculated as the weighted average of the treatment effects estimated in the individual studies. Each study was weighted as the inverse of the variance of the effect estimate (i.e., one over the square of its standard error). Larger studies with smaller standard errors were given more weight than smaller studies with larger standard errors. For the studies which had multiple MTR arms, data from the MTR arms were first pooled within the trials and then between the trials. Dichotomous outcomes were evaluated by making an adjustment to the study weights according to the extent of variation, or heterogeneity, among the treatment effects.

Values for dichotomous outcomes (adherence [based on a threshold measure; yes/no], viral load suppression, safety events, and tolerability) were presented as n/N, where n = subset of sample size; N = total sample size, and the odds ratio (OR) or risk ratio (RR) with 95% CI were calculated. Values for continuous outcomes (CD4 cell counts and adherence [based on pill count or percentage of drug(s) used]) were presented as mean, standard deviation (SD) and N (sample size), with calculated standardized mean differences. For humanistic (qualitative) data, a global approach was adopted to rate the results as negative, neutral or positive based on the change in scores from baseline to the end of the study period. For economic evaluations where studies reported healthcare resource use (HRU), the direct medical costs and incremental cost-effectiveness ratio (ICER) values were summarized.

Results

Study details

The literature search yielded 4002 citations, of which 287 were duplicates, resulting in 3715 unique records. After screening titles and abstracts, 192 potentially relevant studies were identified. Nine additional articles were found from hand searching of bibliographies. Following a careful examination of the 201 full-text articles and clinicaltrials.gov records, a total of 63 studies (34 RCT, 24 observational studies (OS) and five economic studies) met the inclusion and exclusion criteria and were included for qualitative evidence synthesis. The PRISMA flow of the review process is shown in Fig. 1. Nearly half (n = 30) of the studies were conducted in treatment naïve PLWH, 22 studies included treatment experienced PLWH and 11 included both treatment experienced and naïve PLWH.

Twenty-eight of the 63 studies were not included in the previous meta-analysis [11]. Most of the studies not included in the previous review reported efficacy (73%) and safety/tolerability (59%). Adherence was reported in 48% of the added studies. Fewer reported (or assessed) humanistic measures (patient-reported outcomes [PRO]) (14%) and economic endpoints (21%).

Key characteristics of the 63 studies are summarized in Additional file 1: Table S1 Of these 63 studies, only 14 studies reported outcome measures in evaluable format (n/N, mean, standard deviation, N, or median and inter-quartile range) and/or at consistent evaluation time points, with a clear comparison between STR and MTR, and were included for meta-analysis. Baseline demographics of the population in the 14 studies are shown in Additional file 2: Table S2.

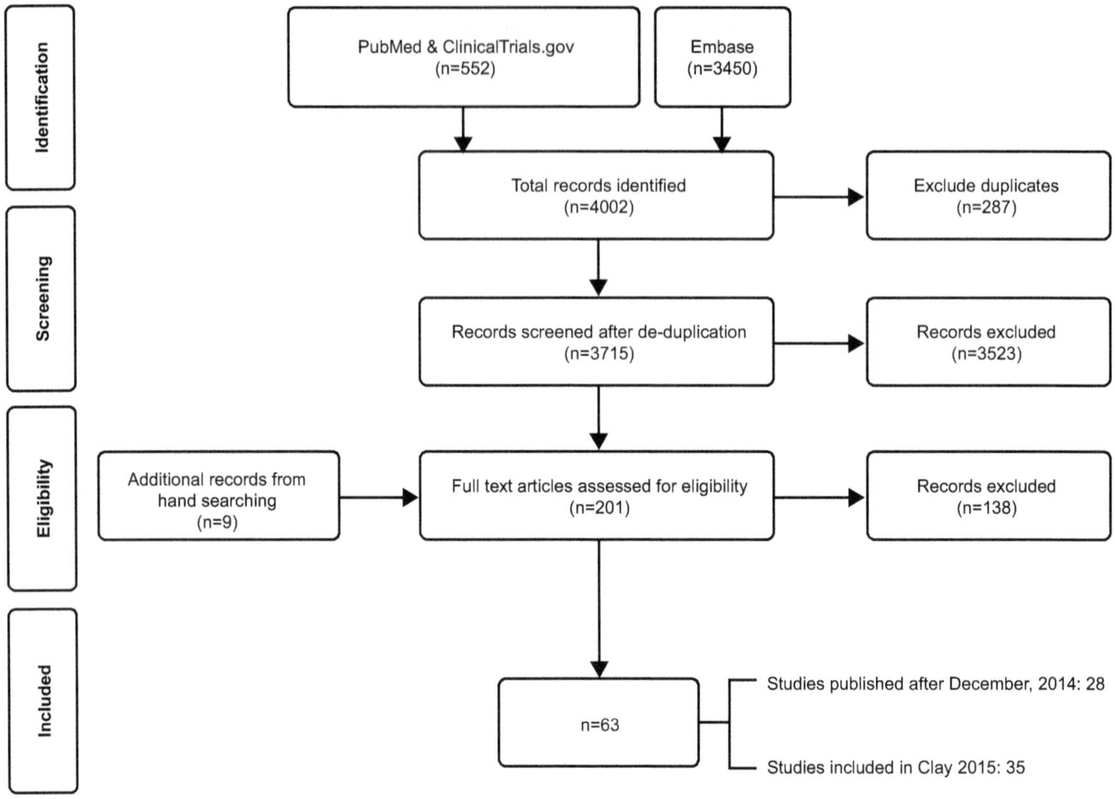

Fig. 1 PRISMA flow diagram for literature search and study selection

The majority of the included RCTs had low risk of bias, with potentially high risk for blinding in treatment allocations. The overall quality of all observational studies was determined as medium and satisfactory. The detailed assessments are presented in Additional file 3: Table S3.

Adherence outcomes

While 30 of the 63 studies reported patient adherence outcomes, only eight studies reported quantifiable data and were included in the meta-analysis [17–24]. Seven of these eight studies [17–23] reported patient adherence as a dichotomous outcome (threshold defined per study protocol), two reported mean difference in medication adherence calculated using pill count and one reported using both formats [17, 24].

In the dichotomous adherence outcome analysis, adherence was significantly better in patients receiving STR than patients receiving once or twice daily MTR: 55.4% (range: 25.7% to 91.6%) versus 42.0% (range: 15.1% to 85.3%), odds ratio (OR) of adherence: 1.96, 95% confidence interval (CI) 1.66–2.33, $p<0.001$. No heterogeneity was observed ($Chi^2=4.91$; $i^2=0.0\%$) (Fig. 2a).

In the sub-analysis of STR versus once daily MTR, adherence was significantly better in patients receiving STR compared with those receiving once daily MTR: 80.5% (range: 76.5% to 85.4%) versus 71.8% (range: 68.0% to 75.0%), OR: 1.66, 95% CI 1.21–2.27, $p=0.002$; Fig. 2a).

In the sub-analysis of STR versus twice daily MTR, adherence was numerically better in patients receiving STR compared with those receiving twice daily MTR: 84.1% (range: 82.6% to 85.4%) versus 66.8% of patients (range: 60.7% to 73.9%), OR: 2.53, 95% CI 1.13–5.65, $p=0.02$; Fig. 2a).

Medication adherence based on "pill count" (two studies) was higher in the STR group (92.1% [range: 86.0% to 98.3%]) compared with 84.8% (range: 73.6% to 95.9%) in the collective MTR groups. The standardized mean difference (SMD) comparing medication adherence was also statistically significantly in favor of the STR group (SMD: 0.68, 95% CI 0.40–0.97, $p<0.001$) in the two studies (Fig. 2b).

Efficacy outcomes

Twenty-four of the 63 studies reported efficacy data for viral load suppression and CD4 count. Eighteen studies were excluded from the meta-analysis since they reported time points other than 48 weeks or parameters not in a quantifiable format. Six studies [22, 25–29]

a

Study name	Subgroup within study	Odds ratio	Lower limit	Upper limit	Z-Value	p-Value	STR	MTR	Relative weight
Bangsberg 2010	STR vs. MTR	2.484	1.166	5.290	2.359	0.018	27/47	25/71	4.97
Fabbiani 2014	STR vs. MTR	2.777	1.525	5.060	3.338	0.001	82/96	310/457	7.89
Skwara 2014	STR vs. MTR	3.886	1.466	10.298	2.730	0.006	24/31	30/64	2.99
Sterrantino 2012	STR vs. MTR	1.623	0.888	2.969	1.573	0.116	71/86	277/372	7.79
Chen 2016	STR vs. MTR	1.607	1.080	2.393	2.337	0.019	127/166	391/584	17.92
Orkin 2017	STR vs. MTR	1.887	0.909	3.916	1.704	0.088	197/215	87/102	5.33
Sutton 2016	STR vs. MTR	1.941	1.540	2.446	5.620	0.000	149/580	241/1594	53.11
		1.964	1.660	2.325	7.853	0.000	677/1221	1361/3244	
Tau²=0.000, Chi²=4.913, df=6 (p=0.555), I²=0.000									
Fabbiani 2014	STR vs. MTR BID	3.798	2.022	7.135	4.148	0.000	82/96	128/211	50.40
Sterrantino 2012	STR vs. MTR BID	1.671	0.875	3.190	1.555	0.120	71/86	136/184	49.60
		2.527	1.130	5.652	2.258	0.024	153/182	264/395	
Tau²=0.231, Chi²=3.175, df=1 (p=0.075), I²=68.508									
Chen 2016	STR vs. MTR Multi-dose	1.689	1.094	2.609	2.364	0.018	127/166	187/284	100.00
		1.689	1.094	2.609	2.364	0.018	127/166	187/284	
Fabbiani 2014	STR vs. MTR once daily	2.060	1.092	3.884	2.233	0.026	82/96	182/246	24.36
Sterrantino 2012	STR vs. MTR once daily	1.578	0.826	3.015	1.380	0.167	71/86	141/188	23.38
Chen 2016	STR vs. MTR once daily	1.532	0.994	2.363	1.932	0.053	127/166	204/300	52.25
		1.658	1.212	2.268	3.166	0.002	280/348	527/734	
Tau²=0.000, Chi²=0.599, df=2 (p=0.741), I²=0.000									

(Statistics for each study: Odds ratio, Lower limit, Upper limit, Z-Value, p-Value; Events/Total: STR, MTR)

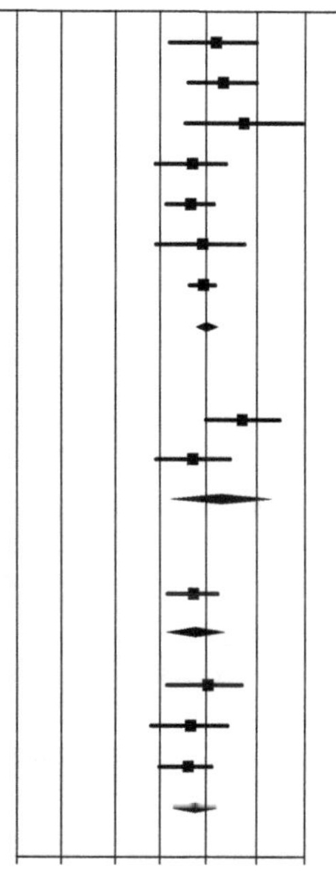

b

Study or subgroup	STR Mean	STR SD	STR Total	MTR Mean	MTR SD	MTR Total	Weight	Std. mean difference IV, random, 95% CI
Bangsberg 2010	86	18	47	73.62	22.05	71	56.6%	0.60 [0.22, 0.98]
Buscher 2012	98.25	2.26	34	95.89	3.25	65	43.4%	0.79 [0.36, 1.22]
Total (95% CI)			81			136	100.0%	0.68 [0.40, 097]

Heterogeneity: Tau²=0.00; Chi²=0.45, df=1 (p=0.5); I²=0%

Test of overall effect: Z=4.73 (p<0.001)

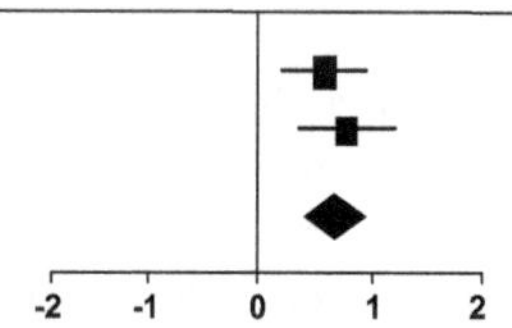

Fig. 2 **a** Adherence rate (dichotomous measure) and **b** adherence per pill count

provided analyzable data for viral load suppression (defined per protocol < 50 copies/ml) at 48 weeks and four studies [25–27, 30, 31] reported change in CD4 cell count at 48 weeks. There was a statistically significant difference in viral load suppression at 48 weeks between the STR and MTR groups (relative risk (RR): 1.05, 95% CI 1.02–1.09, p = 0.002) and low heterogeneity between the studies was observed ($Chi^2 = 7.54$; $i^2 = 33.7\%$) (Fig. 3a). The difference (SMD) in CD4 cell count between STR and MTR was not statistically significant at 48 weeks (SMD: 0.029, 95% CI: − 0.06–0.12, p = 0.51), and no heterogeneity between the studies was observed ($Chi^2 = 1.76$; $i^2 = 0.0\%$, Fig. 3b).

Safety and tolerability outcomes

Of the 63 studies, 37 reported safety outcomes with data relevant to adverse events (AE), laboratory abnormalities, mortality, and tolerability (treatment discontinuation). Six studies [22, 25–28, 32] reported analyzable data for the safety and tolerability outcome parameters. All six studies [22, 25–28, 32] reported rates of discontinuation due to any reason, three reported protocol-defined SAE [22, 25, 26], five reported Grade 3 to 4 AE [22, 25, 26, 28, 32], two reported Grade 3 to 4 laboratory abnormalities [25, 32] and two reported mortality [25, 26].

Meta-analyses of SAE, grade 3 to 4 AE and mortality revealed no statistically significant differences between STR and MTR groups (Fig. 4a) with RR of any SAE (RR:

a

Study name	Subgroup within study	Risk ratio	Lower limit	Upper limit	Z-Value	p-Value	STR	MTR	Relative weight
		Statistics for each study					Events/Total		
Arribas 2014	Viral suppression	1.112	1.028	1.204	2.639	0.008	272/293	121/145	12.70
Pozniak 2014	Viral suppression	1.083	1.006	1.165	2.126	0.034	271/292	126/147	14.25
Dejesus 2009	Viral suppression	1.079	0.967	1.205	1.362	0.173	177/204	82/102	7.45
Choi 2016	Viral suppression	1.061	0.888	1.267	0.649	0.516	40/44	24/28	3.11
Rjinders 2016	Viral suppression	1.055	1.009	1.103	2.356	0.018	390/402	183/199	26.57
Orkin 2017	Viral suppression	1.013	0.982	1.045	0.831	0.406	724/763	354/378	35.91
		1.053	1.019	1.087	3.114	0.002	1874/1998	890/999	

Tau²=0.001, Chi²=7.537, df=5 (p=0.184), I²=33.662

Risk ratio and 95% CI

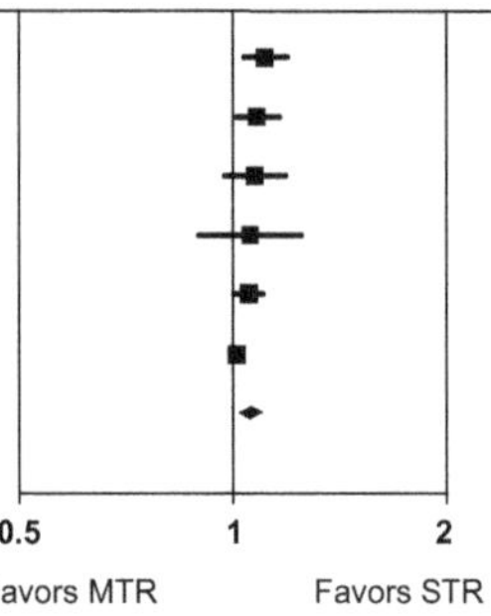

b

Study name	Subgroup within study	Std. diff in means	Std. error	Variance	Lower limit	Upper limit	Z-Value	p-Value	STR	MTR	Relative weight
		Statistics for each study									
Arribas 2014	Change in cell count	0.047	0.103	0.011	-0.155	0.250	0.460	0.646	290	139	18.50
Dejesus 2009	Change in cell count	-0.101	0.123	0.015	-0.343	0.141	-0.814	0.415	203	97	12.91
Pozniak 2014	Change in cell count	-0.013	0.102	0.010	-0.213	0.188	-0.124	0.902	290	143	18.86
Orkin 2017	Change in cell count	0.072	0.063	0.004	-0.052	0.195	1.139	0.255	763	378	49.74
		0.029	0.044	0.002	-0.058	0.116	0.654	0.513	1546	757	

Tau²=0.000, Chi²=1.758, df=3 (p=0.624), I²=0.000

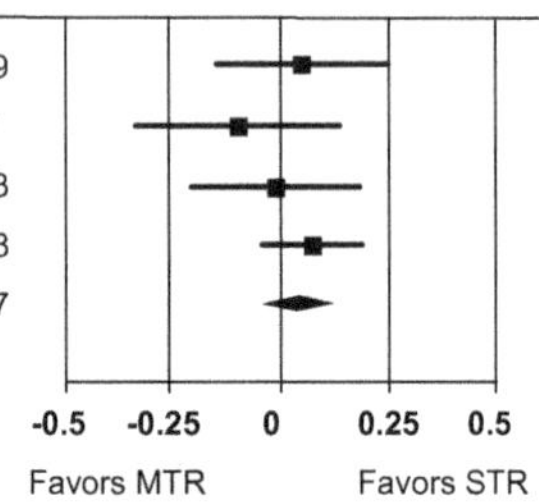

Fig. 3 **a** Viral suppression (<50 copies/ml) at 48 weeks and **b** Increase in CD4 cell count from baseline to 48 weeks

0.96, 95% CI 0.64–1.45, p = 0.86), Grade 3 to 4 AE (RR: 0.83, 95% CI 0.59–1.17, p = 0.29) and mortality (RR: 0.49, 95% CI 0.05–4.65, p = 0.53) and minimal heterogeneity among the studies ($Chi^2 = 0.17–4.55$; $i^2 = 0.00–12.17\%$). Grade 3 to 4 laboratory abnormalities were significantly less likely for the STR group versus the collective MTR groups, RR: 0.68, 95% CI 0.49–0.94, p = 0.02, with no heterogeneity in the studies.

The risk of discontinuation due to any reason was lower in the STR group versus the MTR group, RR: 0.69, 95% CI 0.47–1.00, p = 0.05, —. 4B. Moderate heterogeneity was observed in the tolerability studies ($Chi^2 = 9.71$, $i^2 = 48.49\%$), potentially due to variation in study design and/or population.

Humanistic or patient-reported outcomes (PRO)

Seven [19, 20, 25, 27, 33–35] of the 63 studies reported evaluable results of PRO associated with ART. The most commonly used instruments in the studies included the HIV Treatment Satisfaction Score (HIV-TSQ), HIV Symptom Index (HIV-SI) and the 36-Item Short Form Health Survey (SF-36). Variability among the instruments used meant that the meta-analysis could not include PRO data. Five studies [25, 27, 33–35] reported positive impact with results favoring STR in patient satisfaction, symptom control and overall health status. Among these five studies, the impact of STR or MTR on mental health was rated as neutral. Among the five, only one directly compared STR and MTR [25]. In this study, STR was associated with a higher HIV-TSQ score as compared to MTR at weeks 4 (21.5 versus 13.3, $p < 0.0001$) through week 24 (23.1 versus 14.5, $p < 0.0001$) [25]. Further, STR resulted in lower rates of patient-reported AE such as diarrhea (30% versus 46%, $p < 0.001$) and bloating (33% versus 41%, p = 0.039) compared with MTR ($p < 0.05$ for both) [25]. Similar improvements in the STR and MTR arms in the other two studies, regardless of pill burden [19, 20].

Economic summary

Thirteen [23, 36–47] of 63 studies reported economic outcomes. Ten studies were summarized in the previous review [11]. Three additional studies were identified and are reported in this publication [23, 44, 45]. One study, evaluating overall ART changes in 3850 PLWH, found that modifying therapy resulted in a mean additional cost of €14 (SD €216; range −€528 to +€831) per month per patient [44]. Toxicity and therapy simplifications were cited as the leading causes for regimen changes [44]. Economic outcomes have been modeled using simulations

a

Study name	Subgroup within study	Risk ratio	Lower limit	Upper limit	Z-Value	p-Value	STR	MTR	Relative weight
		Statistics for each study					Events/Total		
Arribas 2014	Any SAEs	0.903	0.413	1.974	-0.257	0.797	17/293	9/140	27.27
Pozniak 2014	Any SAEs	1.147	0.450	2.921	0.287	0.774	14/291	6/143	19.09
Orkin 2017	Any SAEs	0.936	0.536	1.635	-0.233	0.816	34/763	18/378	53.64
		0.963	0.640	1.449	-0.180	0.857	65/1347	33/661	
Tau²=0.000, Chi²=0.170, df=2 (p=0.918), I²=0.000									
Arribas 2014	Grade 3-4 AEs	0.521	0.236	1.152	-1.610	0.107	12/293	11/140	16.74
Pozniak 2014	Grade 3-4 AEs	1.037	0.482	2.235	0.094	0.925	19/291	9/143	17.74
Palella 2014	Grade 3-4 AEs	0.821	0.397	1.696	-0.534	0.594	18/317	11/159	19.58
Choi 2016	Grade 3-4 AEs	9.667	0.574	162.893	1.574	0.115	7/44	0/28	1.47
Orkin 2017	Grade 3-4 AEs	0.842	0.546	1.300	-0.776	0.438	51/763	30/378	44.47
		0.832	0.590	1.173	-1.050	0.294	107/1708	61/848	
Tau²=0.020, Chi²=4.554, df=4 (p=0.336), I²=12.169									
Arribas 2014	Grade 3-4 lab abnormalities	0.627	0.415	0.948	-2.212	0.027	42/293	32/140	64.77
Palella 2014	Grade 3-4 lab abnormalities	0.780	0.445	1.367	-0.868	0.386	28/317	18/159	35.23
		0.677	0.486	0.945	-2.295	0.022	70/610	50/299	
Tau²=0.000, Chi²=0.378, df=1 (p=0.539), I²=0.000									
Arribas 2014	Mortality	0.160	0.007	3.900	-1.125	0.261	0/293	1/140	50.00
Pozniak 2014	Mortality	1.479	0.061	36.091	0.240	0.810	1/291	0/143	50.00
		0.486	0.051	4.654	-0.020	0.502	1/584	1/283	
Tau²=0.000, Chi²=0.932, df=1 (p=0.334), I²=0.000									

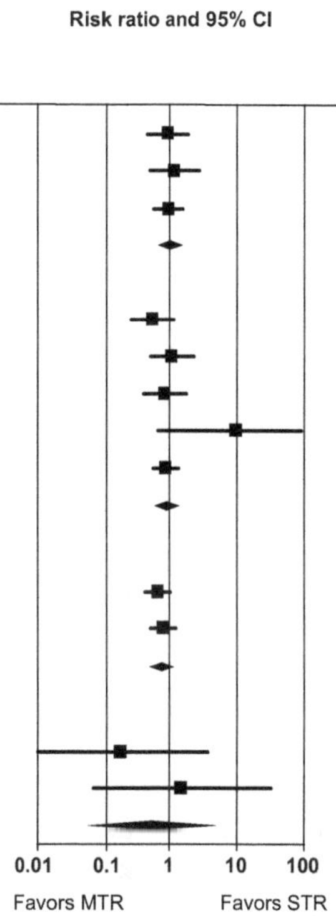

b

Study name	Subgroup within study	Risk ratio	Lower limit	Upper limit	Z-Value	p-Value	STR	MTR	Relative weight
		Statistics for each study					Events/Total		
Arribas 2014	Discontinuation	0.399	0.245	0.650	-3.691	0.000	25/293	31/145	22.66
Pozniak 2014	Discontinuation	0.526	0.304	0.912	-2.288	0.022	23/292	22/147	20.55
Dejesus 2009	Discontinuation	0.876	0.453	1.696	-0.393	0.694	22/203	12/97	17.21
Palella 2014	Discontinuation	1.337	0.637	2.810	0.768	0.443	24/321	9/161	15.10
Choi 2016	Discontinuation	0.636	0.095	4.262	-0.466	0.641	2/44	2/28	3.54
Orkin 2017	Discontinuation	0.842	0.492	1.443	-0.625	0.532	34/763	20/378	20.93
		0.690	0.474	1.006	-1.931	0.054	130/1916	96/956	
Tau²=0.101, Chi²=9.706, df=5 (p=0.084), I²=48.485									

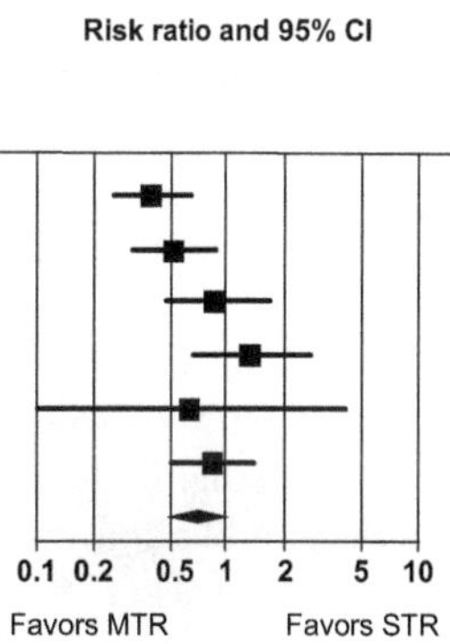

Fig. 4 **a** Safety outcomes and **b** Discontinuation due to any reason

and insurance claims data including comprehensive computer-based microsimulation to compare the cost-effectiveness of STR to MTR for initial treatment and concluded that the ICER of STR to MTR is $26,383 per quality-adjusted life year [45]. A multivariate regression model study using Medicaid medical and pharmacy claims data was completed to determine the impact of ART pill burden in 2174 PLWH [23]. Patients taking STR had a lower risk of hospitalization (HR: 0.71, 95% CI 0.59–0.86, p = NS) and extended time to hospitalization (median: 1508 versus 1032 days, p = 0.0042) [23].

Discussion

The results with respect to adherence, viral load, Grade 3 to 4 laboratory abnormalities favor STR versus MTR. However, in contrast to previous review, the risk of discontinuation due to any reason was lower in the STR group, implying a better tolerability profile. Improved adherence and low discontinuation rates have been seen in other conditions when treatments are simplified that could be attributed to lower pill burdens and dosing frequencies [7]. Although the study was not designed to address the issue, it may be that patient satisfaction with STR may contribute to better adherence and lower rates of discontinuation, leading to improved clinical outcomes. This aspect, rarely reported in clinical trials, should be given enhanced consideration for inclusion.

Improved clinical outcomes could in turn result in lower resource utilization and cost effectiveness of therapy. In fact, the economic studies included in this update indicated lower risk of hospitalization, as well as an ICER of approximately $26,000, which is within the range of willingness to pay thresholds [45]. It should be noted that these economic findings are based on OS and modelling, with inherent selection bias based on variations in patient characteristics and multiple assumptions which may or may not accurately reflect the treatment paradigm in a real-world setting.

We also examined humanistic outcomes based on patient reported data (not included in the meta-analysis), which was not carried out in the previous review. The findings were by and large positive for STR with respect to better patient satisfaction, symptom control and health status, including a lower rate of diarrhea and bloating. Given the weight that humanistic outcomes are gaining with third party payers and government funding bodies, it is worth considering when deciding regimen options. Further, consistent use of assessment tool or inclusion of multiple tools to permit higher order analyses is encouraged.

Similar to the previous review, the strengths of this update are based on the implementation of a well-defined search strategy and the use of a robust random-effects model to assess pooled estimates extracted from both RCTs and observational studies. We only included studies which had quantifiable outcomes that could be included in an analysis. For this reason, we only included open label studies with 48-week outcomes data for the meta-analysis, to enable us to compare STR and MTR. We excluded double blinded, randomized studies where patients on STR would also receive placebo pills (to equal the total number of pills for patients on MTR), since this would not result in an accurate comparison. Authors acknowledge that different classes of medications were compared and factors such as the mechanism of action might also play a role in safety and efficacy results.

Conclusion

Patients on STR have better adherence, lower rates of discontinuation, improved viral load and fewer laboratory abnormalities than those on MTR. Economic and humanistic outcomes favor STR. Additional studies to examine the link between patient satisfaction, adherence and clinical outcomes in PLWH receiving STR or MTR, would provide additional evidence to support STR over MTR. In the meantime, it is important to implement and follow current global and country specific guidelines that specify STR as one of the primary recommended treatments in the management of PLWH. Improving access to STRs for patients, physicians and healthcare systems is critical, in improving the quality of life of PLWH.

Authors' contributions

All authors (PGC, WCY, CHM, ID, KLT, SS, DS) each substantially contributed to the conception or design of the work; the acquisition, analysis, or interpretation of the data for the work; drafting the work or revising it critically for important intellectual content; final approval of the version to be published; and agreement to be accountable for all aspects of the work in ensuring that questions related to the accuracy or integrity of any part of the work are appropriately investigated and resolved. All authors read and approved the final manuscript.

Author details

[1] University of North Texas System College of Pharmacy, 3500 Camp Bowie Blvd, Fort Worth, TX 76107, USA. [2] Jannsen-Cilag GmbH, Johnson & Johnson Platz 1, 41470 Neuss, Germany. [3] Janssen EMEA, Turnhoutseweg 30, 2340 Beerse, Belgium. [4] Janssen-Cilag Polska Sp. Z o.o, Iłżecka 24, 02-135 Warsaw, Poland. [5] Market Access Solutions, LLC, 575 NJ-28, Raritan, NJ 08869, USA.

Acknowledgements

We would like to thank Melissa Stauffer, PhD for her support in developing and running the meta-analysis model.

Competing interests

PGC receives grant funding from Centers for Disease Control and Prevention and National Institute on Minority Health and Health Disparities to conduct practice-based research; is contracted on behalf of University of North Texas Health Science Center by Merck to conduct a Phase III clinical trial; serves on an advisory board or the speaker's bureau for GlaxoSmithKline, NAPO Pharmaceuticals and Merck & Company, Inc; and has been compensated for consultations provided to National Institutes of Health, Agency for Healthcare Research and Quality, Center for Medicare and Medicaid Services, Prime Education, SIGA Consulting, 3D Communications, Market Access Solutions, and Ipsos. CHM, ID, and KLT are employed by Janssen. WCY, SS, and DS have no conflicts of interest.

Funding

This study was financially supported by Janssen EMEA.

References

1. AVERT. Global HIV and AIDS statistics. 2017. https://www.avert.org/global-hiv-and-aids-statistics.
2. U.S. Department of Health and Human Services. FDA approval of HIV medicines; 2016.
3. U.S. Department of Health and Human Services. Guidelines for the use of antiretroviral agents in HIV-1-infected adults and adolescents; 2016.
4. Centers for Disease Control and Prevention. Evolution of HIV/AIDS prevention programs–United States, 1981–2006. MMWR Morb Mortal Wkly Rep. 2006;55(21):597–603.
5. Sepkowitz KA. AIDS-the first 20 years. N Engl J Med. 2001;344:1764–72.
6. World Health Organization. Consolidated guidelines on the use of antiretroviral drugs for treating and preventing HIV infection. 2nd ed. Geneva: World Health Organization; 2016.
7. World Health Organization. Adherence to long-term therapies: evidence for action. Geneva: World Health Organization; 2003.

8. Deeks SG, Lewin SR, Havlir DV. The end of AIDS: hIV infection as a chronic disease. Lancet. 2013;382(9903):1525–33.
9. UNAIDS. Treatment 2015; 2015.
10. U.S. Department of Health and Human Services. HIV/AIDS glossary: boosting; 2017.
11. Clay PG, Nag S, Graham CM, Narayanan S. Meta-analysis of studies comparing single and multi-tablet fixed dose combination HIV treatment regimens. Medicine (Baltimore). 2015;94(42):e1677.
12. Moher D, Shamseer L, Clarke M, Ghersi D, Liberati A, Petticrew M, et al. Preferred reporting items for systematic review and meta-analysis protocols (PRISMA-P) 2015 statement. Syst Rev. 2015;4:1.
13. Higgins JPT GS, eds. Cochrane Handbook for Systematic Reviews of Interventions Version 5.0.2 (updated September 2009). The Cochrane Collaboration 2008.
14. Critical Appraisal Skills Programme (CASP). 12 questions to help you make sense of cohort study. 2017.
15. DerSimonian R, Laird N. Meta-analysis in clinical trials. Control Clin Trials. 1986;7(3):177–88.
16. Higgins JP, Thompson SG. Quantifying heterogeneity in a meta-analysis. Stat Med. 2002;21(11):1539–58.
17. Bangsberg DR, Ragland K, Monk A, Deeks SG. A single tablet regimen is associated with higher adherence and viral suppression than multiple tablet regimens in HIV + homeless and marginally housed people. Aids. 2010;24(18):2835–40.
18. Fabbiani M, Zaccarelli M, Grima P, Prosperi M, Fanti I, Colafigli M, et al. Single tablet regimens are associated with reduced Efavirenz withdrawal in antiretroviral therapy naive or switching for simplification HIV-infected patients. BMC Infect Dis. 2014;14:26.
19. Skwara P, Bociaga-Jasik M, Kalinowska-Nowak A. Adherence to single-tablet versus multiple-tablet regimens in the treatment of HIV infection: a questionnaire-based survey on patients satisfaction. HIV AIDS Rev. 2014;13:95–9.
20. Sterrantino G, Santoro L, Bartolozzi D, Trotta M, Zaccarelli M. Self-reported adherence supports patient preference for the single tablet regimen (STR) in the current cART era. Patient Prefer Adherence. 2012;6:427–33.
21. Chen Y, Chen K, Kalichman SC. Barriers to HIV medication adherence as a function of regimen simplification. Ann Behav Med. 2017;51(1):67–78.
22. Orkin C, DeJesus E, Ramgopal M, Crofoot G, Ruane P, LaMarca A, et al. Switching from tenofovir disoproxil fumarate to tenofovir alafenamide coformulated with rilpivirine and emtricitabine in virally suppressed adults with HIV-1 infection: a randomised, double-blind, multicentre, phase 3b, non-inferiority study. Lancet HIV. 2017;4(5):e195–204.
23. Sutton SS, Hardin JW, Bramley TJ, D'Souza AO, Bennet CL. Single-versus multiple tablet HIV regimens: adherence and hospitalization risks. Am J Manag Care. 2016;22:242–8.
24. Buscher A, Hartman C, Kallen MA, Giordano TP. Impact of antiretroviral dosing frequency and pill burden on adherence among newly diagnosed, antiretroviral-naive HIV patients. Int J STD AIDS. 2012;23(5):351–5.
25. Arribas JR, Pialoux G, Gathe J, Di Perri G, Reynes J, Tebas P, et al. Simplification to coformulated elvitegravir, cobicistat, emtricitabine, and tenofovir versus continuation of ritonavir-boosted protease inhibitor with emtricitabine and tenofovir in adults with virologically suppressed HIV (STRATEGY-PI): 48 week results of a randomised, open-label, phase 3b, non-inferiority trial. Lancet Infect Dis. 2014;14(7):581–9.
26. Pozniak A, Markowitz M, Mills A, Stellbrink HJ, Antela A, Domingo P, et al. Switching to coformulated elvitegravir, cobicistat, emtricitabine, and tenofovir versus continuation of non-nucleoside reverse transcriptase inhibitor with emtricitabine and tenofovir in virologically suppressed adults with HIV (STRATEGY-NNRTI): 48 week results of a randomised, open-label, phase 3b non-inferiority trial. Lancet Infect Dis. 2014;14(7):590–9.
27. Dejesus E, Young B, Morales-Ramirez JO, Sloan L, Ward DJ, Flaherty JF, et al. Simplification of antiretroviral therapy to a single-tablet regimen consisting of efavirenz, emtricitabine, and tenofovir disoproxil fumarate versus unmodified antiretroviral therapy in virologically suppressed HIV-1-infected patients. J Acquir Immune Defic Syndr. 2009;51(2):163–74.
28. Choi JY, Sungkanuparph S, Anekthananon T, Sax P, DeJesus E, Edelstein H, et al. Efficacy and safety of Elvitegravir/Cobicistat/Emtricitabine/Tenofovir Disoproxil Fumarate in Asian subjects with human immunodeficiency virus 1 infection: a sub-analysis of phase 3 clinical trials. Infect Chemother. 2016;48(3):219–24.
29. Rijnders B, Post F, Rieger A. Longer-term renal safety of tenofovir alafenamide vs tenofovir disoproxil fumarate. Conference on retroviruses and opportunistic infections, February 22–25, 2016, Boston 2016.
30. Arribas JR, Thompson M, Sax PE, Haas B, McDonald C, Wohl A, et al. A randomized, double-blind comparison of Tenofovir Alafenamide (TAF) vs. Tenofovir Disoproxil fumarate (TDF), each coformulated with Elvitegravir, Cobicistat, and Emtricitabine (E/C/F) for Initial HIV-1 Treatment: week 144 results. J Acquir Immune Defic Syndr 2017;75:211–8.
31. Koenig E, Orkin C, Clarke A, Podzamczer D, Clotet B, Callebaut C, et al. Improved safety and efficacy of TAF versus TDF single-tablet regimen in HIV-1 treatment-naïve women through week 48. J Int AIDS Soc. 2016;19(Suppl 1):21083.
32. Palella FJ Jr, Fisher M, Tebas P, Gazzard B, Ruane P, Van Lunzen J, et al. Simplification to rilpivirine/emtricitabine/tenofovir disoproxil fumarate from ritonavir-boosted protease inhibitor antiretroviral therapy in a randomized trial of HIV-1 RNA-suppressed participants. Aids. 2014;28(3):335–44.
33. Huhn GD, Tebas P, Gallant J, Wilkin T, Cheng A, Yan M, et al. A Randomized, Open-Label trial to evaluate switching to Elvitegravir/Cobicistat/Emtricitabine/Tenofovir Alafenamide Plus Darunavir in treatment-experienced HIV-1-infected adults. J Acquir Immune Defic Syndr. 2017;74(2):193–200.
34. Airoldi M, Zaccarelli M, Bisi L, Bini T, Antinori A, Mussini C, et al. One-pill once-a-day HAART: a simplification strategy that improves adherence and quality of life of HIV-infected subjects. Patient Prefer Adherence. 2010;4:115–25.
35. Hanna DB, Hessol NA, Golub ET, Cocohoba JM, Cohen MH, Levine AM, et al. Increase in single-tablet regimen use and associated improvements in adherence-related outcomes in HIV-infected women. J Acquir Immune Defic Syndr. 2014;65(5):587–96.
36. Beck EJ, Mandalia S, Sangha R, Youle M, Brettle R, Gompels M, et al. Lower healthcare costs associated with the use of a single-pill ARV regimen in the UK, 2004–2008. PLoS ONE. 2012;7(10):e47376.
37. Grimes RM, Shenouda TA. Using cost as a consideration for antiretroviral regimen selection: an example using average wholesale prices. AIDS Care. 2013;25(11):1380–4.
38. Homar F, Lozano V, Martinez-Gomez J, Oyaguez I, Pareja A, Payeras A, et al. Cost analysis of HIV treatment and drug-related adverse events when fixed-dose combinations of antiretrovirals (FDCs) were stopped, versus continuation with FDCs. Health Econ Rev. 2012;2(1):16.
39. Angeletti C, Pezzotti P, Antinori A, Mammone A, Navarra A, Orchi N, et al. Antiretroviral treatment based cost saving interventions may offset expenses for new patients and earlier treatment start. HIV Med. 2014;15:165–74.
40. Colombo GL, Castagna A, Di Matteo S, Galli L, Bruno G, Poli A, et al. Cost analysis of initial highly active antiretroviral therapy regimens for managing human immunodeficiency virus-infected patients according to clinical practice in a hospital setting. Ther Clin Risk Manag. 2014;10:9–15.
41. Colombo GL, Di Matteo S, Antinori A, Medaglia M, Murachelli S, Rizzardini G. Economic evaluation of initial antiretroviral therapy for HIV-infected patients: an update of Italian guidelines. Clinicoecon Outcomes Res. 2013;5:489–96.
42. Colombo GL, Di Matteo S, Maggiolo F. Antiretroviral therapy in HIV-infected patients: a proposal to assess the economic value of the single-tablet regimen. Clinicoecon Outcomes Res. 2013;5:59–68.
43. Walensky RP, Sax PE, Nakamura YM, Weinstein MC, Pei PP, Freedberg KA, et al. Economic savings versus health losses: the cost-effectiveness of generic antiretroviral therapy in the United States. Ann Intern Med. 2013;158(2):84–92.
44. Sorbino-Jiménez C, Jiménez-Nácher I, Moreno-Ramos F. Analysis of antiretroviral therapy modification in routine clinical practice in the management of HIV infection. Eur J Hosp Pharm. 2017;24:96–100.
45. Sweet DE, Altice FL, Cohen CJ, Vandewalle B. Cost-effectiveness of single-versus generic multiple-tablet regimens for treatment of HIV-1 infection in the United States. PLoS ONE. 2016;11(1):e0147821.
46. Cohen CJ, Meyers JL, Davis KL. Association between daily antiretroviral pill burden and treatment adherence, hospitalisation risk, and other healthcare utilisation and costs in a US medicaid population with HIV. BMJ Open. 2013;3(8):e003028.
47. Juday T, Gupta S, Grimm K, Wagner S, Kim E. Factors associated with complete adherence to HIV combination antiretroviral therapy. HIV Clin Trials. 2011;12(2):71–8.

Permissions

All chapters in this book were first published in AIDS R&T, by BioMed Central; hereby published with permission under the Creative Commons Attribution License or equivalent. Every chapter published in this book has been scrutinized by our experts. Their significance has been extensively debated. The topics covered herein carry significant findings which will fuel the growth of the discipline. They may even be implemented as practical applications or may be referred to as a beginning point for another development.

The contributors of this book come from diverse backgrounds, making this book a truly international effort. This book will bring forth new frontiers with its revolutionizing research information and detailed analysis of the nascent developments around the world.

We would like to thank all the contributing authors for lending their expertise to make the book truly unique. They have played a crucial role in the development of this book. Without their invaluable contributions this book wouldn't have been possible. They have made vital efforts to compile up to date information on the varied aspects of this subject to make this book a valuable addition to the collection of many professionals and students.

This book was conceptualized with the vision of imparting up-to-date information and advanced data in this field. To ensure the same, a matchless editorial board was set up. Every individual on the board went through rigorous rounds of assessment to prove their worth. After which they invested a large part of their time researching and compiling the most relevant data for our readers.

The editorial board has been involved in producing this book since its inception. They have spent rigorous hours researching and exploring the diverse topics which have resulted in the successful publishing of this book. They have passed on their knowledge of decades through this book. To expedite this challenging task, the publisher supported the team at every step. A small team of assistant editors was also appointed to further simplify the editing procedure and attain best results for the readers.

Apart from the editorial board, the designing team has also invested a significant amount of their time in understanding the subject and creating the most relevant covers. They scrutinized every image to scout for the most suitable representation of the subject and create an appropriate cover for the book.

The publishing team has been an ardent support to the editorial, designing and production team. Their endless efforts to recruit the best for this project, has resulted in the accomplishment of this book. They are a veteran in the field of academics and their pool of knowledge is as vast as their experience in printing. Their expertise and guidance has proved useful at every step. Their uncompromising quality standards have made this book an exceptional effort. Their encouragement from time to time has been an inspiration for everyone.

The publisher and the editorial board hope that this book will prove to be a valuable piece of knowledge for researchers, students, practitioners and scholars across the globe.

List of Contributors

George Gachara, Tshifhiwa Magoro, Lufuno Mavhandu and Pascal O. Bessong
HIV/AIDS & Global Health Research Program, Department of Microbiology, University of Venda, Private Bag X5050, Thohoyandou 0950, Limpopo, South Africa

George Gachara
Department of Medical Laboratory Sciences, Kenyatta University, Nairobi, Kenya

Emmaculate Lum and Helen K. Kimbi
Department of Zoology and Animal Physiology, Faculty of Science, University of Buea, Buea, Cameroon

Emmaculate Lum
Department of Biological Sciences, Higher Teachers' Training College, University of Yaounde, Yaounde, Cameroon

Helen K. Kimbi
Department of Medical Laboratory Science, Faculty of Health Sciences, University of Bamenda, Bambili, Bamenda, Cameroon

Roland N. Ndip
Department of Biochemistry and Microbiology, Faculty of Science and Agriculture, University of Fort Hare, Alice, South Africa
Department of Microbiology and Parasitology, University of Buea, Buea, Cameroon

Siyan Yi, Chanrith Ngin, Khuondyla Pals, Sovannary Tuot, Pheak Chhoun, Sok Chamreun Choub and Kolab Chhim
KHANA Center for Population Health Research, No. 33, Street 71, Phnom Penh, Cambodia

Siyan Yi
Center for Global Health Research, Touro University California, Vallejo, USA

Vohith Khol, Sokunmealiny Sau and Penhsun Ly
National Center for HIV/AIDS, Dermatology and STD, Phnom Penh, Cambodia

Gitau Mburu
Division of Health Research, Lancaster University, Lancaster, UK

M. P. Ngogang Djobet, Jeanne Ngogang and Ernest Tambo
LABOREB – Laboratoire de Recherche et d'Expertise Biomédicale, Yaoundé, Cameroon

David Singhe
LANACOME, National Laboratory for Drugs Quality Control, Ministry of Public Health, Yaoundé, Cameroon

Julienne Lohoue
Faculty of Medicine and Biomedical Sciences, University of Yaoundé I, Yaoundé, Cameroon

Christopher Kuaban
Faculty of Medicine, University of Bamenda, Bamenda, Cameroon

Jeanne Ngogang and Ernest Tambo
Université des Montagnes, Bangangté, Cameroon

Ernest Tambo
Africa Disease Intelligence and Surveillance, Communication and Response (Africa DISCoR) Institute, Yaoundé, Cameroon

Kirsten A. M. Donald and Heather Zar
Department of Paediatrics and Child Health, Institute of Child Health Building, Red Cross War Memorial Children's Hospital, 5th Floor, Klipfontein Road, Rondebosch, Cape Town 7700, South Africa

Anne Fernandez, Kasey Claborn and Caroline Kuo
Center for Alcohol and Addiction Studies, Brown University School of Public Health, Providence, RI, USA

Kasey Claborn
Department of Medicine, Rhode Island Hospital, Providence, USA

Kasey Claborn
Department of Psychiatry and Human Behavior, Warren Alpert Medical School of Brown University, Providence, USA

Caroline Kuo
Department of Behavioral and Social Sciences, Brown University School of Public Health, Providence, RI, USA

Caroline Kuo and Dan J. Stein
Department of Psychiatry and Mental Health, University of Cape Town, Cape Town, South Africa

Nastassja Koen and Heather Zar
South African Medical Research Council Unit on Child & Adolescent Health, Cape Town, South Africa

Dan J. Stein
South African Medical Research Council Unit on Risk and Resilience in Mental Disorders, Cape Town, South Africa

Patricia Volkow, Pamela Garciadiego-Fossas and Patricia Cornejo-Juárez
Infectious Diseases Department, Instituto Nacional de Cancerología (INCan), Av. San Fernando No. 22, Col. Sección XVI, Deleg. Tlalpan, 14080 Mexico City, Mexico

Gabriela Cesarman-Maus
Hematology Department, Instituto Nacional de Cancerología (INCan), Mexico City, Mexico

Enrique Rojas-Marin
Radiology Department, Instituto Nacional de Cancerología (INCan), Mexico City, Mexico

Karen M. Hampanda
Department of Community and Behavioral Health, Colorado School of Public Health, 13199 East Montview Boulevard, Suite 310, Mail Stop A090, Aurora, CO 80045, USA

Abigail M. Nimz
University of Colorado School of Medicine, 13001 E 17th Place, Aurora, CO 80045, USA

Lisa L. Abuogi
Department of Pediatrics, University of Colorado School of Medicine and Children's Hospital Colorado, Aurora, CO, USA
Center for Global Health, University of Colorado School of Medicine School of Public Health, 13199 East Montview Boulevard, Suite 310, Mail Stop A090, Aurora, CO 80045, USA

Elizabeth M. Etta, Lufuno Mavhandu, David Rekosh, Marie-Louise Hammarskjold, Pascal O. Bessong and Denis M. Tebit
HIV/AIDS & Global Health Research Program, Department of Microbiology, University of Venda, Thohoyandou 0950, South Africa

Cecile Manhaeve
Bela-Bela HIV/AIDS Prevention Group Wellness Clinic (HAPG), Bela-Bela, South Africa

Keanan McGonigle, Patrick Jackson, David Rekosh, Marie-Louise Hammarskjold and Denis M. Tebit
Department of Microbiology, Immunology and Cancer Biology, Myles H. Thaler Center for AIDS and Human Retrovirus Research, University of Virginia, Charlottesville, VA 22908, USA

Billy Nsubuga Mayanja, Ivan Kasamba, Jonathan Levin, Ivan Namakoola, Patrick Kazooba, Jackson Were, Pontiano Kaleebu and Paula Munderi
MRC/UVRI Uganda Research Unit on AIDS, Entebbe, Ugandas

Ivan Kasamba
MRC Tropical Epidemiology Group, London School of Hygiene and Tropical Medicine, Keppel Street, London WC1E 7HT, United Kingdom

Pontiano Kaleebu
Department of Clinical Research, London School of Hygiene and Tropical Medicine, Keppel Street, London WC1E 7HT, United Kingdom

Joseph T. Ortega, Flor H. Pujol and Hector R. Rangel
Laboratorio de Virología Molecular, Centro de Microbiología y Biología Celular, Instituto Venezolano de Investigaciones Científicas, Caracas, Venezuela

Alirica I. Suárez and Jani Baptista
Laboratorio de Productos Naturales, Facultad de Farmacia, Universidad Central de Venezuela, Caracas, Venezuela

Maria L. Serrano
Unidad de Química Medicinal, Facultad de Farmacia, Universidad Central de Venezuela, Caracas, Venezuela

Rongrong Yang, Hong Zhang, Yong Xiong, Xien Gui, Yongxi Zhang, Liping Deng, Shicheng Gao and Mingqi Luo
Department of Infectious Diseases, Zhongnan Hospital of Wuhan University, 169 Donghu Road, Wuhan 430071, China

Wei Hou and Deyin Guo
Basic Medical College of Wuhan University, Wuhan, China

Awoke Seyoum
Department of Statistics, Bahir Dar University, Bahir Dar, Ethiopia

Principal Ndlovu
Department of Statistics, UNISA, Pretoria, South Africa

Zewotir Temesgen
School of Mathematics, Statistics and Computer Science, University of KwaZulu Natal, Durban, South Africa

Marianne Harris, Bruce Ganase, Birgit Watson, P. Richard Harrigan, Julio S. G. Montaner and Mark W. Hull
British Columbia Centre for Excellence in HIV/AIDS, Vancouver, BC, Canada

Marianne Harris and Bruce Ganase
AIDS Research Program, St. Paul's Hospital, Vancouver, BC, Canada

Marianne Harris
Department of Family Practice, Faculty of Medicine, University of British Columbia, Vancouver, BC, Canada

Marianne Harris, P. Richard Harrigan, Julio S. G. Montaner and Mark W. Hull
Division of AIDS, Faculty of Medicine, University of British Columbia, Vancouver, BC, Canada3

Peter Liu
Department of Internal Medicine, University of Virginia, Charlottesville, VA 22908, USA

Rebecca Dillingham and Kathleen A. McManus
Division of Infectious Diseases and International Health, University of Virginia, Charlottesville, VA 22908, USA

Berhe Beyene Gebrezgabher, Desalegn Tetemke and Mebrahtu Abay
Department of Public Health, Health Science College, Axum University, Axum, Ethiopia

Yigzaw Kebede, Melaku Kindie and Yalemzewod Assefa Gelaw
Department of Epidemiology and Biostatistics, Institute of Public Health, College of Medicine and Health Science, University of Gondar, 196 Gondar, Ethiopia

Guoxian Zhao, Lifeng Liu, Bin Su, Tong Zhang, Peng Chen, Wei Li and Hao Wu
Center for Infectious Diseases, Beijing You'an Hospital, Capital Medical University, Beijing 100069, China

Guoxian Zhao, Lifeng Liu, Bin Su, Tong Zhang, Peng Chen, Wei Li and Hao Wu
Beijing Key Laboratory for HIV/AIDS Research, Beijing 100069, China

Wei Li
Center of Interventional Oncology and Liver Diseases, Beijing You'an Hospital, Capital Medical University, Beijing 100069, China

Jan Weber, Lenka Sácká, Dmytro Strunin, Jan Hodek, Jitka Weberová and Marcela Pávová
Institute of Organic Chemistry and Biochemistry v.v.i., Academy of Sciences of the Czech Republic, Flemingovo n. 2, 166 10 Prague 6, Czech Republic

Richard M. Gibson, David J. Alouani and Miguel E. Quiñones-Mateu
University Hospital Translational Laboratory, University Hospitals Cleveland Medical Center, Cleveland, OH, USA

Robert Asaad, Benigno Rodriguez, Michael M. Lederman and Miguel E. Quiñones-Mateu
Department of Medicine, Case Western Reserve University/University Hospitals Cleveland Medical Center, 10900 Euclid Avenue, Cleveland, OH 44106-7288, USA

Miguel E. Quiñones-Mateu
Department of Pathology, Case Western Reserve University, Cleveland, OH, USA

María Fernanda Álvarez Barreneche, Carlos Andrés Restrepo Castro, Alicia Hidrón Botero, Juan Pablo Villa Franco, Laura Restrepo Carvajal, Alejandro Eusse García and Carlos Andrés Agudelo Restrepo
School of Health Sciences, Universidad Pontificia Bolivariana, Carrera 44 # 18-56, Antioquia, Medellín, Colombia

Carlos Andrés Restrepo Castro and Ivan Mauricio Trompa Romero
Division of Infectious Diseases, Department of Internal Medicine, IPS Universitaria Clínica León XIII, Antioquia, Medellín, Colombia

Alicia Hidrón Botero
Division of Infectious Diseases, Department of Internal Medicine, Hospital Pablo Tobón Uribe, Antioquia, Medellín, Colombia
Division of Infectious Diseases, Department of Internal Medicine, Emory University School of Medicine, Atlanta, GA, USA

Adriana Ocampo Mesa, Lina María Echeverri Toro, Jaime Mauricio Ramírez Rivera and Carlos Andrés Agudelo Restrepo
Division of Infectious Diseases, Department of Internal Medicine, Centros Especializados San Vicente Fundación, Antioquia, Rionegro, Colombia

Lina María Echeverri Toro and Jaime Mauricio Ramírez Rivera
Division of Infectious Diseases, Department of Internal Medicine, Hospital Universitario, San Vicente Fundación, Antioquia, Medellín, Colombia

Porras Fernández de Castro
Department of Internal Medicine, Hospital General de Medellín, Antioquia, Medellín, Colombia

Carlos Andrés Agudelo Restrepo
Division of Infectious Diseases, Department of Internal Medicine, Clínica Universitaria Bolivariana, Antioquia, Medellín, Colombia

Stephen Okoboi, Barbara Castelnuovo, Joseph Musaazi and Andrew Kambugu
Infectious Diseases Institute, College of Health Sciences, Makerere University, Kampala, Uganda

Stephen Okoboi and Annelies Van Rie
Global Health Institute, University of Antwerp, Antwerp, Belgium
Faculty of Medicine and Health Sciences, University of Antwerp, Antwerp, Belgium

David M. Moore
British Columbia Centre for Excellence in HIV/ AIDS, Vancouver, Canada
University of British Columbia, Vancouver, Canada

Josephine Birungi and Mastula Nanfuka
The AIDS Support Organization, Kampala, Uganda

Pontiano Kaleebu
Medical Research Council/ Uganda Virus Research Institute, Kampala, Uganda

Moses R. Kamya
School of Medicine, College of Health Sciences, Makerere University, Kampala, Uganda

Derek J. Chan, Virginia Furner, Don E. Smith, Mithilesh Dronavalli, Rohan I. Bopage and Jeffrey J. Post
Albion Centre, South Eastern Sydney Local Health District, Sydney, NSW 2010, Australia

Derek J. Chan, Don E. Smith and Rohan I. Bopage
School of Public Health and Community Medicine, Faculty of Medicine, University of New South Wales, Sydney, NSW 2052, Australia

Jeffrey J. Post
Department of Infectious Diseases, Prince of Wales Hospital, South Eastern Sydney Local Health District, Sydney, NSW 2010, Australia
Prince of Wales Clinical School, UNSW, Sydney, NSW 2051, Australia

Anjali K. Bhardwaj
University of Sydney, Sydney, Australia

Tamara Nsubuga-Nyombi, Simon Sensalire, Esther Karamagi, Judith Aloyo, John Byabagambi and Mirwais Rahimzai
USAID Applying Science To Strengthen and Improve Systems (ASSIST) Project,USAID, University Research Co., LLC, Plot 40, Ntinda II Road, Kampala, Uganda

Linda Kisaakye Nabitaka
Ministry of Health, Kampala, Uganda

Jacqueline Calnan
United States Agency for International Development (USAID), Kampala, Uganda

Win Min Han, Tanakorn Apornpong, Stephen J. Kerr, Akarin Hiransuthikul, Sivaporn Gatechompol, Tanya Do, Kiat Ruxrungtham and Anchalee Avihingsanon
HIV-NAT, The Thai Red Cross AIDS Research Center, 104 Ratchadamri Rd., Pathumwan, Bangkok 10330, Thailand

Stephen J. Kerr, Kiat Ruxrungtham and Anchalee Avihingsanon
Faculty of Medicine, Chulalongkorn University, Bangkok, Thailand

Lauren A. Saag
Division of Epidemiology, Department of Epidemiology, Vanderbilt University, 2525 West End Ave, Suite 600, Nashville, TN 37235, USA

Ashutosh R. Tamhane, Michael J. Mugavero and Ellen F. Eaton
Division of Infectious Diseases, Department of Medicine, University of Alabama at Birmingham, 845 19th St. South, Birmingham, AL 35294, USA

D. Scott Batey
Department of Social Work, University of Alabama at Birmingham, 900 13th Street South, Birmingham, AL 35294, USA

Patrick G. Clay and Wei C. Yuet
University of North Texas System College of Pharmacy, 3500 Camp Bowie Blvd, Fort Worth, TX 76107, USA

Christiane H. Moecklinghoff
Jannsen-Cilag GmbH, Johnson & Johnson Platz 1, 41470 Neuss, Germany

Inge Duchesne
Janssen EMEA, Turnhoutseweg 30, 2340 Beerse, Belgium

Krzysztof L. Tronczyński
Janssen-Cilag Polska Sp. Z o.o, Iłżecka 24, 02-135 Warsaw, Poland

Sandip Shah and Dong Shao
Market Access Solutions, LLC, 575 NJ-28, Raritan, NJ 08869, USA

Index

CPSIA information can be obtained
at www.ICGtesting.com
Printed in the USA
JSHW060835250523
42126JS00009B/4